ADOLESCENT PSYCHIATRIC NURSING

ADOLESCENT PSYCHIATRIC NURSING

Christina R. Hogarth, *M.S., R.N., C.S.*

Psychiatric Clinical Nurse Specialist
Middletown Regional Hospital
Middletown, Ohio

Private Practice
Middletown, Ohio

Consultant
Dayton, Ohio

Illustrated

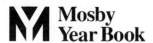

Mosby Year Book

St. Louis Baltimore Boston Chicago London Philadelphia Sydney Toronto

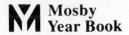
Mosby
Year Book

Dedicated to Publishing Excellence

Editor: Linda L. Duncan
Developmental Editor: Linda Stagg and Teri Merchant

Printed in the United States of America

Mosby–Year Book, Inc.
11830 Westline Industrial Drive
St. Louis, Missouri, 63146

Library of Congress Cataloging in Publication Data

Hogarth, Christina R.
    Adolescent psychiatric nursing / Christina R. Hogarth.
      p. cm.
    Includes bibliographical references and index.
    ISBN 0-8016-3229-3
    1. Adolescent psychiatric nursing.   I. Title.
    [DNLM: 1. Mental Disorders—in adolescence. 2. Psychiatric
Nursing—in adolescence.   WY 160 H715a]
KJ502.3.H64   1991
610.73′68—dc20
DNLM/DLC   91–6888
for Library of Congress   CIP

GW/D/D 9 8 7 6 5 4 3 2 1

Contributors

Patricia Clunn, *Ed.D., A.R.M.P., C.S.*
Professor
School of Nursing
University of Miami
Miamia, Florida

Cary Hatton, *Ed.D., L.P.C.C.*
Director
District II Children's Project
Montgomery County Health Board
Dayton, Ohio

Phyllis A. Johnson, *Ph.D., R.N.*
Associate Professor
Parent–Child Nursing
Georgia State University
Atlanta, Georgia

Norman L. Keltner, *R.N., Ed.D.*
Associate Professor
School of Nursing
University of Alabama at Birmingham
Birmingham, Alabama

Linda A. Mast, *B.S.N., R.N.C.*
Nurse Administrator
South Community, Inc.
Dayton, Ohio

Lawrence R. Schoppe, Jr., *B.S.N., R.N.*
Nurse Manager
Child Mental Health
Vista Hill Hospital
Chula Vista, California

Beatrice Crofts Yorker, *J.D., R.N.*
Chair
Psychiatric Mental Health Nursing
Georgia State University
Atlanta, Georgia

For **Jim**
my love since our own adolescence
and **Laura**
Todd
Brian
and
Rob
whose wonderful and painful adolescence
gave me joy and hope
for you and for all adolescents

Preface

Adolescent Psychiatric Nursing is a book for the nurse with an associate or bachelor's degree in nursing who wishes to begin or improve the practice of psychiatric nursing with adolescents. This book is for the staff nurse in hospital, day treatment, and residential settings. It will also be helpful to clinical specialists and nurses or other managers who have responsibilities for the management, training, or consulting of nurses who work in these settings. School nurses and pediatric nurses who work with adolescents will also find this book useful.

I decided to write this book, because there was no nursing literature available to use in training nurses and technicians to function in a therapeutic milieu for adolescents when I was a manager and administrator in a psychiatric hospital. Because many psychiatric nurses who write or contribute to textbooks have been educated to function as therapists and teachers and consultants in systems, the interventions that are suggested in textbooks often speak heavily to adult psychotherapy, theory, general interventions, medications, and group and family therapy. Strategies for use by staff nurses with adolescents in a moment-to-moment or day-to-day context such as an inpatient unit or at school, were practically nonexistent in the literature. Nurses rarely have an opportunity for educational opportunities in adolescent psychiatric or chemical dependency nursing during their basic programs in nursing; thus they begin their career in this field with limited theory and few if any psychotherapeutic or milieu management skills. Nurses attempt to provide care in settings where the child care workers and technicians have more education and experience in counseling and functioning in the milieu, and the rest of the team is master's or doctorally prepared in social work, psychology, or psychiatry. Adolescent Psychiatric Nursing now provides a theory base and interventions that staff nurses can use in their practice.

As I observed experienced nurses working with adolescents, I began to name the interventions and organize into categories what nurses actually did in their practice. A list of nursing interventions began to emerge. I had used the Adult Standards of Psychiatric Nursing Practice to direct training for some time. I then did the same with American Nurses Association Standards for Child and Adolescent Psychiatric Mental Health Nursing Practice. The literature on therapeutic milieu helped organize my list of interventions into structured and nonstructured ones. These intervention strategies have been helpful to many inpatient units where I consulted and trained nurses and child care workers, and to hundreds of individual nurses who attended seminars on this topic. It is my hope and expectation that many more nurses will begin or improve their practice with the help of this book. Many interventions, especially in chapters 11 and 13, are based on actual care plans used successfully by nurses I have worked with.

Chapters 1, 2, 3, and 4 provide the history of present adolescent problems, an overview of adolescent psychiatric nursing practice as proposed in this book, normal adolescent development, and legal aspects of adolescent psychiatric nursing. Chapter 5 presents the disordered adolescent and family with general interventions relative to each type of disorder. The discussion of posttraumatic stress is quite relevant, with the most recent information being provided by Patricia Clunn. Chapter 6 includes the assessment of the adolescent from the multidisciplinary approach as well as from the nursing approach. Cary Hatton describes the latest thinking in systems of care for children and adolescents in Chapter 7. Dr. Hatton works in the community developing these systems with community mental health systems. Chapter 8 is an overview of all the strategies used by adolescent psychiatric nurses. Chapters 9 and 10 describe interventions used in the community. Chapter 11 describes strategies used in a therapeutic milieu. Chapter 12 includes an overview of the theory and practice of psychotherapy and of expressive therapies. Although staff nurses do not usually provide psychotherapy, nurses must understand the principles of individual, group, and family therapy in order to collaborate with therapists of various disciplines and to increase her skills in individual, group, and family interventions. A section on cultural specific interventions is very relevant. Dr. Norm Keltner provided Chapter 13, which describes psychopharmacology for adolescents, an important area of practice exclusive to nursing and psychiatry. As exciting research in neurochemistry and pharmacology continues to pour out of universities and clinical settings, adolescent psychiatric nurses will need to be active in staying current in this field. At press time, I believe this is the most current thinking in medication management. Chapter 14 describes specific intervention for common problems encountered with adolescents especially in the milieu. This chapter is co-authored with Linda Mast, RNC, a staff nurse who became a nurse manager and now works in a community mental health center with children and adolescents. Finally, Chapter 15, an overview of the strategies for management of the adolescent inpatient unit is provided.

It is my hope that *Adolescent Psychiatric Nursing* will be a practical reference for staff nurses, clinical specialists who train and supervise adolescent psychiatric nurses, and faculty members who introduce students to the wonderful specialty of adolescent psychiatric nursing.

Acknowledgments

So many people contributed to the writing of this book, both directly and indirectly. My husband, Jim, gave unfailing support and encouragement during the whole project, but especially during the third draft. My oldest son, Todd, made many trips to the post office, U.P.S., typists, and the library for me. Linda Duncan, my editor, "hung in there" with the idea of a small interventions-based book for the practicing staff nurse when it was not popular. She also has provided tremendous support by pushing me to improve, making suggestions, and encouraging me. Mahendra K. Mahajan, M.D., my colleague of ten years, introduced me to adolescent psychiatry and supervised my therapy with adolescents in the early years and provided the initial conceptualization of the phases of goal setting with adolescents. Grayce Sills assisted me with reorganizing the book contents so that it is more valuable to educators and linked me with leaders in the field. Brenda Wagner provided a thoughtful manuscript review which drove the third draft. Eric Rothman also provided a helpful review. Pat Clunn provided long distance intellectual and emotional support, as well as contributing or co-authoring several chapters. Pat Givens typed the first and second draft with quiet skill. Of course, all of the hundreds of adolescents and families that have brought their problems and strengths to programs I have supervised or to my private practice, gave me my life work and the motivation to practice, consult, and write. Finally, the nurses I have worked with in the "trenches," especially Linda Mast, Jeanine Clausi, Larry Schoppe, Greg Walters, a child care worker, at Detmer Hospital in Troy, Ohio, and Nancy Williams, RN, MS, school nurse at Kettering Fairmont High School, demonstrated superb adolescent psychiatric nursing skills and assisted me in various ways to spell out very specifically the tenets of that practice.

Christina R. Hogarth

Contents

Part I

Overview of adolescent psychiatric nursing

1   The Challenge of Adolescent Psychiatric Nursing, 3

2   Historical Development of Current Adolescent Problems, 15

3   Development of the Healthy Adolescent and Family, 27
     Linda A. Mast
     Lawrence R. Schoppe
     Christina R. Hogarth

4   Legal Issues in Adolescent Psychiatric Nursing, 51
     Phyllis Johnson
     Beatric Yorker

5   Disordered Adolescents and Families, 69
     Patricia Clunn
     Christina R. Hogarth

6   Assessment of the Adolescent, 133
     Patricia Clunn

7   A System of Care for Emotionally Disturbed Children and
     Adolescents, 187
     Cary Hatton

Part II

Strategies for adolescent psychiatric nursing

8   Intervention Strategies for Adolescent Psychiatric Nurses:
     an Overview, 215

9   Strategies for Prevention, 245

10   Strategies for Crisis Intervention, 259

11   **Strategies for the Therapeutic Milieu, 273**

12   **Psychotherapy and Expressive Therapies, 311**
Patricia Clunn
Christina R. Hogarth

13   **Psychopharmacology, 351**
Norman L. Keltner

14   **Nursing Interventions for Common Adolescent Psychiatric Problems, 373**
Linda A. Mast
Christina R. Hogarth

15   **Management of the Adolescent Psychiatric Unit, 417**

Appendix A   DSM-III-R Diagnoses and Codes, 424

Appendix B   Classification of Human Responses of Concern for Psychiatric Mental Health Nursing Practice, 432

Appendix C   Graduate Programs in Psychiatric Mental Health Nursing, 441

Part I

Overview of Adolescent Psychiatric Nursing

Chapter 1

The Challenge of Adolescent Psychiatric Nursing

The ultimate challenge of adolescence is to achieve capable adulthood (Glenn and Warner, 1982). Reaching capable adulthood requires developing the attributes of a capable adolescent. The capable or competent adolescent possesses a variety of social, cognitive, and psychological assets including (1) consistent values, (2) interpersonal sensitivity, (3) cooperativeness, (4) curiosity, (5) verbal communication skills, (6) the capability for abstraction and self-reflection, (7) responsibility, (8) self-control, (9) autonomy, (10) self-esteem, (11) achievement, and (12) physical health. (Garmezy, 1981, 1984; Werner and Smith, 1982). For these areas of competence to emerge, the adolescent must be exposed to appropriate experiences throughout life.

The challenge and focus of adolescent psychiatric–mental health nursing is to facilitate the development of these competencies and provide for adolescents' needs. Adolescent psychiatric nurses "intervene with the adolescent as he/she develops— socially, emotionally, cognitively, and physically—within the adolescent's significant social systems including family, school, community, and institution(s)." (American Nurses Association, 1985). There are eight basic categories of needs that adolescents require for growth. These needs are supplied first by the family and then by other adults who come into the adolescent's life (see box on p. 4), such as nurses, teachers, coaches, ministers, and scout leaders.

Adolescent Needs

LOVE AND COMMITMENT

A critical ingredient in the growth and development of adolescents is *love*. Love is a feeling that moves people toward relationships with others. Fromm (1956) states that in a loving relationship, "one can act, help, heal, educate, raise, redeem, and forgive. . . . Love is characterized by four basic elements: care, responsibility, respect and knowledge." *Care* is the "active concern for the life and growth of that which we love." It is "helping another grow and actualize himself . . . a process, a way of relating to someone that involves development . . . through mutual trust" (Mayeroff, 1971). Although parental love especially comes to mind with this definition, concern about growth in a broad sense applies to all close relationships—marriage,

3

Adolescent Needs for Growth to Capable Adulthood

Love and commitment
Surveillance
Structure
Opportunity to develop social, cognitive, and psychological skills
Opportunity to learn to make good decisions in the presence of caring adults
Increasing freedom and responsibility
Adequate physical health
Safe, responsive community

---

friendship, nurse-client, and therapist-client. Adolescents need others to have an active interest in their growth, development, and well-being. *Responsibility* is the ability to respond to another. Having responsibility for an adolescent requires being physically present for the young person who is in need. The parent, teacher, or nurse who is elsewhere or preoccupied cannot know what is happening with an adolescent. Being responsible also means observing and listening actively and empathetically in order to understand the context of a young person's life. Adults involved with adolescents have a responsibility to assess the environment adolescents must negotiate at school, in social activities, and at home. *Respect* is an element of love that refers to valuing the uniqueness, privacy, and independence of others. Adolescents' temperaments, growth and development patterns, talents, and abilities vary from those of their parents and other children in the family and community. Respect for these differences is a key factor in helping adolescents to grow and mature. *Knowledge* of self and others and of the nature of adolescence is critical in caring for adolescents.

To provide these four basic elements, the act of loving someone—especially a child—requires *commitment* and *sacrifice*. These two values have been out of style during the past 2½ decades, when individual rights have been in the forefront. Families and children are more successful when parents make a commitment to marriage and to parenting, are loving and competent, and share a consistent value system (Block and Block, 1980). In the process, a parent may sacrifice a great deal of personal time, freedom, and occupational achievement. When nurses choose psychiatric nursing, especially with adolescents, they commit themselves to forming caring relationships with troubled young people and their families. Those relationships are the basis of healing, just as the loving relationship of parent and child is the basis of growth.

SURVEILLANCE

Another activity that is required in the art of caring for and about adolescents is *surveillance*. The term is found in Leininger's (1981) taxonomy of caring constructs. Although the word is often associated with spying, surveillance in the context of health care means watching over a person who is ill or in need. With children and adolescents—or even adults who are unable to protect themselves—surveillance means monitoring with love and concern. Close, even strict, supervision enhances self-control in adolescents and reduces crime in communities (Rutter, 1979, 1980).

STRUCTURE

Structure is a "set of believable and attainable expectations and standards from the community (and the family) to guide movement from child to adult status" (Ianni, 1989). Consistency in the values of both family and community and clear and consistent guidelines are essential to adolescents (Ianni, 1989). The adolescent's family provides specific structures such as routines and rules. Adolescents need regular, scheduled times for nutritious meals, sleep, activities, homework, chores, and family interaction. They also need some unstructured time. *Rules and consequences* provide safety and develop conscience and self-control. The adolescent should know the rules and understand the consequences if a rule is broken. Rules must be enforced, and consequences should be applied consistently by appropriate adults.

The adolescent's structure includes beliefs about behavior, achievement, and morals. Adolescents need to observe the congruent expression of *values and beliefs* taught by their parents, and they should have the opportunity to discuss different value systems. The child who has a clear set of values will be better able to compare value systems and take a stand when confronted with an ethical or moral decision. The adolescent's clear and predictable structure provides a safe haven from which to explore new ideas and situations. The more secure the home structure is, the less likely the adolescent is to seek fundamental security in a peer group.

OPPORTUNITY TO DEVELOP SOCIAL, COGNITIVE, AND PSYCHOLOGICAL SKILLS

The adolescent and family values system is heavily influenced by the community. Communities have a "youth charter" (Ianni, 1983), which reflects the community's beliefs about adolescents' behavior and roles as they progress from childhood to adulthood. The charter also reflects adults' attitudes, roles, and behavior toward youth. Schools are particularly influential in introducing and modifying structures relevant to adolescents.

Adolescents need a variety of social, cognitive, and psychological skills to succeed in today's complex environment. Capable adolescents have several social abilities that enable them to succeed. Friendliness and cooperativeness (Garmezy, 1981) are important; so is curiosity about people, situations, and different roles (Murphy and Moriarity, 1976). Interpersonal sensitivity is an asset in building relationships. The capacity to work and to engage in alternative social roles during adolescence is associated with mental health in adulthood (Long and Vaillant, 1984).

A capable adolescent possesses several cognitive abilities. Adequate intelligence and the ability to abstract are prerequisites for success (Garmezy, 1984). The adolescent must have good verbal communication skills, a sense of responsibility, and achievement that conforms to community standards (Werner and Smith, 1982). Under-average intelligence and poor academic achievement predispose children and adolescents to a variety of personal, social, and career problems.

The psychological skills possessed by a competent adolescent include self-esteem—an acceptance of one's self academically, socially, and physically—and an internal locus of control (Werner and Smith, 1982). Impulse control and a sense of personal power or control over the environment are also marks of competence (Garmezy, 1981). Special talents, such as artistic, musical, or athletic ability or some special academic ability, provide a sense of achievement, confidence, and self-esteem. Capable adolescents have an awareness of themselves and are able to introspect.

The traits listed in this section, along with a reliance on positive social support systems either in the family or community (Garmezy, 1983; Werner and Smith, 1982; Rutter, 1979), are characteristics of capable adolescents, even those who endure severe stress. Adolescent psychiatric nursing is heavily focused on assisting adolescents to develop or enhance these skills.

OPPORTUNITY TO LEARN TO MAKE GOOD DECISIONS IN THE PRESENCE OF CARING ADULTS

Children and teenagers learn to make good decisions and develop good judgment by observing, discussing, and practicing the decision-making process with adults who are responsible for and who truly care for the child (Glenn and Warner, 1982). Ideally, the caring adults should be parents and a network of other caring adults. An adolescent needs a good relationship with one parent; even if the other parent is dysfunctional or absent, the adolescent benefits from a solid relationship with one. That single parent fares even better with a network of supportive adults (Werner and Smith, 1982). The adult's communication should be "enabling" (facilitating). Enabling communication accepts the child's ideas, focuses the direction of the conversation, and explains concepts, ideas, and customs to the adolescent (Hauser and others, 1984). If caring adults are not readily available, the adolescent learns to make decisions in other ways, usually using a peer group as a model. In this era of dual-earner and single-parent families, providing adequate time for and attention to children is difficult but critical.

INCREASING FREEDOM AND RESPONSIBILITY

Children and adolescents learn to become responsible when responsibilities that are appropriate for their age and level of cognitive, emotional, and physical development are assigned to them. When the child demonstrates responsible behavior, additional freedoms or privileges are earned. For example, if the teenager's household chores are completed, the afternoon may be spent with friends. Logical consequences for responsible, appropriate behavior or for irresponsible, inappropriate behavior provide children and adolescents with a clear structure on which to base decisions. (Dreikus and Grey, 1970; Adler, 1963).

For appropriate consequences to be applied and additional freedom to be established, adolescents must have close supervision or surveillance, as noted earlier. However, the family must permit autonomy for teenagers that is appropriate to the adolescent's developmental level (Ianni, 1989; Beavers, 1977). Adolescents need encouragement to pursue their own interests and abilities and to explore new roles and opportunities.

ADEQUATE PHYSICAL HEALTH

Adolescents need nutritious meals and snacks to meet rapid growth needs; adequate sleep and exercise are necessary as well. Adolescents also need education about and protection from many things: mind-altering drugs, especially alcohol and marijuana; early and promiscuous sexual activity; and risky activities such as car racing, overly-vigorous athletic competition, obsessive dieting, and dare taking. An adolescent with a health problem or handicap needs appropriate care. Adolescence was at one time relatively free of health concerns, but during the last 2 decades adolescents have become the only age-group with an increase in health problems.

SAFE, RESPONSIVE COMMUNITY

Ideally, the communities in which adolescents and their families live are safe from crime and physical hazards; community government and associations are responsive to the educational and social needs of children and adolescents, and the citizens take an active stance in dealing with issues and problems in that area.

The community's value system regarding adolescence, or the "youth charter" (Ianni, 1983, 1989), should reflect attitudes that encourage competence in youth. The whole community, including business and industry, should be concerned with the development of youth. Schools make a difference in changing adolescents' patterns of learning and valuing (Rutter, 1979). Schools should enhance academic achievement and inculcate the values of achievement and family involvement. The community should provide capable role models for young people (Murphy and Moriarity, 1976). Government, school, business, social, and activity group leaders can all be role models; and when normal role models are not available, social service agencies can provide them.

The Nature of Psychiatric Nursing with Adolescents

Adolescent psychiatric nursing is the nursing process with emphasis on the psychosocial aspects of assessment and intervention. The theory base for adolescent psychiatric nursing includes a thorough understanding of all aspects of growth and development for ages 11 through 19. Cognitive development is especially important because of the differences in cognition during early middle and late adolescence. Knowledge of the principles of "acting out" (as opposed to normal adolescent behaviors expressing the adolescent's ambivalence toward dependence and independence) are necessary for the nurse's background. Study of family systems theory—and the value systems and behaviors of families in different socioeconomic and cultural groups—are equally necessary. An effective adolescent psychiatric nurse is familiar with peer cultures and with curriculum, discipline, and extracurricular activities at school. Knowledge of community functioning, types of power bases, resources for youth (including social service agencies), and community value systems are vital for nurses who work in the community and helpful for nurses in inpatient settings. Techniques for evaluating interventions are becoming very important.

The assessment of adolescents requires communication skills that are compatible with the overly sensitive and easily embarrassed adolescent. Families of troubled teenagers require sensitivity and empathy. Families are essential for data collection, so nurses must learn basic family and group interviewing techniques. The ability to work with families is critical. Nurses serve as liaisons between the school, hospital, or agency and the parents. The nurse must instill a sense of trust and cooperation and intervene directly with families. Parental reliability regarding problems and strengths of the adolescent decreases as the age of the child increases, so it is important to gather data from other sources, especially school, and often juvenile court, child protection services, and case managers.

Planning for the care of adolescents requires collaborating with other disciplines and services and with the family. Interventions with adolescents will certainly include talking therapies, but a creative approach using a variety of strategies is necessary. The use of various media — visual, audio, art, and activity — helps the adolescent learn new skills. The evaluation of nursing care should be outcome oriented. Although time and resources are limited in most settings, determining the effectiveness of individual interventions and programs is sorely needed.

CHARACTERISTICS OF THE NURSE

The nurse who works with adolescents must possess certain characteristics to be successful. Foremost are the capacity to love and *empathize* with teenagers and their families, and the ability to *let go* of attachments to them when care is completed. Another trait of adolescent nurses is the belief that *everyone has the capacity to grow and change.* This conviction gives families and adolescents hope. The other characteristic a nurse working with adolescents must have is the ability to *set limits.* Underlying the capacity to love, a hopeful attitude, and the ability to set limits is a high level of *self-esteem.*

A sense of humor is essential. Adolescents usually have more humor than adult psychiatric patients and enjoy joking and fun activities even when seriously disordered. Flexibility is an attribute of an adolescent psychiatric nurse; adolescents' moods and interests change quickly and their vulnerability to changes in the family and other milieus require the nurse to adjust schedules and adapt treatment strategies. The adolescent psychiatric nurse must be willing to explore and work through his or her own unresolved developmental issues through introspection, clinical supervision, and personal therapy.

ANA STANDARDS FOR THE NURSING PROCESS WITH ADOLESCENTS

The Standards of Child and Adolescent Psychiatric and Mental Health Nursing Practice (American Nurses Association, 1985) direct the practice of adolescent psychiatric nursing (see box on p. 9). The first standard states: *The nurse applies appropriate, scientifically sound theory as a basis for nursing practice decisions.* The adolescent nurse draws especially on developmental theory, systems and family theory, and theories of mental health and illness.

The second standard relates to assessment: *The nurse systematically collects, records, and analyzes data that are comprehensive and accurate.* Systematic assessment of the adolescent in conjunction with other professionals, parents, and school is performed by the nurse. The assessment includes health status, physical and developmental history, daily activities, social and cultural information, normal behavior, status of development problems, and mental status.

Professional Practice Standards*

Standard I. Theory

The nurse applies appropriate, scientifically sound theory as a basis for nursing practice decisions.

Standard II. Assessment

The nurse systematically collects, records, and analyzes data that are comprehensive and accurate,

Standard III. Diagnosis

The nurse, in expressing conclusions supported by records assessment data and current scientific premises, uses nursing diagnoses and/or standard classifications of mental disorders for childhood and adolescence.

Standard IV. Planning

The nurse develops a nursing care plan with specific goals and interventions delineating nursing actions unique to the needs of each child or adolescent, as well as those of the family and other relevant interactive social systems.

Standard V. Intervention

The nurse intervenes as guided by the nursing care plan to implement nursing actions that promote, maintain, or restore physical and mental health, prevent illness, effect rehabilitation in childhood and adolescence, and restore developmental progression.

Standard V-A. Intervention: therapeutic environment

The nurse provides, structures, and maintains a therapeutic environment in collaboration with the child or adolescent, the family, and other health care providers.

Standard V-B. Intervention: activities of daily living

The nurse uses the activities of daily living in a goal-directed way to foster the physical and mental well-being of the child or adolescent and family.

Standard V-C. Intervention: psychotherapeutic interventions

The nurse uses psychotherapeutic interventions to assist children or adolescents and families to develop, improve, or regain their adaptive functioning; to promote health; prevent illness; and facilitate rehabilitation.

Standard V-D. Intervention: psychotherapy

The child and adolescent psychiatric and mental health specialist uses advanced clinical expertise to function as a psychotherapist for the child or adolescent and family and accepts professional accountability for nursing practice.

Standard V-E. Intervention: health teaching and anticipatory guidance

The nurse assists the child or adolescent and family to achieve more satisfying and productive patterns of living through health teaching and anticipatory guidance.

*From American Nurses Association (1985) Standards of child and adolescent psychiatric and mental health nursing practice, Kansas City, Mo, The Association.

Continued.

Professional Practice Standards — cont'd

Standard V-F. Intervention: somatic therapies

The nurse uses knowledge of somatic therapies with the child or adolescent and family to enchance therapeutic interventions.

Standard VI. Evaluation

The nurse evaluates the response of the child or adolescent and family to nursing actions in order to revise the data base, nursing diagnoses, and nursing care plan.

Standard VII. Quality assurance

The nurse participates in peer review and other means of evaluation to assure quality of nursing care provided for children and adolescents and their families.

Standard VIII. Continuing education

The nurse assumes responsibility for continuing education and professional development and contributes to the professional growth of others studying children's and adolescents' mental health.

Standard IX. Interdisciplinary collaboration

The nurse collaborates with other health care providers in assessing, planning, implementing, and evaluating programs and other activities related to child and adolescent psychiatric and mental health nursing.

Standard X. Use of community health systems

The nurse participates with other members of the community in assessing, planning, implementing, and evaluating mental health services and community systems that attend to primary, secondary, and tertiary prevention of mental disorders in children and adolescents.

Standard XI. Research

The nurse contributes to nursing and the child and adolescent psychiatric and mental health field through innovations in theory and practice and participation in research, and communicates these contributions.

Standard 3 discusses diagnoses: *The nurse, in expressing conclusions supported by recorded assessment data and current scientific premises, uses nursing diagnoses and/or standard classifications of mental disorders for childhood and adolescence.* Adolescent psychiatric nurses have a working knowledge of the revised edition of the *Diagnostic Statistical Manual of Mental Disorders,* or *DSM III-R* (American Psychiatric Association, 1987), which is used by all mental health disciplines. There are two classifications of nursing diagnoses available for psychiatric nurses: *The Classification of Nursing Diagnoses* by the North American Nursing Diagnosis Association (NANDA) (McLane, 1987) and *The Taxonomy of the Classification of the Phenomena of Concern for Psychiatric Mental Health Nursing (PMH)* (O'Toole and Loomis, 1989). The former is in widespread use in medical-surgical nursing but has only a few nonspecific diagnoses for psychiatric nursing. The latter is more relevant to psychiatric nursing. Nurses may use these classifications or use behavioral descriptions that are understood by the treatment team, the adolescent, and the family. The *DSM-III-R* and the *PMH* are used in this book. The complete listings may be found in Appendixes A and B.

The fourth standard gives direction for the planning of care: *The nurse develops a nursing care plan with specific goals and interventions delineating nursing actions unique to the needs of each child or adolescent, as well as those of the family and other relevant interactive social systems.* In most mental health treatment settings the written nursing and multidisciplinary treatment plan is mandated by the state, the Joint Commission on Hospital Accreditation, or both. The individualized treatment plan indicates specific goals and objectives (strategies) designed to alleviate client problems. The team member responsible for the intervention is identified, as is the date by which each objective is to be achieved. The plan is evaluated at specified intervals, and written notations are made as to whether the objectives have been met. The plan is developed with the help of the adolescent and the family.

The fifth standard describes the nursing intervention practiced by psychiatric–mental health nurses: *The nurse intervenes as guided by the nursing care plan to implement nursing actions that promote, maintain, or restore physical and mental health, prevent illness, effect rehabilitation in childhood and adolescence, and restore developmental progression.* The intervention standard is expanded to cover six areas of nursing interventions: (A) therapeutic environment, (B) activities of daily living, (C) psychotherapeutic interventions, (D) psychotherapy, (E) health teaching and anticipatory guidance, and (F) somatic therapies.

A *therapeutic environment* or milieu is a treatment setting, usually inpatient, residential, or partial hospitalization, in which the nurse provides, structures, and maintains a goal-directed, safe, therapeutic program and atmosphere in collaboration with other mental health disciplines. *Activities of daily living* are used "in a goal-directed way to foster the physical and mental well-being of the child or adolescent and family." *Psychotherapeutic interventions* assist "adolescents and families to develop, improve, or regain adaptive functioning; to promote health; prevent illness; and facilitate rehabilitation." Psychotherapeutic interventions include using principles of communication and human development, interviewing techniques, group process, problem solving, and crisis intervention to assist adolescents and families in developing intellectual, coping, and social skills. *Psychotherapy* with adolescents and families is an intervention practiced by the clinical specialist in psychiatric nursing. *Health teaching and anticipatory guidance* are often used. Teaching can be formal or informal and includes physical health, medications, parenting, coping, social skills, and developmental information. The intervention of *somatic therapies* refers to psychopharmacological treatment and the role of the nurse in administering and monitoring response to medication, and educating the adolescent and family about specific medications.

The standards also include *evaluation* as an element of nursing practice. There are five professional performance standards stating that participation in *quality assurance, continuing education,* and *research* is necessary and that *interdisciplinary collaboration* and the *use of community health systems* are also expected of the adolescent psychiatric nurse.

Strategies Used by Adolescent Psychiatric–Mental Health Nurses

To meet the standards described by the ANA and to serve the needs of adolescents and their families, psychiatric nurses develop a repertoire of intervention techniques (see box). Some of the techniques are common in all types of nursing, but others are specialized techniques used in psychiatric settings or situations. These strategies, used by staff nurses or other nurses with undergraduate degrees, include caring; therapeutic relationships; therapeutic communication; role modeling; self-esteem building; teaching; crisis intervention; limit setting and anger management; surveillance; somatic therapy; goal setting; and social, psychological and coping skills, and cognitive skill training. Also included are advocacy, referral, community action, and multidisciplinary collaboration.

This intervention strategies list, which is the focus of Chapter 8, has been developed in response to the need to explain to nurses themselves and to other members of the treatment team what psychiatric nurses actually *do* in their work settings, especially in therapeutic milieus. Most related textbooks and literature focus on theory, assessment, the therapeutic relationship, or even psychotherapy with clients who have certain diagnoses or problems. The literature on therapeutic environments provides a better direction for understanding the nursing *actions* of psychiatric nurses. The ANA's standards clearly state what psychiatric nurses should be doing, and this book describes the skills and strategies nurses need to live up to those standards in the various work settings where they serve adolescents and their families.

Strategies Used by Nurses Who Care for Adolescents

Caring
Therapeutic relationships
Therapeutic communication
Role modeling
Self-esteem building
Teaching
Crisis intervention
Limit setting and anger management
Surveillance
Somatic therapy
Goal setting
Social, psychological, coping, and cognitive skill training
Advocacy
Referral
Community action
Multidisciplinary collaboration

REFERENCES AND SUGGESTED READINGS

Adler A (1963) The problem child, New York, Capricorn Books.

American Nurses Association (1985) Standards of child and adolescent psychiatric and mental health nursing practice, Kansas City, Mo, The Association.

American Psychiatric Association (1987) Diagnostic and statistical manual of mental disorders III-R, Washington, DC, The Association.

Beavers WR (1977) Psychotherapy and growth: a family systems perspective, New York, Brunner-Mazel Publishers, Inc.

Block JH and Block J (1980) The role of ego control and ego resiliency in the origins of behavior. In Collins WA, editor, Development of cognition. Minnesota symposia on child psychology, vol 13, Hillsdale, NJ, Erlbaum Associates.

Buber M (Translated by W Kaufman) (1970) I and thou, New York, Scribner Book Companies, Inc.

Dreikus R and Grey L (1970) A parent's guide to child discipline, New York, Hawthorne Books, Inc.

Dugan TF and Coles R (1989) The child in our times and studies in the development of resilience, New York, Brunner-Mazel Publishers, Inc.

Fromm E (1956) The art of loving, New York, Harper & Row Publishers, Inc.

Garmezy N (1981) Children under stress: perspectives on antecedents and correlates of vulnerability and resistance to psychopathology. In Rabin AI, Aronoff J, Barclay AM, and Zucher RA, editors, Further explorations in personality, New York, John Wiley & Sons.

Garmezy N (1983) Stressors of childhood. In Garmezy N and Rutter M, editors, Stress coping and development in children, New York, McGraw-Hill Book Co.

Garmezy N (1984) Stress-resistant children: the search for protective factors. In JE Stevenson, editor, Recent research in developmental psychopathology, Journal of Child Psychology and Psychiatry Book Supplement No 4, Oxford, Pergamon Press.

Garmezy N, Masters A, and Tellegen A (1984) The study of stress and competence in children: a building block for developmental psychopathology, Child Development 55:97-111.

Glenn S and Warner J (1982) Developing capable young people, Houston, Humansphere, Inc.

Hauser SJ, Powers SI, Noam GG, Jacobson AM, Weiss B, and Follansbee DJ (1984) Family contexts of adolescent ego development, Child Development 55:195-213.

Ianni FAJ (1983) Home, school and community in adolescent education, New York, ERIC Clearing House on Urban Education, Teachers College, Columbia University.

Ianni FAJ (1989) The search for structure: a report on American youth today, New York, The Free Press.

Leininger M (1981) Caring: an essential human need, Thorofare, NJ, Slack, Inc.

Long J and Vaillant G (1984) Natural history of male psychological health. XI. Escape from the underclass, American Journal of Psychiatry, 141:341-346.

Marcel G (Translated by M Harari) (1949) The philosophy of existence, New York, Books for Libraries Press.

Mayeroff M (1971) On caring, New York, Harper & Row Publishers, Inc.

McLane A (1987) Classification of nursing diagnoses: proceedings of the seventh conference of the North American Nursing Diagnosis Association, St Louis, The CV Mosby Co.

Murphy CB and Moriarity AC (1976) Vulnerability, coping and growth from infancy to adolescence, New Haven, Conn, Yale University Press.

Naisbitt J (1984) Megatrends: ten new directions transforming our lives, New York, Warner Books, Inc.

O'Toole AW and Loomis ME (1989) Revision of the phenomenon of concern for psychiatric mental health nursing, Archives of Psychiatric Nursing 3(5):288-299.

Rutter M (1979) Protective factors in children's responses to stress and disadvantage. In Kent MW and Rolf SE, editors, Primary prevention of psychopathology, vol 3: Social competence in children, Hanover, Penn, University Press of New England.

Rutter M (1980) Changing youth in a changing society, Cambridge, Mass, Harvard University Press.

Werner EE and Smith RS (1982) Vulnerable but invincible: a study of resilient children, New York, McGraw-Hill Book Co.

Chapter 2

Historical Development of Current Adolescent Problems

During the past 60 years a dramatic social and cultural revolution has taken place in the United States. In the 1930s a young child had some responsibility for the family's welfare, had extensive interpersonal contact with and worked alongside adult family members, and was surrounded by an extended family who shared and passed on the same values. Logical and natural consequences occurred if a child failed to fulfill his or her obligations: for instance, a child learned very clearly that if eggs were not gathered, the family could not eat breakfast. Family members spent many hours a day in direct contact with each other. A child had capable adults with whom to explore ideas — adults who provided directions and served as role models for functioning in real life. Moreover, this contact gave a child validation as a competent person.

The youngster was taught similar values at school and church because parents in small communities carefully chose teachers and clergy who shared their value system. This life-style may seem idyllic today; it provided opportunities to learn problem solving, decision making, and responsibility, and it produced competent, creative adults. Young adults who had the ability to solve problems and make good decisions and who had a sense of responsibility to something greater than themselves were free to pursue the numerous opportunities available in this country (Glenn, 1982).

Since the mid-1930s several major events have had an impact on family life in America (see box on p. 16). The first event was a rapid shift in population. In 1935 70% of persons lived in rural areas; in 1950 70% lived in or near cities. This movement separated the workplace from in or near the home to a location away from the home. Work became less visible, and parents became increasingly separated from their children during the day. The family unit became smaller, with few if any extended family members living in the home. Education also became centralized, and parents had little control over the selection of teachers. Soon husbands and fathers were working far from home, earning money to purchase goods and services previously produced at home. Wives and mothers became isolated at home. They had less physical labor, less interpersonal interaction, and more free time. Children became passive recipients of the fruits of their parents' labor rather than active participants and learners in the adult work world.

An event of equal impact was the invention of television. This device has many

---

Social Revolution

Urbanization
Television and media
Civil rights movement
Women's rights movement
Children's and other personal rights movements
Divorce
Substance abuse
Child abuse

---

positive effects, such as education and entertainment, but its presence in every household has had many negative effects on family life. Television exposes youngsters to undesirable values, including violence and other criminal activity, and to political and moral attitudes that conflict with the family's beliefs. Stereotypes of the "American dream" that are portrayed have little to do with reality. Exposure to new and different ideas is not negative, but overexposure is confusing, especially when television viewing takes the place of personal interaction with capable, caring adults. Most Americans spend many hours a day watching television. Sophisticated advertising on TV instills yearning for material goods to fill the void caused by isolation and the loss of personal interaction.

A series of events—the rights movements—has also significantly affected family life in the last 40 years. The civil rights movement was concerned with eliminating discrimination against black Americans. This movement, characterized by both nonviolent and violent protest, stretched from the mid-1950s into the mid-1970s. The idea that all individuals have a right to participate fully in American life kindled the women's rights struggle for equality with men at work and at home. Both of these movements resulted in legislation that prohibits discrimination based on race or sex. The rights of other groups have become the focus of policy changes in the United States, for instance, the rights of persons charged with or convicted of crimes, of handicapped people, the elderly, and the mentally ill. Finally the rights of children to make certain decisions affecting their lives regarding such things as curriculum, custodial parents, and life-styles, were emphasized. Superimposed on all of these struggles and changes was the Vietnam War. The years between 1960 and 1980 were filled with protest against abuses of civil rights and against the conduct and existence of the Vietnam War. The values behind American life were reviewed, examined, and sometimes rejected; the focus shifted from commitment to family, work, and school to the individual self. Paradoxically, there was a strong emphasis on providing services and money to assist lower-income people, the arts, schools and universities, and natural resources.

Additional factors have contributed to the changes in society. The introduction of birth control pills and the legalization of abortion resulted in unprecedented sexual freedom for women. The extensive use of illegal mood-altering drugs by all levels of society has yielded problems of enormous magnitude, which are yet unsolved.

Unfortunately, the emphasis on individual rights and privileges did not include an emphasis on individual or family responsibility. The chaos of those decades resulted in people who, although unsure of their values and commitments, have unprecedented freedom to do as they wish. If those who lived through those tumultuous times are uncertain, it is no surprise that their children have often fared poorly (see box). In fact, the increase in treatment programs for adolescents, including school intervention, psychiatric hospitals, juvenile detention centers, group homes, and chemical dependency treatment programs gave rise to the need for this book.

Adolescent Problems

There are currently over 35 million adolescents in the United States (see box on p. 18). The increase of 10% expected by 1990 will be predominantly made up of minority youth. This adolescent segment of the population is the only group to show an increase in mortality. The mortality rate is 100 per 100,000; accidents, suicide, and homicide are the three leading causes of death (U.S. Department of Health, Education and Welfare, 1979; National Center for Health Statistics, 1986; Kovar, 1978).

Accidents are the leading cause of death among adolescents. Over 16,500 young people between 15 and 24 years of age died in 1980 as a result of automobile accidents (National Highway Traffic Safety Administration, 1981). Approximately 40% to 60% of fatal accidents involving a teenage driver are alcohol related (Douglass, 1981).

Suicide in the 15 to 19 age-group has increased 300% in the last 3 decades (Centers for Disease Control, 1985). Approximately 5000 young people commit suicide every year, and 50 to 100 adolescents attempt suicide for each suicide completed (Garfinkel and others, 1982). These are conservative estimates because suicide is underreported for various reasons. Suicide is the second most frequent cause of death among 15- to 19-year-olds.

Alcohol and drug abuse among adolescents increased significantly during the past decades, with a leveling off noted in the first half of the 1980s. By age 18, 92% of males and 73% of females drink alcohol. Approximately 16% drink heavily (Zucker and Harford, 1986). An estimated 3.3 million 14- to 17-year-olds are problem drinkers

---

Major Adolescent Problems in the 1990s

Accidents
Suicide
Substance abuse
Teen pregnancy
Sexually transmitted diseases
Abuse
Juvenile crime
Poverty
Runaways
Poor academic performance

One Day in the Lives of American Children

17,051	women get pregnant
2,795	of them are teenagers
1,106	teenagers have abortions
372	teenagers miscarry
1,295	teenagers give birth
689	babies are born to women who have had inadequate prenatal care
719	babies are born at low birthweight (less than 5 pounds, 8 ounces)
129	babies are born at very low birthweight (less than 3 pounds, 5 ounces)
67	babies die before 1 month of life
105	babies die before their first birthday
27	children die from poverty
10	children die from guns
30	children are wounded by guns
6	teenagers commit suicide
135,000	children bring a gun to school
7,742	teens become sexually active
623	teenagers get syphilis or gonorrhea
211	children are arrested for drug abuse
437	children are arrested for drinking or drunken driving
1,512	teenagers drop out of school
1,849	children are abused or neglected
3,288	children run away from home
1,629	children are in adult jails
2,556	children are born out of wedlock
2,989	see their parents divorced
34,285	people lose jobs

From Children's Defense Fund (1981) Children 1990: a report and briefing book and action primer, Washington, DC, The Fund.

(Dusek and Girdano, 1980). About 30% of seventh graders have tried alcohol. Other illicit drug use by adolescents peaked in 1979 and 1980, when 60% of high school seniors reported using marijuana, 15% had tried hallucinogens and/or cocaine, 26% had used stimulants, 15% had used sedatives, 15% had tried tranquilizers, and 74% used cigarettes. In 1985 and 1986 there was an increase in the use of cocaine in powder and crack forms (Institute for Social Research, 1987). Surveys conducted in the southwest Ohio area indicate that about 70% to 80% of youth in grades 7 through 12 use alcohol once a week. Parental chemical abuse and dependence is associated with family conflict, physical and sexual abuse, and adolescent runaways.

Among adolescents, 50% have begun *sexual intercourse* by age 16 and 70% by age 19. Two thirds of adolescent girls use ineffective contraception or none at all (Zelnick and Kanter, 1980).

Teen pregnancy has increased to 1,005,000 pregnancies in adolescents in 1984, resulting in 470,000 births, 400,000 abortions, and approximately 134,000 miscarriages (Hayes, 1987). In 1978, one teenage girl in ten became pregnant. In 1985, there were almost 10,000 births to teenagers under age 15 (U.S. Department of Health and Human Services, 1988). Over 1.3 million children live with teenage mothers, and another 1.6 million children under age 5 live with mothers who gave birth as teenagers (Leepson, 1982). These birth statistics have enormous implications for a whole generation of children.

Sexually transmitted diseases occur at higher rates in adolescents than in adults. *Chlamydia trachomatis* has been found in 15% of sexually active females and *Neisseria gonorrhoeae* was found in 4% (Shaffer, 1988). At present 17% of AIDS cases are found in adolescents. Adolescents are at particular risk for increased incidence of disease (and pregnancy) because of the widespread failure to use condoms. It is important to note that adolescent sexual activity is correlated with alcohol and drug use (Jessor, 1977; Jessor and Jessor, 1984).

Almost half of all marriages end in *divorce,* and a third of all children under age 18 experience the divorce of their parents (Furstenberg, 1983). At the time of separation and divorce, children and adolescents experience crisis, loss, and grief. Longitudinal studies have shown that children never fully recover from this painful experience (Wallerstein, 1983, 1987).

There were 1,712,614 cases of child *physical abuse* (American Humane Association, 1985) and 123,000 cases of child *sexual abuse* reported by November, 1984; an increase of 9% per year was noted (National Committee for the Prevention of Child Abuse, 1985). In 1986 2.1 million reports of child abuse and neglect were reported (American Humane Association, 1988). Of the 737,000 confirmed cases, 27.6% were determined to be physical abuse, 15.7% sexual abuse, 54.9% neglect, 8.3 emotional maltreatment, and 7.9% other types of abuse. In 1987 2.2 million reports were documented, with 686,000 confirmed — about 38% (American Humane Association, 1989). Confirmation means that the case met all of the state's criteria for abuse. The American Humane Association estimates that for every reported case, there are two or three unreported cases. Violence causing injuries to siblings is the most common form of abuse. Four out of five children (3 to 17 years old) are the victims of sibling violence an average of once per year (Straus and others, 1980).

Juvenile crime steadily increased from 1964 to 1978, with a decline beginning in 1983. There is, however, a significant increase in alcohol-related offenses and fraud (Kratcoski and others, 1986). Of all the murders in the United States, 8% are committed by juveniles under the age of 19 (Federal Bureau of Investigation, 1985); 30% of rapes and 56% of child molestations are perpetrated by adolescents under 18 (Fehrenbach and others, 1986). Juvenile delinquency used to be associated with unstable inner-city families and high unemployment, but rural and suburban crime increased dramatically by 1978. The decline since then in adolescent suburban crime is related in part to the passage of the "baby boom" cohort through the teen years. Adolescents remain unsupervised because of working mothers and commuting parents, greater teen use of cars, impersonal shopping centers (popular gathering places), and increasing alcohol and drug use (Kratcoski and Kratcoski, 1986).

One in five American children lives in *poverty.* The proportion of children living in poverty increased 23% between 1979 and 1988. More than 12 million children have no health insurance. Poor teenagers are three times more likely than other teens to drop out of school and four times more likely to have below-average basic skills.

Teenagers with below-average academic skills and from poor families are five to seven times more likely to be parents. When young men make low wages, they are less likely to marry. Since 1973 marriage rates among young men have declined by one third, and out-of-wedlock births have doubled. Median incomes for young families dropped 24% between 1973 and 1987 (Children's Defense Fund, 1990). Because the number of young adults from age 18 to 24 entering the work force is significantly declining, it is essential that all youth be prepared for the work world.

About 12% of American teenagers *run away* from home for a period of time (Garbarino and others, 1986). In 1985, 60,500 youths were provided shelter in 271 facilities, 305,000 teens were provided drop-in services, and 250,000 teens used hotlines (House Committee of Education and Labor, 1985). Runaway youth are usually running away from a family environment severely conflicted by parental chemical dependencies and physical and sexual abuse (Janus and others, 1987).

Satanism — cults in which believers worship the devil or Satan and engage in ritualistic seduction, torture, substance abuse, animal and sometimes human sacrifices — is an increasing problem for youth. Although no reliable statistics of membership in such cults are available, one study demonstrated that 67% of psychotherapists had treated adolescents involved in Satanism (Wheeler and others, 1988). Adolescents who become involved in this phenomena range from those having very few symptoms to those who experience posttraumatic stress disorder, psychosis, dissociative states, and multiple personality disorder. Substance abuse and dependency are frequently associated with Satanism.

Poor academic performance is reflected in the drop in average scores in college entrance examinations; one half million youth drop out of school each year. The number of teenagers with severe behavior disorders has increased (as has the number of classrooms providing special services for them).

Services and Professional Help Available

Adolescents who are experiencing any of the problems described in the preceding section draw attention to themselves because of their symptomatic behaviors, which are often disturbing to others. It was estimated in 1986 that almost 12% of children and youth experience some psychiatric disorder; this amounts to approximately 7.5 million children under the age of 18. About 6% of that number were receiving treatment in 1986 (Office of Technology Assessment, 1987). Recent studies have demonstrated that the incidence of a DSMIII Axis I disorder was present in 34% of youth aged 8, 12, and 17 (Kashani and others, 1989) and 22% of children aged 7 to 11 (Costello, 1988). None of these studies identify children at risk because of poverty or other conditions. In both studies around 10% of parents did not notice their child's problem. The number of adolescents and families who are experiencing these behaviors have overwhelmed the existing structures for dealing with them and have given rise to new programs.

Adolescent and child admissions to *inpatient treatment programs* have increased 38% between 1980 and 1986 from 81,532 to 112,215 admissions (Manden, Scheid, and Barrett, 1987). The distribution of the admissions in 1986 was 16,612 to state facilities, 16,735 to private psychiatric hospitals, and 48,185 to general hospitals. All of these admissions represent 0.19% of the population of children under 18 that year (National Association of Private Psychiatric Hospitals, 1988).

There have been several media exposés about this increase (Schiffman, 1989). In these stories reporters interview families who say that their adolescent was unnecessarily hospitalized in a for-profit hospital, with the direct or indirect inference that the adolescent was exploited for financial profits. Although the professional associations connected with psychiatric care providers were exposed in the public media, there have been several commentaries in professional journals (Pruitt and Weiner, 1989; Lewis, 1989; Pothier, 1989). No studies have been done to determine if these admissions are indeed appropriate. Furthermore, there is a dearth of outcome studies on whether inpatient treatment is effective.

The American Academy of Child and Adolescent Psychiatry has developed a fact sheet for families (1988) and criteria for admission, utilization review, and quality assurance for practitioners (Stevenson, 1987). Both The American Nurses Association and the Advocates for Child Psychiatric Nursing have been silent on this issue.

During the past decade, there have been changes in reimbursement patterns for public and private psychiatric mental health care. Because expenditures by insurance companies for inpatient care have risen dramatically, the industry has moved to control this cost by limiting benefits and by strictly and intrusively managing cases and care systems. This results in problems with patient and family confidentiality; increased costs for utilization review, photocopying, and mailing of patient records to the company; increased paperwork to meet criteria of Medicare or Medicaid; and increased time spent on documentation. The work of psychiatrists and other professionals is questioned and reviewed by unseen nurses and others over the telephone. HMOs are particularly apt to limit both inpatient and outpatient mental health and substance abuse services. Public reimbursement by state and local governments for these services is extremely limited. As the number of teens needing intensive treatment rises, states are decreasing the number of beds and services to teens. The reduction in treatment days and dollars results in recidivism, inability to establish new coping skills before discharge, lower staff-to-patient ratios, more aggression, and greater burnout of nursing personnel (Jemerin and Philips, 1988). Some of the inpatient admissions may have been directed to partial-hospitalization programs, but third-party reimbursement for such service is rare. Publicly financed outpatient services are inadequately funded and understaffed; this results in waiting lists and inadequate treatment. The new role of case manager is emerging to provide relief. Private practitioners may not have skills in both individual adolescent and family therapy, and they may not devote enough resources to networking with the schools and courts. A comprehensive system of psychiatric mental health care is desperately needed. A model is described in Chapter 7.

Juvenile court systems are overwhelmed with cases. In many larger metropolitan areas, juvenile courts operate their own counseling services. Because of the case load, some juvenile detention facilities can handle only felony cases, thereby permitting lesser offenses to go essentially unpunished and untreated. Offenses related to chemical dependence rarely reach an intervention situation until felony charges are filed.

Child protection services for abused and neglected children and teens have caseloads so high that in many areas only the most severe situations receive attention. The qualifications and compensation for caseworkers vary but are often inadequate, resulting in high burnout and turnover rates.

School systems provide treatment within the schools. Many school systems have hired crisis and substance abuse–intervention specialists to train counselors and teachers to identify and refer students to appropriate assessment and treatment. Often serving as the crisis coordinator, the school nurse is usually actively involved in identification, referral, and treatment of adolescent problems. Besides crisis intervention, many schools provide support groups for chemically dependent adolescents, children of chemically dependent parents, and abused adolescents.

Nurses in many communities and some high schools provide free or low-cost *contraceptive* counseling and devices to reduce teenage pregnancy and sexually transmitted disease.

There are severe shortages of personnel to serve the needs of adolescents and their families. In 1980 the Graduate Medical Education National Advisory Committee indicated that 9000 child psychiatrists would be needed within the next 10 years. At that time there were 3000 child psychiatrists. Currently there are about 6000 child/adolescent psychiatrists (Academy of Child and Adolescent Psychiatry, 1990). In a study of child and adolescent psychiatric nurses, 240 Master's-prepared nurses were identified as working in the field; 17% of the respondents to the survey were employed in schools of nursing and only 39.5% of their time was spent in direct service (Pothier and others, 1985).

There are 11 graduate programs in child and adolescent psychiatric nursing (see Appendix C). Master's- and doctorate-prepared nurses tend to work as therapists, educators, and administrators. A minimum of data is available on the number of BSN- and AD-prepared nurses serving adolescents. Of those working as staff nurses, most reported receiving no curriculum content or practice related to this specialty. It is hoped that this book will fill that gap for the staff nurse and for those nurses who practice in schools and pediatric clinics.

Although the numbers and severity of adolescent problems and the lack of resources and research-based information needed to prevent and treat problems seem overwhelming, some recent events evince some hope for success. The so-called war on drugs has focused attention on the substance abuse epidemic, and through the Drug-Free Schools Executive Initiative sponsored by former President Reagan, some new monies have become available for prevention and intervention in the schools. The Institute of Medicine (1989) published a report commissioned by the National Institute of Mental Health (NIMH) recommending that NIMH establish a national plan for child mental health research. The plan calls for the following goals:

1. Provide support and incentives at each stage of career development, including research training and career stability, for an expanded pool of (child mental health) research scientists.
2. Increase support for individual project, program project, and center grants (in child mental health research).
3. Increase funding for (child mental health) research in the areas of epidemiology; assessment, diagnosis, and treatment; prevention and special

populations; services and systems of care; basic behavioral and social sciences; neurosciences; and the NIMH intramural research program.
4. Establish an institute-wide consortium concerned with child and adolescent mental health research to implement this national plan.

Although this plan focuses on research, it is an indication that the national attention is now directed toward adolescents, their families, and those who provide mental health services.

REFERENCES AND SUGGESTED READINGS

American Academy of Child and Adolescent Psychiatry (1988) Eleven questions to ask before psychiatric hospital treatment of children and adolescents. In Facts for families, No 32, Washington, DC, The Academy.

American Academy of Child and Adolescent Psychiatry (1990) Phone conversation with Public Information Department, Washington, DC, The Academy.

American Humane Association (1985) Statistics collected for the National Center for Child Abuse and Neglect as of November, 1984, Aurora, Ill, The Association.

American Humane Association (1988) Highlights of aggregate official child neglect and abuse reporting, 1986, Denver, The Association.

American Humane Association (1989) Highlights of aggregate official child neglect and abuse reporting, 1987, Denver, The Association.

Centers for Disease Control (1985) Suicide surveillance 1970-1980, Atlanta, US Department of Health and Human Services, Public Health Services, Violent Epidemiology Branch, Center for Health Promotion and Education.

Children's Defense Fund (1990) Children: a report card, briefing book and action primer, Washington, DC, The Fund.

Costello E (1988) Child psychiatric disorders and their correlates: a primary care pediatric sample, Journal of the American Academy of Child and Adolescent Psychiatry 28(6):851-855.

Douglass P (1981) Alcohol, youth and traffic accidents. In National Institute on Alcohol Abuse and Alcoholism: Special population issues, Alcohol and health monograph, No 4, Rockville, Md, The Institute.

Dusek D and Girdano DA (1980) Drugs: a factual account, Reading, Mass, Addison-Wesley Publishing Co, Inc.

Federal Bureau of Investigation (1985) Uniform crime report, Washington, DC, The Bureau.

Fehrenbach PA, Smith W, Monastersky C, and Beisher B (1986) Adolescent sex offenders: offender and offense characteristics, American Journal of Orthopsychiatry 56:225-233.

Furstenberg FF (1983) The life course of children of divorce, American Sociological Review 48:656-668.

Garbarino J, Wilson J, and Garbarino A (1986) The adolescent runaway. In Garbarino J and Sebes J, editors: Troubled youth, troubled families, New York, Aldine Publishers.

Garfinkel B, Fraese A, and Hood J (1982) Suicide attempts in children and adolescents, American Journal of Psychiatry 139:1257-1261.

Glenn S (1982) Developing capable young people, Houston, Humansphere, Inc.

Graduate Medical Education National Advisory Committee (1980) Present and future supply and requirements for physicians, US Department of Health and Human Services, Washington, DC, US Government Printing Office.

House Committee of Education and Labor, Subcommittee of Human Resources (July 25, 1985) Runaway & homeless youth, 99th Congress, second session, Y4Ed 8/1, 99-23.

Institute of Medicine (1989) Research on children and adolescents with mental, behavioral, and developmental disorders, Washington, DC, National Academy Press.

Institute for Social Research (1987) Press release, University of Michigan at Ann Arbor: Monthly vital statistics report: advance report of final mortality statistics — 1984, 35(4)(suppl).

Janus MD, McCormack A, Burgess A, and Hartman C (1987) Adolescent runaways: causes and consequences, Lexington, Mass, DC Heath & Co.

Jemerin JM and Philips I (1988) Changes in inpatient child psychiatry: consequences and recommendations, Journal of the Academy of Child and Adolescent Psychiatry 27(4):397-403.

Jessor R (1984) Adolescent problem drinking: psychosocial aspects and developmental outcomes. Presented at The Carnegie Conference on Unhealthful Risk-Taking Behavior Among Adolescents, Stanford, Calif.

Jessor R and Jessor SL (1977) Problem behavior and psychosocial development: a longitudinal study of youth, New York, Academic Press, Inc.

Kashani J, Orvaschel H, Rosenberg T, and Reid J (1989) Psychopathology in a community sample of children and adolescents: a developmental perspective, 28(5)701-706.

Kovar MG, editor (1978) Adolescent health status and health-related behavior in adolescent behavior and health, Institute of Medicine Pub No 78-004, Washington, DC, National Academy of Sciences.

Kratcoski PC and Kratcoski LD (1986) Juvenile delinquency, Englewood Cliffs, NJ, Prentice Hall.

Leepson M (1982) Sex education. In Editorial Research Reports: Youth problems, Washington, DC, Congressional Quarterly, Inc.

Lewis JE (1989) Are adolescents being hospitalized unnecessarily? Journal of Child and Adolescent Psychiatric–Mental Health Nursing 2(4):134-138.

Manderscheid RW and Barrett S, editors (1987) Mental health — United States, 1987, Rockville, MD, US Department of Health and Human Services, National Institute of Mental Health, DHAS Pub No (ADM) 87-1518.

National Association of Private Psychiatric Hospitals (1988) In perspective: child and adolescent psychiatric hospitalization, Washington DC, The Association.

National Center for Health Statistics (1986) Vital statistics of the US — 1981, vol II, Part B: Mortality, Department of Health and Human Services 1102, Public Health Service, Washington, DC, US Government Printing Office.

National Committee for the Prevention of Child Abuse (1985) Survey data for 1984. In Stuart GW and Sundeen SJ (1987) Principles and practice of psychiatric nursing, ed 3, St. Louis, Mosby–Year Book, Inc.

National Council on Alcoholism (1982) Facts on teenage drinking, New York, The Council.

National Highway Traffic Safety Administration (1981) Fatal accident reporting system, 1980: an overview of US traffic fatal accident and fatality data collected in FARS for the year 1980, Pub No DOT HS 805 953, Washington, DC, US Department of Transportation.

Office of Technology Assessment (1987) Children's mental health: problems and services, Durham, NC, Duke University Press.

Pothier P (1989) The impact of privatization of psychiatric care on children and adolescents, Archives of Psychiatric Nursing 9(3):123-137.

Pothier P, Norbeck J, and Laliberte M (1985) Child psychiatric nursing: the gap between need and utilization, Journal of Psychosocial Nursing 23(7):11-21.

Pruitt DB and Weiner JM (1989) The AACAP and hospitalization for children and adolescents [letter to the editor] Journal of the American Academy of Child–Adolescent Psychiatry 28:136-137.

Schiffman JR (February 3, 1989) Children's wards: teenagers end up in psychiatric hospitals in alarming numbers, The Wall Street Journal, pp A1, A6.

Shaffer MA (1988) The problem of sexually transmitted disease education of adolescents: a current view. In Schinazi EF and Nahmias AJ, editors: AIDS in children and adolescents and heterosexual adults, New York, Elsevier.

Stevenson K and Maholick M (1987) Child and adolescent psychiatric illness: guidelines for treatment resources, quality assurance, peer review, and reimbursement, Washington, DC, American Academy of Child and Adolescent Psychiatry.

Straus M, Coules R, and Steinmitz S (1980) Behind closed doors: violence in the American family, New York, Anchor Books.

US Department of Health, Education and Welfare (1979) Healthy people: the Surgeon General's report on health promotion and disease prevention, Department of Health, Education, and Welfare Pub No 79-55071, US Government Printing Office.

Wallerstein JS (1983) Children of divorce: the psychological tasks of the child, American Journal of Orthopsychiatry 53:230-242.

Wallerstein JS (1987) Children of divorce: report of a ten-year follow-up of latency age children, American Journal of Orthopsychiatry, 57:199-211.

Wheeler BR, Wood S, and Hatch RJ (1988) Assessment and intervention with adolescents involved in satanism, Social Work (November-December):547-550.

Zelnick M and Kanter JF (1980) Sexual activity, contraceptive use and pregnancy among metropolitan teenagers—1971-1979, Family Planning Perspectives 12:230-237.

Zucker R and Hartford T (1986) National study of the demography of adolescent drinking practices in 1980. In Felstead C, editor: Youth and alcohol abuse: readings and resources, Phoenix, Oryx Press.

US Department of Health and Human Services, Public Health Service. National Center for Health Statistics (1988). Vital statistics of the United States (1986) vol 1, Natality Table p. 1-60.

Chapter 3

Development of the Healthy Adolescent and Family

Linda A. Mast
Lawrence R. Schoppe
Christina R. Hogarth

Adolescents experience extensive biological, social, psychological, and spiritual changes during the period between ages 12 and 18. Through those years the adolescent is a part of a family whose individual members, as well as the family as a whole, progress through various stages of development. Adolescents and families live in communities that influence their growth and development and determine which services are available. In this chapter the healthy adolescent family and community is discussed.

The Adolescent as an Individual

PSYCHOSOCIAL DEVELOPMENT

The nurse applies appropriate, scientifically sound theory as a basis for nursing practice decisions. Erik Erikson's prototype of psychosocial development is such a theory; it includes eight general age groupings with a set of orderly, acquired behaviors for each stage from infancy to old age (Erikson, 1963). Erikson sees each stage as a conflict between opposing values, with accomplishment of that stage being determined by a resolution of the conflict. The stages most appropriate to the adolescent are *middle childhood,* which sets the stage for the development of the adolescent, *adolescence,* and the goal toward which the adolescent is strives, *adulthood.* Progression through the earlier stages should be considered because it may have an impact on how the child develops.

Erikson describes the major task of middle childhood as *industry versus inferiority.* The age range of this stage is 6 to 12 years, when the child begins moving from the confines of the nuclear family to experiment with the larger social setting. Activities that are concurrent with this stage are the beginning of formal education and participation in organized sports and social activities; with these comes a greater dependence on self in relation to peers. *Industry* in this context is the child's appropriate practice of new skills in a social setting and the consequent perception of success. *Inferiority,* then, is the self-perception of failure or inadequacy. Accomplishment leads to the acquisition of *competence.*

Adolescence is the stage that resolves the conflict of *identity versus role confusion.* Familial bonds are further loosened as the adolescent moves into the social realm occupied by the *peer group.* The adolescent seeks an appropriate present role and clues to future roles. Since adolescents cannot see themselves clearly and they seek more independence from their families' direction and values, they turn to the peer group to test their views of themselves. They receive confirmation and comfort from their peers if their self-perceptions correspond with those of their peers. If they make choices that are in conflict with their peer groups, they risk ostracism. Adolescents' fluctuations between dependence and independence and their choices based on family or peer group values cause confusion within them and within those who care for them.

There is a certain rigidity and lack of tolerance for peers who do not conform to the group, which is one reason adolescents in a certain group may dress similarly, have common interests, and feel obligated to try whatever the others in the group may attempt. If the choice of a peer group is a poor one and the adolescent has few other resources for support, identity may be confirmed in a detrimental manner. When adolescents cannot get a positive message confirming their views of themselves and for some reason cannot problem solve for better choices, then role confusion may occur. Consequently, the adolescent feels lost, separate, and abandoned. It is not surprising that there is so much perceived loneliness during adolescence (Moore and Schultz, 1983; Mahan and Yarcheski, 1988). The loneliness, confusion, and striving for independence prompt some acting out or rebellious behavior in most teenagers. Adolescents require a great deal of tactful support and assistance with decision making and problem solving.

Erikson says *fidelity* is the virtue gained by attaining a sense of identity. In this context fidelity corresponds with the term *loyalty.* As a product of gaining a comfortable self-image, adolescents learn to trust their choices and to stand by commitments. These commitments may be to others (as in personal relationships), to the successful acquisition and continuation of productive employment, or to the planning and sacrifice necessary to continue educational goals. Because of self-trust, adolescents can be loyal to their own needs.

Young *adulthood* is the ultimate goal of adolescence. The drama of this stage is *intimacy versus isolation.* The acquisition of *love,* or the ability to form comfortable intimate relationships, is the accomplishment of intimacy. If emotional isolation occurs at this stage, Erikson's theory questions whether the adolescent had acquired fidelity.

The adolescent and adult stages have related tasks dealing with separation, consolidation of the self, and formation of increasingly intimate relationships. In contemporary American society the transition from adolescence to adulthood is protracted. Real independence, including financial independence, is often difficult to achieve because of the limited opportunities offered in unskilled jobs and the need for higher education.

PSYCHOANALYTIC THEORIES OF ADOLESCENT DEVELOPMENT

Major psychoanalytic contributors to the interpretation of adolescent psychodynamics began with the theories of Anna Freud (1965), whose extensive studies of normal adolescent development and adolescent pathology are major contributions, as are the separation-individuation theories of Melanie Kline and Margaret Mahler (1971). Freud (1953) divided adolescence into 4 periods with related developmental tasks:

1. Preadolescence, around 9-13 years of age, marked by resurgence of libidinal and aggressive drives, striving toward strengthening sexual identification, with regression a common reaction during this time, seen in fighting, gang activity, temper outburst, and depression.
2. Early adolescence, around 12-15 years of age, associated with the emergence of a definite genital drive, more varied emotional life, and slightly less regression than during preadolescence. There are increased peer relations with same sex, dissolution of family ties, attachment to peers, and work interests. Acting out, regression, depression, feelings of isolation, and running away are common reactions during this time.
3. Middle adolescence, around 14-18 years of age, marked by increased efforts toward mastery of heterosexual relationships and object relationships. Hero worship, social group identification strong, with concerns about social/political issues, values, religion are reactions of this period.
4. Late adolescence, around 18-20 years of age, marked by resolution of the separation-individuation conflict. Character formation via identification is completed, and parental ideas and attitudes rejected during earlier adolescent phases are reintegrated.

Anna Freud identified three ego defenses that predominate adolescence: 1) asceticism, defined as adolescent idealism and a mistrust of pleasure; 2) intellectualization, characterized by adolescents achieving mastery of impulses and drives through thinking and imagination, and 3) identification, characterized by the adolescent isolating himself from and abandoning his family and his superego. Adolescents idealize adults other than their parents to desexualize their parents and yet they learn about adult sexuality.

Blos, an adolescent analyst, emphasizes the psychological shift that begins at puberty and the biological changes that are behaviorally manifested in a surge toward maturation that replaces the passivity of earlier years with activity (Blos, 1962). Adolescence is a period when there is a resurgence of instinctual drives brought about by biological and physical changes of puberty and reflects the transition period from childhood to adulthood. Behavioral manifestations include elements of both stages. Generally there is little stability as the adolescent moves from crisis to crisis, which are brought about by various libidinal drives.

Dynamic explanations of adolescents are described as having unpredictable behaviors, for example, strong and mature at times, yet regressing to using defenses used in childhood. The child's ego, by nature of development, is fluid in comparison to the ego of the adult, and is constantly shifting and regressing with fluid ego boundaries, especially in times of stress.

Assessment of the adolescent's level and quality of object relations and ego's ability to relinquish old object ties provide important guidelines for structuring interventions from these psychodynamic orientations. The quality of object relations can be assessed from both dependency expectations and reactions to actual disappointments. Relinquishing old object ties is seen in adolescent development of crushes and hero worship, indicating reinvestment of libidinal energy into outside objects. Adolescents often retreat from family involvement in an exaggerated manner reflecting ambivalent feelings and attachment to parental figures.

The major defense mechanisms adolescents use to counteract strong attachment to objects include regression, a preoccupation with the self in the form of grandiose fantasies, displacement, and withdrawal. Adolescents live out their pleasures and anxieties and play out their disorders by direct actions, similar to those of younger children, who rely on play for development (Anthony, 1982; Freud, 1969). The natural tendency for children is bodily discharge for all discomfort and tension. Small children play alone, in pairs or in small groups; adolescents play in teams with highly organized rules and roles.

There is an intensification of drives as the psychological equilibrium of childhood partially disintegrates and the maturing adolescent learns how to deal with basic conflicts that are different from those of earlier childhood. The new adaptations progressively emerging are more compatible with adult role expectations. The transition to mature self-reliance is a process of individuation, and according to Blos (1962), the accomplishment of adolescent tasks is achieved through successful separation-individuation.

Contemporary psychoanalytic theories stress the following developmental tasks that are of significance during adolescence: separation and individuation from the family structure; promotion of significant peer relations; development of a positive self-esteem and sexual identity; and control of sexual drives and adaptation to sexual norms.

SOCIAL DEVELOPMENT

Social development is a key activity during the stages of development from middle childhood through adulthood. Havighurst (1953) identifies tasks to be accomplished for healthy social development. He was influenced by Erikson's theory of psychosocial developments, and his six *developmental tasks of life phases* are in many ways analogous to Erikson's eight stages. Havighurst says that each task develops out of a combination of physical developments, cultural expectations, and individual values and goals. When the appropriate time comes for a task to be accomplished and all factors or influences are present, a special period of readiness or sensitivity will make the task attainable. Havighurst (1972) calls this a "teachable moment." If adolescents successfully accomplish their tasks, they feel competent and ready to move on to another task or phase. If they fail or the conditions in the situation do not permit accomplishment, then they experience unhappiness, social disapproval, and difficulty with later tasks.

The life phases most relevant for this book are middle childhood, adolescence, and adulthood. Erikson's tasks should be compared and contrasted with the behaviors described by Havighurst (Table 3-1). The progression through those stages requires

Text continued on p. 33.

Table 3-1   Comparison of Erikson's and Havighurst's Developmental Stages and Tasks

Developmental Stage	Erikson	Havighurst
Infancy	*Trust vs. mistrust* 1. Oral needs of primary importance 2. Adequate mothering necessary to meet infant's needs 3. Acquisition of hope	1. Learning to walk 2. Learning to take solid foods 3. Learning to talk 4. Learning to control elimination of body wastes 5. Learning sex differences and sexual modesty
Toddler years	*Autonomy vs. shame* 1. Anal needs of primary importance 2. Father emerges as important figure 3. Acquisition of will	6. Achieving physiological stability 7. Forming simple concepts of social and physical reality 8. Learning to relate oneself emotionally to parents, siblings, and other people 9. Learning to distinguish right and wrong and developing a conscience
Early childhood	*Initiative vs. guilt* 1. Genital needs of primary importance 2. Family relationships contribute to early sense of responsibility and conscience 3. Acquisition of purpose	
Middle childhood	*Industry vs. inferiority* 1. Active period of socialization for child moving from family into society 2. Acquisition of competence	1. Learning physical skills necessary for ordinary games 2. Building wholesome attitudes toward self as a growing organism 3. Learning to get along with age mates 4. Learning an appropriate sex role 5. Developing fundamental skills in reading, writing, and calculating

From Sundeen SJ and others (1989) Nurse-client interaction: implementing the nursing process, ed 4, St Louis, The C.V. Mosby Co.   *Continued.*

Table 3-1   Comparison of Erikson's and Havighurst's Developmental Stages and Tasks — cont'd

Developmental Stage	Erikson	Havighurst
		6. Developing concepts necessary for everyday living
		7. Developing conscience, morality, and scale of values
		8. Developing attitudes toward social groups and institutions
Adolescence	*Identity vs. identity diffusion* 1. Search for self in which peers play important part 2. Psychosocial moratorium is provided by society 3. Acquisition of fidelity	1. Accepting physique and accepting a masculine or feminine role 2. New relations with age mates of both sexes 3. Emotional independence of parents and other adults 4. Achieving assurance of economic independence 5. Selecting and preparing for an occupation 6. Developing intellectual skills and concepts necessary for civic competence 7. Desiring and achieving socially responsible behavior 8. Preparing for marriage and family life 9. Building conscious values in harmony with adequate scientific world picture
Adulthood	*Intimacy vs. isolation* 1. Characterized by increasing importance of human closeness and sexual fulfillment 2. Acquisition of love	1. Selecting a mate 2. Learning to live with a marriage partner 3. Starting family 4. Rearing children 5. Managing a home 6. Getting started in an occupation 7. Taking on civic responsibility 8. Finding a congenial social group

Table 3-1   Comparison of Erikson's and Havighurst's Developmental Stages and Tasks—cont'd

Developmental Stage	Erikson	Havighurst
Middle age	*Generativity vs. self-absorption* 1. Characterized by productivity, creativity, parental responsibility, and concern for new generation 2. Acquisition of care	1. Achieving adult civic and social responsibility 2. Establishing and maintaining an economic standard of living 3. Assisting teenage children to become responsible, happy adults 4. Developing adult leisure activities 5. Relating to spouse as a person 6. Accepting and adjusting to physiological changes of middle age 7. Adjusting to aging parents
Old age	*Integrity vs. despair* 1. Characterized by a unifying philosophy of life and a more profound love for mankind 2. Acquisition of wisdom	1. Adjusting to decreasing physical strength and health 2. Adjusting to retirement and reduced income 3. Adjusting to death of spouse 4. Establishing explicit affiliation with age group 5. Meeting social and civic obligations 6. Establishing satisfactory physical living arrangements

physical maturation (the development of gross and fine motor skills) and leads to experiences that are based, first, on societal expectations and then on personal choices.

Middle childhood focuses, as it does with Erikson, on the beginning of separation from the family and experimentation with others not within the family group. Tasks in this phase help pubescent children to discover and become more comfortable with themselves as physically growing and changing beings. At the same time, they are learning skills that help them function within society, such as reading, writing, and independent living skills. They also develop an awareness of their own emerging values as distinguished from those of social groups and institutions.

The *adolescent* phase further defines the individual with regard to sex-role orientation and differentiation and greater independence from the family. Physical maturation is occuring rapidly, and the male or female sex role is defined more clearly. Cultural expectations push the adolescent into even more sophisticated interactional patterns and force choices as to career and economic usefulness. Values identification begins to include views originating not only in the self but also in the social and intellectual environment.

Havighurst's tasks reflect a middle-class orientation. This shows up most clearly in his life phase of *early adulthood.* The tasks do not reflect the prevalent cultural differences and changing education, work, marriage, and family patterns; however, they are useful criteria for social skill development.

MORAL DEVELOPMENT

Kohlberg (1976) examines yet another component of development. His *cognitive theory of moral development* is an attempt to define progressive levels of moral/ethical decision making. Moral development in this model is divided into three levels of morality, each with two stages (see box on p. 35). Progress from the lower to the higher stages is influenced by both increasing intellectual-cognitive development and the awareness of others as described by Erikson. These stages are not directly related to age. However, when viewed as moral *behaviors,* they can be related to the judgments expected of a child, adolescent, or adult.

Level 1 is called *preconventional morality* or *premoral.* This is a concrete level at which limits are established externally. *Stage 1* is *punishment and obedience.* The motivation here is to conform to those in authority to escape punishment. This can be illustrated most clearly by a parent saying "No!" or "Don't touch!" in a sharp tone to a toddler. The child learns to stop a behavior to avoid parental disapproval. *Stage 2* is *instrumental and hedonistic.* Modification of behavior is still externally controlled, but children are more aware of their own needs and wants (hedonistic) and will manipulate the authority figure to get them fulfilled. The child will do something to get something in return.

Level 2 is *conventional morality.* At this level external control gradually fades. *Stage 3* is called *good boy morality.* Here, decision making differs from the earlier stages in that rather than being directed by the seeking of pleasure or the avoidance of punishment, it is based on an awareness of others in relation to the self. The individual seeks to please others and conforms to elicit approval. The child still needs others for assistance in determining appropriate behaviors and decisions and mimics what is perceived as the right thing to be done. *Stage 4* is formal *law and order* orientation. Making moral decisions is based on the conventions of society rather than other individuals approval. This is roughly comparable to Erikson's task of moving away from the nuclear family to the greater society. The adolescent recognizes what is right, wrong, lawful, and unlawful and adheres to or disputes these concepts somewhat rigidly. The adolescent is continuously concerned with what is "fair" or what "rights" of his or hers have been violated.

Level 3 is *postconventional morality.* Morality is defined by principles that have become accepted by the individual. This differs from the earlier stages because there is greater flexibility in the interpretations and the variety of ideals used when making

---

Kohlberg's Stages of Moral Development

Level 1   Preconceived morality

Stage 0: The good is what I want and like
Stage 1: Punishment-obedience orientation
Stage 2: Instrumental hedonism and concrete reciprocity

Level 2   Conventional morality

Stage 3: Orientation to interpersonal relations of mutuality
Stage 4: Maintenance of social order, fixed rules, and authority

Level 3   Postconventional morality

Stage 5A: Social contract, utilitarian law-making perspective
Stage 5B: Higher law and conscience orientation
Stage 6: Universal ethical principle orientation

---

moral judgments. *Stage 5* moves into *social contract* and *democratically accepted law.* Whereas there was a rigid adherence to one's own rights and laws during stage 4, there is now greater flexibility and consideration of rights as they influence more than one party. For example, contracting involves an agreement on the rights of each individual involved and defines the relationship these individuals have with each other. Parents have an informal contract to set a consistent limit or consequence for their child, but to reach this consensus they may take into consideration each other's different views. Law is structured with regard to democratic consensus among individuals; it may be modified when the law no longer meets the need of the majority. The last of Kohlberg's stages is also the most abstract and most difficult to attain. *Stage 6* is the *morality of universal ethical principles.* People in this stage might have a conflict with the principles of their society because of their belief in a greater justice and higher moral or ethical values. Morality is no longer attached to the individual's needs or rights but is based on ideals, concepts, and abstractions. Civil disobedience is based on this principle.

The adolescent psychiatric nurse will see moral development at stage 3 or below. One must keep in mind that Kohlberg's stages are based on research with boys. Gilligan (1982) studied girls' responses to Kohlberg's research questions and obtained different results. Girls and women generally base moral judgments on the nature of the relationships of people involved and on the responsibilities of those involved to each other. Girls tend to consider multiple possibilities for solving a problem, whereas boys choose one solution and defend it staunchly.

BIOLOGICAL DEVELOPMENT

Biophysical maturation of the adolescent sets the stage for the broad variety of other changes that occur during this period. Hormonal fluctuations that lead to physical growth and the formation of primary and secondary sexual characteristics lead to newer perceptions of the self as an individual, a member of a group, and finally as a member of the larger community. The many physical modifications will influence self-image, self-concept, and role performance. Any attempt to understand adolescents' behaviors out of the context of biological growth will certainly lead to a fragmented approach to meeting their needs.

The term *puberty* is used frequently to describe the entire transition from childhood to young adulthood. More correctly, puberty can be thought of as the biological changes that lead to sexual maturity (the ability to reproduce). The chronological boundaries of *adolescence* can be fixed loosely at ages 11 to 19 years; however, *pubescence* — the beginning of the pubertal period — starts shortly after 7 or 8 years of age. The distinction in terminology is subtle. The physical changes associated with pubertal development will occur at some point concurrent with the psychosocial event of adolescence. Individual variation dictates the time of onset and completion of puberty. There is no set time when these developmental tasks may occur in all individuals — a significant fact to anyone observing the behaviors of same-age adolescents. Prepubertal and postpubertal adolescents will differ physically, cognitively, and emotionally despite being the same chronological age (Miller, 1986).

During pubescence the hypothalamus triggers the anterior pituitary gland, stimulating the endocrine glands. At age 7 to 8 years this gradually increases the hormones *estrogen* for females and *androgen* for males. These hormones do not increase exclusive of each other but in a ratio depending on the sex of the individual. Two other hormones are stimulated by the anterior pituitary: the *pituitary growth hormone* (PGH) and *thyroid-stimulating hormone* (TSH). PGH appears to be responsible for hyperplastic cell growth, or the normal increase of cells in the growing adolescent body. TSH is responsible for increased metabolism, which is important to both hyperplastic and hypertrophic (enlargement of existing cells) cell development in the organs and skeletal and nervous systems (Schuster and Ashburn, 1986). The increase of these hormones is responsible for both *primary* sexual development, including development of organs responsible for sexual reproduction, and *secondary* sexual development, such as breast development and hip enlargement in the female and lowering of the voice, growth of the beard, and broadening of the shoulders in the male (Kalat, 1984). The first visible evidence of pubertal change in the female is the emergence of breast buds; for the male it will be enlargement of the testicles. *True puberty* is indicated in the female by the attainment of *menarche* (the first menstrual period), which is analogous with the onset of nocturnal emissions ("wet dreams") in the male (Malasanos and others, 1990). Note the normal variation in ages of onset and completion of these changes in Table 3-2.

Young adolescent females may need reassurance that the changes they experience are normal. The pubertal female may have premenstrual and postmenstrual discharges of varying color and consistency; the color can range from yellow to pinkish to brown, and the consistency may vary from watery to viscous. The cycle is initially irregular and eventually stabilizes. Amenorrhea during the first year after menarche is not unusual; however, if amenorrhea occurs after the establishment of a consistent menstrual cycle, pregnancy or health problems may be suspected.

Female clients may complain about a variety of discomforts related to the menstrual cycle. *Premenstrual syndrome* may be responsible for constipation,

Table 3-2   Selected Pubertal Milestones

Change	Age at Onset (Years)	Age at Completion (Years)
Female		
Breast buds	8-13	13-18
Menarche	9-14	14-18
Male		
Testicular enlargement	10-13	13-17
Nocturnal emissions	11	13

Data from Malasanos L and others, (1990) Health assessment, ed 4, St Louis, Mosby–Year Book, Inc.

diarrhea, nausea, fatigue, dizziness, and weakness, as well as mild hypoglycemia, irritability, restlessness, emotional lability, and mild depression. *Menstrual water retention* may cause discomforts such as headache, breast enlargement and tenderness, and urinary frequency. *Cramps* and *backache* may occur because the decreased blood flow to the uterus causes it to contract and pull on the uterine ligaments connected to the spine (Schuster and Ashburn, 1986).

The pituitary stimulates the release of testosterone in the adolescent male. One of the first noticeable signs of this hormonal stimulation is testicular enlargement, with subsequent tenderness and sensitivity. A year after onset of testicular growth the penis may grow to maturity. Scrotal support may help to decrease discomfort, particularly during physical activities. Another potential source of anxiety for males is gynecomastia (slight, transient breast enlargement or tenderness).

Musculoskeletal growth occurs similarly in males and females. During pubescence or prepuberty the feet, hands, and facial features begin to develop, followed by long-bone growth. Torso growth occurs during puberty; there is a difference in the amount and character of this development for boys and girls. Boys average an eight-inch height gain, and girls average a three-inch gain (Tanner, 1978). Adolescent growth and development begin 2 years earlier for females, starting at the age of 9½ and ending at age 14. Boys begin growth and development at age 10½ and end at age 16 (Malasanos and others, 1990).

Muscular development occurs concomitantly with skeletal development. Females tend to develop greater fatty tissue mass than males, giving them rounder, softer features. Note that secondary sexual development, including breast development, pelvic enlargement, vocal change, and growth of axillary and pubic hair is occurring at this time. Males may develop twice the muscular density, allowing them to be two to four times stronger than females (Cooke, 1968). The nurse may observe a need in the male to exhibit his newfound strength and power. However, because of his immature emotional development, this can result in the male inadvertently harming himself or others. Gross motor awkwardness and continuing maturation of the central nervous system may lead to adolescents requiring support as they master finer physical skills.

To meet the increased demands of an enlarging musculoskeletal system, growth also occurs in the cardiovascular and respiratory systems. The heart enlarges before puberty, with an increase of both muscular and cardiac mass (Schuster and Ashburn, 1986). The vessels of the vascular system mature later, accommodating the heart's enlargement. One effect of the difference of maturational growth between the heart and vessels is an increase in intensity of the pulse. Murmurs may also be present but may not indicate a pathological abnormality. The nurse should be aware of any cardiovascular deviations, particularly if medications are involved. Respiratory development also occurs in conjunction with increased physical growth. Lung capacity increases relate to physical stature. The respiratory rates of males is slower than that of females (Shuster and Ashburn, 1986).

The Family*

DEVELOPMENTAL STAGES

Development implies an orderly evolution of events moving from simple to complex. Human development has been studied extensively in all spheres of human experience, including biological, psychological, (that is, cognitive and emotional,) social, and spiritual realms. The family is both an assemblage of individuals in varying stages of development and a unified group in its own stage of development.

Duvall (1971) lists the basic tasks and development stages of families as the following:
1. Physical maintenance
2. Allocation of resources — meeting family needs and costs; apportioning goods, facilities, space, and authority
3. Division of labor
4. Socialization of family members
5. Reproduction, recruitment, and release of family members
6. Maintenance of order
7. Placement of members into the larger society.
8. Maintenance of motivation and morale — providing encouragement and affection, meeting personal and family crises, refining a philosophy of life, and developing a sense of family loyalty through rituals.

Friedman (1981) ascribes Duvall's eight stages of family development to the following types of family:
1. Beginning families (married couples)
2. Early childbearing families (oldest child: infant to 30 months)
3. Families with preschool children (oldest child: 2½ to 5 years)
4. Families with school children (oldest child: 6 to 13 years)
5. Families with teenagers (oldest child: 13 to 20 years)
6. "Launching center" families (children leaving home)
7. Families of middle years (from stage 6 through retirement)
8. Family in retirement and old age (retirement to death of both spouses)

---

* This section is reprinted from Johnson BS, editor (1988) Psychiatric mental health nursing: adaptation and growth, Philadelphia, JB Lippincott Co.

Table 3-3 on p. 40 further describes Duvall's eight stages of family development and their tasks.

Stevenson (1977) identifies four stages of family development based on the length of the couple's relationship:
Stage I   — Emerging family
Stage II — Crystallizing family
Stage III — Integrating family
Stage IV — Actualizing family

The *emerging family* encompasses the first 7 to 10 years of the relationship. The couple initiates work and career paths, and children often are born during this stage. Both developments are stressful, as are the beginning stages of the relationship. By the end of this period, family life patterns are established.

The *crystallizing family* stage extends from 10 to 25 years of cohabitation. This period of family life is usually calm until the children reach adolescence. There is considerable contact between children and parents before the children are launched from the family. The adults continue to grow and begin to participate in community life.

The *integrating family* stage lasts from about the twenty-fifth year of the relationship until the fortieth. Usually the children are young adults by this time, and the parents renew and enhance their relationship. Although work roles continue to be important, increased humanistic tendencies appear and leisure is significant to the couple. The grown children may need to adjust to aging parents.

The *actualizing family* period is the time after 40 years of living together. The couple continues to grow, or if one partner dies, the remaining partner grieves and continues to grow. Family members deal with aging, chronic illness, and dying parents.

VALUE SYSTEMS

The value systems of families include basic beliefs about man, nature, the supernatural, time, and family relationships. Value systems tend to coincide within any single socioeconomic status or ethnic group.

Families of lower economic brackets, for example, tend to have a present-time orientation and view themselves as subjugated to the environment and the supernatural—a fatalist perspective. Family relationships tend to be disrupted by spousal desertion and early emancipation of children caused by economic difficulties. Families cope, however, by taking in other extended family members' children and often by the grandmother's direct assistance to family members. Power is usually authoritarian or absent.

Families at the middle socioeconomic level generally espouse the "Protestant work ethic" that is prevalent in this country. This philosophy dictates the importance of work and planning for the future and includes the belief that people are somewhat evil but changeable by hard work. Financial stability and success are viewed as the rewards of hard work. Family relationships center around the nuclear family, with socialization occurring among neighbors or work-related friends. Power is more egalitarian in middle-class families than in poorer families but becomes more male dominated as the economic level of the family rises. Middle-class families see

Table 3-3   Stage-Critical Family Developmental Tasks Through the Family Cycle

Stage of the family life cycle	Positions in the family	Stage-critical family developmental tasks
Married couple	Wife Husband	Establishing a mutually satisfying marriage Adjusting to pregnancy and the promise of parenthood Fitting into the kin network
Childbearing	Wife–mother Husband–father Infant daughter or son	Having, adjusting to, and encouraging the development of infants Establishing a satisfying home for both parents and infant(s)
Preschool-age	Wife–mother Husband–father Daughter–sister Son–brother	Adapting to the critical needs and interests of preschool children in stimulating, growth-promoting ways Coping with energy depletion and lack of privacy as parents
School-age	Wife–mother Husband–father Daughter–sister Son–brother	Fitting into the community of school-age families in constructive ways Encouraging children's educational achievement
Teenage	Wife–mother Husband–father Daughter–sister Son–brother	Balancing freedom with responsibility as teenagers mature and emancipate themselves Establishing postparental interests and careers as growing parents
Launching center	Wife–mother–grandmother Husband–father–grandfather Daughter–sister–aunt Son–brother–uncle	Releasing young adults into work, military service, college, marriage, and so on with appropriate rituals and assistance Maintaining a supportive home base
Middle-aged parents	Wife–mother–grandmother Husband–father–grandfather	Rebuilding the marriage relationship Maintaining kin ties with older and younger generations
Aging family members	Widow/widower Wife–mother–grandmother Husband–father–grandfather	Coping with bereavement and living alone Closing the family home or adapting it to aging Adjusting to retirement

From Duvall E (1971) Family Development, ed 4, Philadelphia, JB Lippincott Co.

themselves as able to work for and attain some mastery over the environment.

Families in the upper income brackets are accustomed to success and control of the environment. They usually purchase high-quality goods and services. When a child or other family member is in a difficulty, the adults attempt to purchase the solution—for instance, the best mental health care available. They sometimes have a difficult time dealing with the idea that the solution to a child's problem requires their physical and emotional presence rather than their simply paying for treatment. It is especially hard for families of high social and economic standing to accept that their children have problems, especially if academic failure or acting out is involved.

These statements are broad generalizations of social class values and do not consider cultural differences. For example, many ethnic groups place great importance on extended family relationships.

FAMILY SYSTEMS THEORY

Family systems theory developed during the 1950s on both the east and west coasts of the United States. The west coast group of Jackson, Haley, and others in Palo Alto explored the notions of communications theory and homeostasis applied to families with a schizophrenic member (Bateson and others, 1968; Satir, 1967; and Watzlawick and others, 1963). Jackson, Watzlawick, Haley, Beaven, and Satir have become well known for their contributions to the understanding of double-bind communication and family dynamics in schizophrenia, and for their pioneering (and still relevant) efforts in family therapy. These researchers and practitioners state that the child learns and develops by responding to verbal and nonverbal communication. The child's interpretation of self and the environment depends on messages received from parents. The messages are powerful because the child depends on the parents for survival.

On the East coast, Bowen (1978) in Washington, DC, based his family systems concepts on a biological systems model. In Philadelphia, Minuchin (1976) used the systems model in his research with families exhibiting psychosomatic disorders. Most recently Lewis and others (1976) and Beavers (1977) have explored both disturbed families and healthy families from a systems viewpoint.

A *system* is a whole that consists of more than the sum of its parts; that is, although a system can be divided into subsystems, the subsystems do not represent the whole. Human beings are complex organisms who respond, grow, and change in the context of relationships with others and in response to the environment. To study family research, theory, and therapy, the nurse must understand the basic characteristics of living systems.

CHARACTERISTICS OF LIVING SYSTEMS

One's *boundaries* are limits, or imaginary lines drawn to define the limits, past which another may intrude. A system as a whole, as well as subsystems within it, may have boundaries. One example of a physical boundary is the use or nonuse of bedroom doors. Boundaries exist between individuals, between subsystems, and between the family system and the environment. The family's values, style, and self-worth determine the permeability of the boundary to outside influences such as the media, friends, school, and church. Boundaries may be clearly defined but open to change and input, so poorly defined that confusion and chaos exist, or so rigid that little input can permeate.

Negentropy is a tendency toward openness to the environment, both inside and outside the family. Living, open systems tend to become more complex over time; this increase in complexity is called *differentiation.* An example of differentiation is human growth and development. The child grows from a totally dependent infant into a child who feels safe at home and possesses concrete thinking and a short attention span, to a young adult who has abstract thinking and a lengthy attention span and who is capable of living independently in a complex environment. *Entropy* is the tendency of a system to be closed to the environment. A person who remains closed to others, tends to develop distorted and peculiar perceptions, thoughts, and feelings.

The concept of *time* in families is important because systems change with the passage of time as people age and children are born, grow up, and leave home. *Stresses* and *strains* occur within family systems and are normal and inevitable as change occurs. Adolescence is a common developmental stressor. *Conflict,* another normal and common phenomenon, often results from stress and change. A family's ability to manage change and conflict is termed *adaptation;* this ability may range from failure to adapt, to mere survival, to growing and changing into a highly differentiated system.

The concept of *change* is central in family systems theory. Because people and children constantly grow and change and because the social environment changes so rapidly and drastically, families discover their lives and the environment to be in a continual flux. Change causes stress within the system. Every system, though, works to maintain *homeostasis* — that is, some kind of balance between what is valued and desired and the disruptive changes.

It is useful to view families on a continuum from most negentropic to most entropic, or from more to less growth oriented. The most negentropic families are open and growth-oriented and produce the most personally and interpersonally capable people. The most entropic families are least open and growth-oriented and produce less capable people, who often come to the attention of health care workers, mental health care providers, educators, and law enforcement personnel.

PRODUCING COMPETENT PEOPLE: OPTIMAL FAMILIES

Beavers (1977) describes nine critical variables for producing competent people (see box on p. 43). Optimal families have an *open system orientation.* This orientation assumes that an individual needs a group from which to derive satisfaction and personal definition, and that life is complex, with experience resulting from many causes.

Optimal families have *permeable boundaries.* They view the world positively and use input from society and the environment to enrich their lives; subsystems within the family, such as the parent-child relationship, permit privacy and aloneness but allow for the inclusion of others.

The optimal family experiences contextual *clarity,* which means that verbal and nonverbal communication is congruent and clear and that generational lines are clear, with a strong parental coalition. Oedipal issues in these families are resolved appropriately.

Power in optimal families is shared and flows from the parental couple. The parental pair have an egalitarian partnership that consists of role behaviors that are complementary rather than shared; for example; one partner is more aggressive and

---

Family Variables for Producing Capable People

Open system orientation
- Multiple causation of events
- Need for each other and other people

Boundaries
- Touching
- Interaction
- Allocation of space in household
- Links to society

Contextual clarity
- Resolution of oedipal issues
- Clear generational lines
- Strong parental coalition
- Communication—Clear, direct, honest, specific, congruent

Power
- Flow from parental coalition
- Delegation to children appropriate to age
- Clear role definition
- Lack of sex definition
- Rules

Encouragement of autonomy
- Acceptance of differentness

Affective issues
- Warmth and caring
- Empathy
- Attention to feelings
- Amount of conflict
- Resolution of conflict
- Self-esteem of members

Negotiation and task performance
- Input from all members
- Leadership from parents
- Little amount of conflict

Transcendent values
- Expectation of loss
- Ability to prepare for, recover from loss
- Hope
- Altruism

Health measures
- Healthy diet
- Freedom from drugs and chemicals
- Regular exercise and recreation
- Concern for the environment
- Abstinence from dangerous activities

---

complementary rather than shared; for example; one partner is more aggressive and the other is more supportive. These complementary roles exist without sexual stereotyping but follow the prevalent social patterns of the time. Sex does not determine overt power in optimal families. Neither do people in these families lose their power when they become close and intimate. Children do not assume parental responsibilities, and parents use authoritarian approaches when needed.

Optimal families *encourage autonomy*. They consciously realize that children will need to leave the family and live interdependently, and they progressively encourage independent thinking and behaviors. Individual views are respected, and each member claims responsibility for and clearly communicates his or her thoughts, feelings, and actions. People from optimal families possess a high degree of initiative and performance.

The *affective tone* in optimal families is caring, warm, empathic, and hopeful. Members ask about and attend to each others' feelings; they are involved with one another. Conflict, which is inevitable, is dealt with and resolved. The family members believe that they are able to survive difficult or unpleasant situations and occurrences. Their management or resolution of conflict strengthens their relationships and increases their confidence in the relationships. *Negotiation* and *task performance* are accomplished with input from all members and attention to the developmental capabilities of children. No one is excluded. Parents lead the negotiations, typically in *family meetings*.

The optimal family has *transcendent values;* that is, the family has a belief system that tolerates and transcends the pain of loss and change. This belief system may be based in part on conventional religious beliefs but is usually an intrinsic belief that love is a worthwhile risk even though the loved one may be lost. The family has an altruistic bent toward society. Children, of course, cannot conceptualize these notions until they near adulthood. Nevertheless, parents set the tone for the family with their ability to transcend inevitable losses, deaths, and change.

Satir (1988) views families as people-making factories with the parents acting as the engineers or architects. Satir states that *communication* is the way members "work out to make meaning with one another." In optimal families, communication is congruent, "direct, clear, specific, and honest." *Self-worth* is high in nurturing families; the family members all have positive feelings about themselves. *Rules* are norms for how people in the family should think and act. In nurturing families the rules are "flexible, human, appropriate, and subject to change." *Links to society* are the ways family members relate to the community. The linking in nurturing families is "open and hopeful."

PRODUCING CAPABLE PEOPLE: ADEQUATE FAMILIES

According to Beavers (1977), adequate families produce people who do not have mental health problems. The adequate family maintains an *open systems orientation:* the family is flexible and open, does not believe the causation of events is linear, and expresses the need for each other and other people. The intrasystem *boundaries* are clearly defined but open. Members of the family respect each other's privacy, but considerable face-to-face interaction and touching occur.

The family's *links to society* are numerous and are viewed positively. They are likely to include work, schools, church, friends, extended family, family physician, and community service organizations. The family is not likely to have connections with social welfare agencies. *Contextual clarity* is present in these families. Oedipal issues are resolved as appropriate to the age of children. The parents provide strong leadership and maintain their relationship as a couple. *Communication* is clear, direct, honest, specific, and congruent.

Power in adequate families flows from the parents, who use authoritarian measures when necessary. Parents delegate responsibility to children as appropriate for their age and stage of development. Roles are clear; family members know and agree on their functions and performance of activities. Family members understand and generally respect family rules. Power and authority are not determined by sex, although the mother in the family generally has less power than her husband for two reasons: she earns less money, and she is more likely to set aside her goals, including career goals, to meet the needs of the children (Bohen, 1981). The truly egalitarian family with equally divided family and work responsibilities is rare. Achievement of an egalitarian relationship necessitates an enormous output of energy and probably occurs with paid help or extended family providing some of the nurturing of children and performing household chores (Rapoport and Rapoport, 1971, 1976). For children's needs to be met in an adequate manner, at least one of the marital partners must sacrifice some aspect of self-realization, and in this era that person is more likely to be the mother.

An adequate family *encourages autonomy* by encouraging the children and adults to try new activities and express their ideas, even when they are divergent with the family's values. Family members are valued for their differentness and for their similarities with others. Idiosyncracies are tolerated with good humor.

The *affective tone* in adequate families is warm and caring. Members are empathic, often at early ages. Members consider and ask about others' feelings. Although more conflict occurs in the adequate family than in the optimal family, it is resolved without loss of self-esteem. Self-esteem is high in these families. The mother may experience more stress, loneliness, or depression than other family members.

Negotiation and *task performance* are accomplished with considerable ease, but not as easily as in optimal families. Decisions are often reached at family meetings; parents lead the discussions and have the final say in decisions. Some conflict over household work exists, and the mother is likely to assume a disproportionate share of the work, which may be self-imposed or undone because of the many activities of the other family members. The adequate family, however, can usually find ways to prevent the overload of one person. Family members are competent and excel in some areas. The adeqate family is less likely than the optimal family to be uniformly high achievers. There is no significant deviance in school or work performance or in relationships with others.

Transcendent values include a hopeful, positive outlook; the expectation of and preparation for retirement and loss of children; and an altruistic bent toward neighbors. These families also practice adequate *health* measures and do not usually suffer significant health problems.

The Community

Adolescents and their families need good communities in which to live. To provide appropriate services to families, the effective adolescent psychiatric or school nurse must understand the structure and function of the community. Warren (1978) defines a community in the following way:

> . . . [a] combination of social units and systems that perform the major social functions having locality relevance. In other words . . . the organization of social activities to afford people daily local access to those broad areas of activity that are necessary in day-to-day living.

These activities can be grouped into five major functions: (1) production, distribution, and consumption of goods and services; (2) socialization; (3) social control; (4) social participation; and (5) mutual support (Warren, 1978). *Production, distribution,* and *consumption* summarize the economic situation, and refer to the processes by which products and services are made available to and purchased or used by the citizens. *Socialization* is the process by which the community passes on knowledge, values, and behaviors, particularly to children. The school system is the primary institutional vehicle for this practice, with churches playing a significant role.

Of course the family is the first and most influential source in this area. *Social control* refers to the regulation of the society through government, including the police and courts. Family, church, and other social groups and agencies play a significant part in regulating and protecting citizens. *Social participation* is the way citizens interact with one another for pleasure or the accomplishment of social goals. The church and school are central to social activity. Many formal and informal groups provide opportunities for socializing and community involvement. *Mutual support* implies the provision of assistance to people in need. This assistance can be person-to-person, family-to-family, or organized by volunteers.

Although all communities have these major functions, they vary in several dimensions. Strengths or weaknesses occur in (1) local autonomy, (2) coincidence of service areas, (3) psychological identification with the locality, (4) the horizontal pattern, and (5) the vertical pattern (Warren, 1978). *Local autonomy* is defined by how much the community depends on systems outside itself to fulfill the five functions. The *coincidence of service areas* refers to the distance between the various service units in the community. *Psychological identity* is the strength of the sense of belonging in the community. The *horizontal pattern* implies strength of the relationship of individuals, families, and other subsystems to the systems providing the five functions of the community. The *vertical pattern* is the system of extracommunity subsystems that relate to the five functions.

The structure and functions of communities are useful concepts by which nurses can examine communities, but they do not address the quality of life. Lyon (1987) believes that the quality of life depends in great part on the community and that a "good" community has the "potential for meaningful change and improvement." He proposes five basic and seven subjective components of a good community (see box on p. 47). A community may disagree on how much money to allocate for the basic services or what level of education should be provided, but there is no argument about the need. The subjective components, on the other hand, may be nonexistent. *Individual liberty* refers to the community's tolerance for individual differences. A balance somewhere between total conformity and extreme social deviance seems ideal. *Categorical equality* means the willingness of the community to grant equal status to various groups of citizens, especially with regard to age, sex, and race. *Communal fraternity* is the "regard for the whole and a compassion for the individual, a way in which we can treat others as brothers, a sense of caring and being cared about" (Warren, 1970). *Representative, responsive government* is founded on leaders who act in the community's best interest and respond efficiently when the community needs action. Community viability refers to the economic stability and potential for stability and growth. *Local identification* means the citizens think of themselves as community residents, care about what happens, and extend themselves to improve the community. *Resident heterogeneity* implies that a community has a cross-section of economic, ethnic, and racial groups and that cultural diversity is viewed as enriching.

Of course communities vary considerably in their desires concerning the subjective variables. A community's "goodness" is not necessarily determined by the judgment of the nurse; it is based on the members' opinions about the 12 criteria. To intervene in communities successfully, nurses must assess these various aspects; only then can

---

Components of a "Good" Community

Basic components	Subjective components
Public safety	Individual liberty
Strong economy	Categorical equality
Health care	Communal fraternity
Educational opportunities	Representative, responsive government
Optimal population size	Community viability
	Local identification
	Resident heterogeneity

Modified from Lyon L (1987) The community in urban society, Chicago, The Dorsey Press.

---

they determine how best to achieve goals on behalf of adolescents and their families.

REFERENCES AND SUGGESTED READINGS

Anthony J (1982) The comparable experiences of child and adult psychoanalysis, Psychoanalytic Study of the Child 37:339.

Bateson G, Jackson D, Haley J, and Weakland J (1968) Toward a theory of schizophrenia. In Jackson D, editor, Communication, family, and marriage, Palo Alto, Calif, Science & Behavior Books.

Beavers WR (1977) Psychotherapy and growth: a family systems perspective, New York, Brunner-Mazel, Inc.

Blos P (1962) On adolescence: a psychoanalytic interpretation, New York, Free Press of Glencoe.

Bohen HH and Viveros-Long A (1981) Balancing jobs and family life, Philadelphia, Temple University Press.

Bowen M (1978) Family therapy in clinical practice, New York, Jason Aronson, Inc.

Cooke RE, editor (1968) The biologic basis of pediatric practice, New York, McGraw Hill Book Co.

Duvall E (1971) Family development, ed 4, Philadelphia, JB Lippincott Co.

Erikson E (1963) Childhood and society, ed 2, New York, WW Norton & Co, Inc.

Freud A (1969) Adolescence as developmental disturbance. In Kaplan G and Lebovici S, editors, Adolescence: psychobiological perspective, New York, Basic Books.

Freud A (1965) Normality and pathology in childhood, New York, International Universities Press.

Friedman MM (1981) Family nursing: theory and assessment, New York, Appleton-Century-Crofts.

Gilligan C (1982) In a different voice: psychological theory and women's development, Cambridge, Mass, Harvard University Press.

Griffith JW and Christensen PJ (1982) Nursing process: application of theories, frameworks, and models, St Louis, The CV Mosby Co.

Havighurst RJ (1953) Human development and education, New York, Lowgrians, Green.

Havighurst RJ (1972) Development tasks and education, ed 3, New York, David McKay Co, Inc.

Hetherington EM and Parke RD (1979) Child psychology: a contemporary viewpoint, ed 2, New York, McGraw-Hill Book Co.

Kalat JN (1984) Biological psychology, ed 2, Belmont, Calif, Wadsworth Publishing Co.

Kaplan HI and Sadock BJ, editors (1985) Comprehensive textbook of psychiatry, ed 4, Baltimore, Williams & Wilkins Co, Inc.

Kohlberg L (1976) Moral stages and moralization: the cognitive-developmental approach. In Lickman T, editor, Man, morality and society, New York, Holt, Rinehart & Winston.

Lewis JM, Beavers WR, Gossett JT, and Phillips VA (1976) No single thread: psychological health in family systems, New York, Brunner-Mazel, Inc.

Lyon L (1987) The community in urban society, Chicago, The Dorsey Press.

Mahan NE and Yarcheski A (1988) Loneliness in early adolescents: an empirical test of alternate explanations, Nursing Research 37(6)330-335.

Mahler M (1971) A study of the separation-individuation process and its possible application to borderline phenomena in the psychoanalytic situation, Psychoanalytic Study of the Child 26:404.

Malasanos L, Barkauskas V, Moss M, and Stoltenberg-Allen K (1990) Health assessment, ed 4, St Louis, Mosby–Year Book, Inc.

Miller D (1986) Attack on the self: adolescents behavioral disturbances and their treatment, Northvale NJ, Jason Aronson, Inc.

Minuchin S (1976) Families and family therapy, Cambridge, Mass, Harvard University Press.

Moore D and Schultz NR (1983) Loneliness at adolescence: correlates, attributions and coping, Journal of Youth and Adolescence (12)95-100.

Rapoport R and Rapoport R (1971) Dual-career families, Baltimore, Penguin Books.

Rapoport R and Rapoport R (1976) Dual-career families re-examined, New York, Harper Colophon Books.

Satir V (1967) Peoplemaking, Palo Alto, Calif, Science & Behavior Books.

Satir V (1988) The new peoplemaking, Palo Alto, Calif, Science & Behavior Books.

Schuster C and Ashburn S (1986) The process of human development: a holistic approach, Boston, Little, Brown & Co.

Stanhope M and Lancaster J (1988) Community health nursing: process and practice for promoting health, ed 2, St Louis, The CV Mosby Co.

Stevenson J (1977) Issues and crises during middlescence, New York, Appleton-Century-Crofts.

Stuart GW and Sundeen SJ (1989) Principles and practice of psychiatric nursing, ed 3, St Louis, The CV Mosby Co.

Sundeen SJ, Stuart GW, Rankin EAD, and Cohen SA (1989) Nurse-client interaction: implementing the nursing process, ed 4, St Louis, The CV Mosby Co.

Tanner JM (1978) Foetus into man: physical growth from conception to maturity, London, Open Book.

Warren R (1970) The good community—what would it be? Journal of the Community Development Society (1)1:14-23.

Warren R (1978) The community in America, ed 3, Chicago, Rand-McNally & Co.

Watzlawick P, Beaven J, and Jackson D (1963) Pragmatics of human communication, New York, WW Norton & Co, Inc.

Wicks-Nelson R and Israel AC (1986) Behavior disorders of childhood, Englewood Cliffs, NJ, Prentice-Hall.

Chapter 4

Legal Issues in Adolescent Psychiatric Nursing

Phyllis Johnson
Beatrice Yorker

The law governing rights and responsibilities of adolescents is generally vague and confusing. Adolescence has only recently received recognition as a unique period that requires a separate legal discussion. Unfortunately, most of the law dealing with psychiatric health care barely acknowledges any adolescent demarcation. Instead, most juvenile law simply divides persons into two categories: adults and minors. In the context of an overly simplistic legal background, this chapter highlights the critical cases that provide guidance for professionals working with adolescents, and comments on the need for a legal recognition of this age group.

Sources of Law

CONSTITUTIONAL LAW

The Constitution of the United States is the supreme law of the land. If any conflict exists between enacted laws and the fundamental rights identified in the Constitution, the laws must be changed so that their enforcement abridges no constitutional guarantees. The federal courts generally determine if laws or regulations violate any individual's constitutional rights. The courts typically balance competing interests in a dispute. For example, the interests of the state in enforcing mandatory seat belt laws are weighed against the potential for the infringement of an individual's liberty. The Supreme Court is the final tribunal that determines the validity of laws challenged on constitutional grounds.

COMMON LAW

Common law evolved from English tradition; it essentially declares that a decision made in a court of law should be followed in the future by judges faced with similar disputes. This is also known as *case law,* or *judge-made law.* Much of the current understanding of malpractice is derived from case precedent. Vestiges of English common law and the doctrines derived from it still remain in health care law. For example, hospitals have historically been found liable for nurses' negligence under the doctrine of *respondeat superior* (let the master answer), which holds the employer responsible for acts of the employee (Northrop and Kelly, 1987). Modern technology and a move away from paternalism in health care have rendered many such doctrines irrelevant to current nursing practice.

STATUTORY LAW

Statutory law is the most definitive kind of law because it is made by the legislature and recorded in code books. Nurses often seek legal guidance exclusively from the written law in state or federal codes; unfortunately, the codified laws cannot possibly specify the correct course of action for every potential nursing issue.

There are, however, some very important statutes, or codified laws, of which nurses should be aware. Each state has a *Nurse Practice Act* (NPA). These laws typically define the scope of nursing practice in relation to medicine or psychology. NPAs also provide general definitions of nursing activities, including diagnostic reasoning. Some NPAs defer to the professional standards of practice published by various nursing specialty groups as the appropriate source of guidance for nursing practice (Chally and Yorker, 1989). Many state nurses' associations have worked with their legislatures to update their NPAs to include specified advanced practice roles such as midwifery, anesthesia, or clinical specialties.

Two federal laws enacted in the 1970s have a profound impact on adolescent mental health and education. The first, PL 94-142, better known as the *Mainstreaming Act,* entitled handicapped children to a "free appropriate education" in the "least restrictive environment" (Davis and Schwartz, 1987). As a result, many needs of emotionally disturbed children should be met in regular classrooms. Although there are stressful aspects of implementing this law, the benefits far outweigh the burdens. Nurses should be aware of the mental health implications of PL 94-142. Educational facilities and funds have become available for psychoeducational services. The schools are now required to provide services for children with special needs, including psychiatric or mental health services. Some schools are even hiring clinical specialists in child and adolescent psychiatric nursing to meet the emotional needs of students (Bonham, 1989).

The other law is the *Rehabilitation Act of 1973,* which states: "No otherwise qualified handicapped individual . . . shall solely by reason of his handicap, be excluded from the participation in, be deprived the benefits of, or be subjected to discrimination under any program or activity receiving Federal financial assistance" (US Code, 1982). This act must be implemented by psychiatric hospitals if they are to receive any funding from the government.

Adolescence and the Law

Although the law has drawn a line between childhood and adulthood in terms of rights and responsibilities, adolescence was largely unrecognized as a separate stage until the 1970s. But problems remain; as Melton and Schmechel (1989) state, "Even today, the law is unsettled in regard to many practical problems of adolescent mental health law and policy. . . . The current state of the law is a conflict-laden and sometimes incoherent array of assumptions and doctrines that often leave considerable ambiguity about the correct answer to legal problems of adolescent mental health practice."

What little juvenile law existed during the first half of the twentieth century was formulated in response to juvenile offenders. Common law assumed that any attempts to regulate minors were equally beneficial to the child, the family, and the state. Issues such as child abuse and civil rights have forced the creation of a new framework in juvenile law that realizes the potential conflicts between the interests of parents, child, and state and balances the competing factors accordingly.

ADOLESCENTS' RIGHTS

Melton and Schmechel (1989) describe two types of legal advocates for youth. The "child savers," or the protectionist group, consider minors a vulnerable group entitled to education, good parenting, and health care. This group is not particularly concerned with the rights of minors to self-determination; rather, children are viewed as requiring protection from their own underdeveloped decision-making capacities.

The other group, labeled "kiddie libbers" by Melton and Schmechel (1989), are concerned with the autonomy and civil liberties of adolescents. These advocates have gone as far as the Supreme Court in their attempts to give adolescents equal standing with adults. For example, minors have successfully challenged restrictions on the following rights: to protest the Vietnam war (*Tinker v Des Moines Independent School District*, 1969); to stop formal education for religious reasons (*Wisconsin v Yoder*, 1972); to due process, such as a formal hearing before detention or prolonged suspension from school (*In Re Gault*, 1967; and *Goss v Lopez*, 1975); to obtain an abortion without parental consent, which is on tenuous ground in 1990, (*Planned Parenthood of Central Missouri v Danforth*, 1976); and to confidential contraceptive services (*Carey v Population Services International*, 1977).

On the other hand, minors have not achieved the following constitutional rights: to purchase "obscenity" (*Ginsberg v New York*, 1968); to drink alcohol; to engage in lewd speech at school (*Bethel School District v Fraser*, 1986); or to be free from corporal punishment in the schools. Although many states and school districts prohibit corporal punishment, the Supreme Court allows schools to determine the acceptability and procedures for administering corporal punishment (*Ingraham v Wright*, 1977). The libertarian adolescent advocates "emphasize the significance of civil liberties in the lives of children as well as their parents, and thus they believe minors are entitled to protection of privacy and the basic freedoms of self-expression, even when such rights bring them into conflict with their parents as well as the state" (Melton and Schmechel, 1989).

Nurses who provide care for adolescents can find some guidance in two landmark Supreme Court decisions involving the rights of adolescents. The case of *In Re Gault* (1967) represents the first direct attempt by the Supreme Court to deal with questions of the constitutional rights of adolescents. This case involved a 15-year-old who was accused of having made an obscene phone call and was taken into custody without parental notification. On the basis of an improper hearing, Gault was committed to a juvenile correctional facility for an indefinite period. The Supreme Court overturned the juvenile court's decision and ruled that children in delinquency proceedings have a right to the same procedural protections provided adult defendants. This was the Court's first recognition of minors as "persons," as described in the Bill of Rights and the Fourteenth Amendment. The Court made clear that minors do possess fundamental rights by law but nevertheless raised other questions that have yet to be answered concerning the scope of minors' autonomy and appropriate emphasis regarding such rights. For example, the Court wanted to preserve the minor's rights, but it also expressed concern that juveniles might be taken advantage of during the legal process because of their ignorance, fear, or despair (*In Re Gault*, 1967). The Court decision failed to address the separate interests of child, family, and state. Evidence of this is seen in the Court's statement that "there must be [Court] notice to the child and his parents" of the child's right to counsel. The statement raises the question of who is the focus of notification (Melton and Schmechel, 1989).

The second case involves the legal differentiation between minors who should be considered incompetent to make certain decisions regarding their own self-determination and minors who possess the developmental and reasoning skills necessary to make decisions about their own lives. In *Bellotti v Baird* (1976), a case in which a minor was seeking an abortion, the court articulated the "mature minor" exception to the general requirement of parental consent. This ruling has been applauded by child development experts: "The Court appears to be saying that although parents still possess substantial control over their children, the importance of parental rights decreases as their child's capacity to make mature decisions increases" (Wilson, 1978). The Supreme Court further articulated this recognition of development as they concluded that "Constitutional rights do not mature and come into being magically only when one attains the state-defined age of majority" (*Planned Parenthood of Central Missouri v Danforth*, 1976). Thus, whether parental or minors' interests are upheld depends as much on the content of the right as on the age of the minor.

PARENTAL AND STATE'S RIGHTS

The deference to parental rights has its origin in English common law that emerged between the twelfth and fourteenth centuries. Common law relating to juveniles is generally based on the assumption that parents always act in the best interest of their child.

The laws recognize duties that parents owe children: "to maintain, educate and protect"; duties that children owe their parents: "to honor and obey"; and the power of parents over their children. Common law recognized children as persons and not merely property of an adult (Blackstone, 1765).

Laws that protected children included English common law, which regarded certain ages of childhood as a rebuttable defense in criminal and tort law. To protect the estates of families, the law as *parens patriae* (sovereign parent) assumed the role of benevolent overseer in ensuring that dependent, incompetent minors were supervised by adult guardians.

Wald (1979) categorizes children's rights into those that protect children and those that emancipate them. Although few would argue that children need protection, the limitations placed on children's rights represent diverse opinions based on the assumptions that children lack the capacity to make decisions for themselves, that parents must make decisions for them, and that parental control and authority are necessary to preserve the family unit as a social structure. In this context, parental rights may be viewed as a form of constitutional liberty protected by the Fourteenth Amendment (*Meyer v Nebraska,* 1923). Family privacy has traditionally been an area that the courts hesitate to scrutinize, as emphasized in *Prince v Massachusetts,* 1944): "It is cardinal with us that the custody, care and nurture of the child reside first in the parents, whose primary functions and freedom include preparation for obligations the state can neither supply nor hinder. . . . And it is in recognition of this that these decisions have respected the private realm of family life which the state cannot enter." However, the growing awareness of child abuse, neglect, and incest has prompted the courts to seek a balance between family privacy and child protection.

There are cases in which the state's interest in child welfare outweighs family autonomy. For example, when parents refused a blood transfusion for their child on religious grounds, the court appointed a *guardian at litem* to consent to the treatment despite the parent's objections. "Under these circumstances the court felt intervention by the state, pursuant to its strong interest in preserving the well-being of its children, was proper even against the important individual interests of religious freedom and parental authority" (Davis and Schwartz, 1987).

Access to Mental Health Services

ADMISSION TO PSYCHIATRIC FACILITIES

There are three ways that adolescents can enter inpatient psychiatric facilities. The first is through voluntary admission. This should include documented evidence of (1) an informed consent, (2) absence of coercion, and (3) competence to make the decision (Laben and McLean, 1989); all three of these elements are problematic with minors. For example, parents actually retain the right to serve as a proxy for a minor's consent. Additionally, many adolescents enter psychiatric facilities under obvious coercion from parents or juvenile authorities. The element of competence is also problematic. The law in many states assumes adolescents to be incompetent by virtue of their status as minors, and psychiatric admissions are often for impaired mental states that would preclude the competence of any psychiatric patient. However, nurses should be aware that competence is a legal determination made by a court; it is not a psychiatric status.

The second option for admission to an inpatient facility is emergency commitment. "When an individual is unwilling to seek treatment and poses an immediate threat of serious harm to self or others as a result of mental illness, state statutes provide for emergency involuntary admission to a psychiatric facility" (Laben and McLean, 1989). This type of admission allows temporary involuntary detention for evaluation. In current practice the threat of imminent harm is generally a strict requirement for this type of commitment.

The third and most controversial type of admission is indefinite confinement to a psychiatric facility, also called "civil commitment."

Adolescent commitment. In 1966 a federal court ruled that persons confined to mental health facilities have a right to treatment (*Rouse v Cameron,* 1966). Since that time, one of the major questions addressed by the courts has been whether persons, both children and adults, also have the right *not* to be treated. During the last decade, federal courts mandated a number of rights for confined persons such as prisoners (*Lessard v. Schmidt*, 1972). These decisions apply equally to confined children (*Horowitz and Davidson*, 1984). Nevertheless, even though the statutes rule that adults and children alike can be admitted to residential care by either voluntary, involuntary, or emergency methods, there are frequently two essential differences. Voluntary admissions of children are not, in most cases, made through the request and consent of the minor but by the parent. Furthermore, the ability of voluntarily placed children to leave the facility, unlike their adult counterparts, is predicated upon more than their own desire to leave. Thus, during the establishment of a child's rights, not only the interest of the state but also the rights of the parents must be considered.

Right to refuse. That medical treatment cannot be administered to a patient without informed consent, except in an emergency, has long been established in this country's common law. Because of the idea that children lacked the capacity to provide consent for purposes of avoiding battery (discussed later in this chapter), courts held that the parent or legal guardian should give consent for medical treatment (Prosser, 1971). The principle is based on the First Amendment (freedom of speech), the Eighth Amendment (freedom from cruel or unusual punishment), and the Fourteenth Amendment (the right to equal protection and due process) (Miller, 1987). Until recently, the one exception to this rule has been that the involuntarily committed psychiatric patient had no right to refuse any appropriate psychiatric treatment employed to improve the patient's mental disability—particularly since the reason for commitment was, after all, treatment.

Notwithstanding other forms of treatment for psychiatric patients, psychotropic medications have in the past 20 years become the treatment of choice for many forms of mental illness (Miller, 1987). Thus the phrase "right to refuse treatment" has become almost synonymous with the right to refuse psychotropic medication. Considering the potentially dangerous side effects of antipsychotic drugs, it is not surprising that many mental health patients refuse to take drugs. The following experience (Opton, 1974) illustrates this concern:

> There is no other feeling like it. Nothing to relate it to, no experience anyone would normally go through in their life. It affects you mentally and physically and you feel suicidal. The spasms, predominantly in the legs, but also in other parts of the body including your facial muscles. You get lockjaw; you can't control your tongue; you get leg cramps. You get so tired (as if you had been up three days in a row) that you lie down. But you can't stay down for more than three or four minutes because your knees begin to ache, an itching type of ache.
>
> Your thoughts are broken, incoherent; you can't hold a train of thought for even a minute. You're talking about one subject and suddenly you're talking about another. You start to roll a cigarette, drop it, pick up a book, . . . Your mind is like a slot machine, every wheel spinning a different thought.

The mental patient's right to refuse treatment with anti-psychotic drugs has been debated in the courts, based in part on the issue of mental patients' competence to give or withhold consent to treatment and their status under the civil commitment statutes.

The first two landmark cases involving the right to refuse treatment in a mental facility arose in federal courts in New Jersey and Massachusetts. In *Rennie v Klein*

(1979) the federal district court ruled that the standard of clinical practice, including the prescription of medications, at a state mental hospital was unacceptable. The judge granted the plaintiff's request for the right to refuse treatment, except in emergency situations (subject to review by a judicial patient advocate). On appeal, the court held that rather than a judicial review, a review by the hospital medical director would suffice (*Rennie v Klein*, 1981), (*Rennie v Klein*, 1983).

In *Rogers v Okin* (1979) the request for a right to refuse treatment came from six mental patients at Boston State Hospital, a well-staffed university teaching institution. The court ruled that patients involuntarily committed are not incompetent and are protected by the constitution from being forced to receive medication without their consent or the consent of the patient's guardian. This right could be overridden only in an emergency; the court ruled that forcible administration of medication is justified when the "need to prevent violence outweighs the possibility of harm to the medicated individual" (*Rogers v Okin*, 1979).

The Court of Appeals (*Rogers v Okin*, 1980) upheld the patient's right to refuse treatment but also maintained that the state's interest in preventing violence and the parent's or guardian's interest in protecting the patient (from deteriorating health) could override the patient's right to refuse medication. The patient also had to be ruled incompetent by judicial finding. The First Circuit Court instructed the district court to rule that the statutory procedural rights of involuntarily committed patients (first, to advice about the proposed treatment, its risks and benefits, and any alternative treatments; second, to a review by the patient's treatment team; and third, to a review by the hospital director or his designee) (*Rogers v Commissioner of the Department of Mental Health*, 1983) are protected by the Fourteenth Amendment. Currently, Massachusetts prohibits the nonconsensual, nonemergency, forced psychotropic drug treatment of involuntarily committed patients.

In 1985, 41 states had no explicit statutory provisions for a right to refuse treatment by institutionalized patients, and 10 states required consent before medicating in nonemergency situations (Lindsay, 1988). The United States Supreme Court has yet to rule on the issue of the involuntarily committed mental patient's right to refuse medication, so such cases will continue to have different outcomes in different states.

Many courts and statutes require that the committed person receive treatment in the "least restrictive appropriate environment" (*O'Connor v Donaldson*, 1975). The client should retain as much freedom as particular circumstances permit. Under this principle, hospitalization should not be ordered if outpatient treatment might be effective. Also, outpatient treatment should not be ordered if the respondent will accept such treatment on a voluntary basis. The definition of what is restrictive presents problems and can be interpreted in various ways. In general, a restrictive environment deprives the client of liberty or the treatment alternative the client would choose. If the client must be removed from home, the placement should be as close to home as possible (Lindsay, 1988).

Outpatient commitment.   The movement toward deinstitutionalization of psychiatric patients and mentally retarded children and the "least restrictive environment" standard have led to the creation of several alternative treatment settings in nursing homes, halfway houses, therapeutic foster care, home care, support groups, and one-to-one counseling with a therapist. Other alternatives include medication monitoring and, more recently, outpatient commitment. Some states are modifying their statutes to include this latter disposition. In states that permit the client to be "committed" to or compelled to accept outpatient care, debate is underway as to what due process protections and standards should be provided the proposed patient. The American Psychiatric Association supports a variation of outpatient commitment, one that removes the prerequisite of dangerousness as a requirement for involuntary civil commitment and requires only a finding that the client is in need of treatment. The client thus can be committed to outpatient treatment but cannot be committed to a hospital without proof of danger. Adaption of this proposal would require a change of statutes in most states (Lindsay, 1988).

A 1985 survey of state mental health program directors revealed that 42 states permitted commitment to outpatient treatment; 19 states reported that medication can be required as a condition of the court order. In most states in which medication could be required, noncompliance would result in rehospitalization (Miller, 1987).

Case law—the Parham decision. After *In Re Gault* was decided in 1966, the Supreme Court continued handing down decisions in favor of adolescents' civil rights. In 1979, however, the *Parham v J.R.* decision signaled a change in this projuvenile direction. The Parham case was a class action suit filed by two unrelated boys, ages 12 and 13, on behalf of the approximately 140 children in the state of Georgia who were confined indefinitely to state mental hospitals. The two boys named as plaintiffs had been confined to the hospital for over 5 years despite recommendations by hospital personnel for foster care. Both children had a history of social service intervention and placement. The state admitted that many of the children in state hospitals were there because they were wards of the state, and that they could be treated in less restricted settings (Melton, 1984). The advocates on behalf of the hospitalized children argued that the constitutional rights of liberty and due process were violated by the Georgia commitment procedures. The Supreme Court acknowledged the independent liberty interest of the minors involved; however, the Court concluded that the "natural bonds of affection" parents have for their children together with a review by the admitting mental health professional provided sufficient due process to safeguard the rights of the minors in commitment proceedings. The Supreme Court's decision was based on an idealistic notion of family rather than on the reality of the number of hospitalized children with few or no treatment options.

Legislative response. After the *Parham* decision many states enacted laws that provided much more stringent civil commitment policies for adolescents. The Supreme Court did emphasize the need for due process in admission procedures; however, their standard in *Parham* simply represents a level of protection below which the states or psychiatric institutions may not fall.

Another recent federal law has implications for the provision of mental health services. The National Institute of Mental Health issued a document, *Model Treatment Plan* (1987), from which the following excerpt is taken:

On November 14, 1986, President Reagan signed Public Law 99-660, The Mental Health Planning Act of 1986, which authorizes grants to States to develop and implement State comprehensive mental health plans for persons with severe, disabling mental illness.

Section 502 of PL 99-660 amends Title XIX of the Public Health Service Act and affirms the Federal leadership role in providing technical assistance to States in establishing and implementing mental health plans for services to persons with severe, disabling mental illness. States are required to submit their annual plans to the Federal Government for 3 years beginning in fiscal year 1988.

The plans developed by States must reflect evidence of having responded to a number of specific actions required by the legislation. These include: (1) the establishment and implementation of an organized, comprehensive community-based system of care for severely mentally ill individuals; (2) specification of quantitative targets to be achieved; (3) the description of services to be provided to enable these individuals to have access to mental health services, including treatment, prevention, and rehabilitation; (4) the description of services to be provided to enable these individuals to function outside of inpatient institutions; (5) the reduction of the rate of hospitalization of these individuals; (6) the provision of case management to each individual with severe, disabling mental illness who receives substantial amounts of public funds; (7) the provision of a program of outreach to persons who are mentally ill and homeless; (8) the provision for consultation with representatives of employees of various long-term care facilities; and (9) the use of State mental health planning councils for advice on the development of the mental health services plan.

Adolescents such as the plaintiffs in the *Parham* case will benefit tremendously from this federal mandate. Nurses should ask to see the part of their state's mental health plan that relates to child and adolescent services. A very encouraging aspect for nurses is the inclusion in a state plan of in-home crisis intervention as a specific intervention (Georgia Department of Human Resources, 1989).

INFORMED CONSENT

In general the law does not discriminate between children and adolescents, so any discussion of minors refers to both. Moreover, the law regards the parent or legal guardian as the person able to provide consent for a minor, irrespective of the actual competence of the adolescent. Although parental consent is generally the rule, exceptions are based on the recognition that the withholding of treatment from minors who need it is deleterious to the minor and/or to society. Legal issues of mental health services are often related to issues of informed consent. Components of informed consent include the following: (1) the health professional must disclose any information that might affect the patient's decision, including the nature, risks, and benefits of proposed treatment and any alternatives; (2) patients must meet standards of competence to consent (as defined by courts and legislatures); and (3) consent must be given voluntarily.

According to general rule of law, minors do not have unrestricted access to medical care or mental health services. They must have parental consent before undergoing most outpatient treatments and all inpatient treatments. This is based on the following rationale: (1) it protects minors who may be too immature to make wise decisions and thus may be taken advantage of by others; and (2) since parents are legally responsible for the support and maintenance of their children, they should be able to control factors that might increase their child-rearing costs (Wilson, 1978).

Exceptions to the general rule of required informed consent include (1) emergency situations; and (2) the (controversial) therapeutic privilege, whereby the physician may decide to withhold essential information from the patient if, in the physician's opinion, the information would be detrimental. This policy has lost acceptance as a justification for not obtaining informed consent (Melton and Schmechel, 1989); and (3) the patient's waiver of the right to treatment decisions to a proxy. This last exception may create a conflict of interest if the proxy (usually the parent) has a stake in the decision, and brings into play other related legal issues of autonomy and right to privacy.

Other court and legislative exceptions to parental consent apply to those minors the state considers emancipated and thus independent of parental control. Requirements for emancipation vary from state to state but generally include marriage, parenthood, enlistment in the armed forces, or living alone or otherwise self-supporting. Some statutes merely state that emancipated minors may consent to treatment; others define specific terms. In general, the statutes are designed to address issues of financial responsibility rather than issues associated with the recognition of adolescent autonomy and right to privacy (Melton and Schmechel, 1989).

The "mature minor" rule, which is based on a combination of considerations of emancipation exceptions and privacy, protects health professionals from liability in treating obviously competent, older minors without parental consent; unlike most general emancipation statutes, the mature minor rule applies to consent for health services only. Almost all states incorporate statutes exempting parental consent with regard to medical services such as the dispensation of contraception and treatment for sexually transmitted diseases or drug dependence. In issues regarding liability, courts have generally not held physicians liable for treating, without parental consent, minors who have been emancipated from parental control (*Smith v Seibly,* 1967). The Supreme Court found physicians justified in relying on the consent of mature minors in the case of abortion (*Bellotti v Baird,* 1976).

In addition to these exceptions, child rights advocates have proposed the adoption of a special exception to permit minors to consent independently to mental health treatment. "Child savers" advocate from the position that children who need such services may not receive them if parental permission is required. Child libertarians advocate independent access to treatment from the fundamental perspective of autonomy and individual privacy (Melton and Schmechel, 1989). Although some research supports the argument that adolescents are as competent as adults in providing consent (Adelman and others, 1984), to date no such laws exist, other than the exceptions cited. Reasons for the failure to enact such laws stem in part from the fact that such rulings often raise more questions than they answer.

The Nurse's Role

ADVOCACY

Nurses who care for adolescents must be conversant not only in the principles of pediatrics but also in the principles of adult care. In addition, they must incorporate the emerging knowledge base that applies specifically to issues of adolescent development. Because nurses in a psychiatric setting have firsthand knowledge of the many legal and ethical issues that can arise, they must become involved in policy-making at a variety of levels. They can participate in the facility where they are employed, and they can be active in local and state organizations that advocate for youth. Nurses should communicate with legislators about changes in the laws affecting minors; nursing organizations often submit *amicus curiae* (friend of the court) briefs when critical issues reach the courts. Briefs submitted by the American Nurses Association and other professional groups have been supportive of the right to privacy in recent Supreme Court abortion decisions. Commentators suggest that this form of professional input can actually influence the courts.

Autonomy is the concept of self-determinism. Although nursing practice places great value on patient autonomy, maintaining a belief in that value becomes difficult when confronted with an anorexic or a suicidal youth. Individual freedom must always be balanced against societal good. In cases of self-destructive individuals, society determines the limits of personal freedom. When a nurse deals with any persons who are "dangerous to themselves," the law empowers psychiatric treatment to restrict personal liberty temporarily. In the case of a minor, the issue of patient autonomy becomes more difficult to balance, since minors have little legal standing to make decisions independent of their parents. Thus nurses may feel quite uncomfortable when they enforce restrictions on minors during the course of psychiatric treatment that adults could legally refuse. Clear institutional policies should exist regarding adolescent treatment and restrictions. Nurses can be instrumental in raising concerns that should be addressed by policies or procedures, and they can be valuable participants in formulating new guidelines.

Adolescent psychiatric nurses may also be advocates if they believe patients are being "dumped" in institutions because of inadequate placement resources. The *Parham* decision brought the issue of appropriate placement to the attention of legislators. More funding for less restrictive placement options can be allocated with nursing input.

Another area of advocacy may be explored when a nurse believes that the adolescent's rights are being jeopardized by the parents or the family. This can occur outside the hospital in cases of abuse or neglect, or it can occur in the hospital in cases of parental consent for treatment that is too harsh or restrictive given the patient's condition. Although the courts have hesitated to interfere with parental control and discretion, support is growing among legal and ethical bodies for limits on parental actions that could adversely affect the health and welfare of a minor.

Nurses should provide adolescents with the same degree of confidentiality that adult patients receive. Nurses may feel pressured by parents to reveal information gained during therapy. Although the legal protection of this information is somewhat limited regarding parental access, nurses should ethically reveal information only in cases of danger to the patient or others or as required by state reporting statutes. Criminal behavior is not protected by confidentiality guidelines, except in cases of treatment for chemical dependence.

Principles of confidentiality provide a strong argument in favor of family therapy as a form of treatment for minors. It is often preferable for secrets to emerge in the context of the family group, than for a nurse or therapist to be in the awkward position of knowing information that the adolescent is keeping from the parents. Nurses should seek supervision when confronted with such difficult issues.

LIABILITY FOR ADOLESCENT PSYCHIATRIC CARE

The types of psychiatric lawsuits that result in substantial monetary awards are typically suicide or physical injury in the hospital setting, sexual misconduct (on the part of the treating professional) and suicide, or homicide in the outpatient setting. The following elements must exist for a nurse to be liable for malpractice:

1. Duty to the patient
2. Breach of that duty
3. Causation
4. Damages

For example, for a nurse to be held responsible for an inpatient suicide, the nurse would have to have been accountable to the patient in some way—that is, as charge nurse, primary nurse, or nurse assigned to the patient at the time of death. The nurse would have to have acted below the standard of care, that is, not following hospital procedures or the American Nurses Association (ANA) *Standards of Child and Adolescent Psychiatric and Mental Health Nursing Practice* (1985). The behavior (or omission of duty) on the part of the nurse would have to have caused the patient's injury, and the negligence would have had to result in some type of damages. In a comprehensive review of inpatient suicides, 10% could be attributed to negligence on the part of health professionals (Perr, 1985).

The most problematic issue after suicide is homicide by a psychiatric patient. Until the mid-1970s, the standard of psychiatric care mandated a determination of dangerousness followed by detention if the risk of harm was imminent. The landmark case of *Tarasoff v Regents of the University of California* (1976) added a new dimension to the duty of the mental health professional. This case involved a male student at the University of California at Berkeley who revealed to a psychologist in the student counseling center his intentions of killing a girl who had rejected him romantically. The psychologist requested a detention hearing; the patient was hospitalized for the statutory period and then released by a psychiatrist. The student ultimately shot and killed the girl, Ms. Tarasoff. The court held that the psychologist not only had a duty to detain a dangerous patient (which he did) but also a *duty to warn a third-party intended victim* i.e., the girl or her family. Nurses who care for adolescents must know this duty, and if a patient threatens an identifiable victim, notification procedures should be followed.

Nurses are also bound by the mandatory child abuse reporting statutes in their states. Nurses must report any *suspected* or known abuse to the appropriate state agencies. It is imperative that nurses adhere to the reporting laws because failure to report abuse can lead to criminal penalties—fine or imprisonment in many states—or civil liability if a child advocate sues the health care provider for negligence. Nurses who fear retribution for reporting their suspicions of child abuse should be aware that most reporting laws include a provision of immunity from libel or slander suits unless they have willfully provided false information (Northrop and Kelly, 1987).

INTENTIONAL TORTS

The primary legal principles governing the relationship of health professionals to their adult patients are found in the tort law of battery and negligence. For the most part the standard of care is unaffected by whether the patient is an adult or a minor.

Assault, battery and false imprisonment are examples of intentional torts. An *intentional tort* requires a voluntary act and an intent to bring about a physical consequence. In the most basic terms, a voluntary act is a voluntary movement of the body. The requirement for intent is met when the defendant acts purposefully to achieve a result or is substantially certain that the result will occur. If the second party (the patient) consents to an act, there can be no intentional tort. Similarly, self-defense and the defense of others are justified and can be used to defend successfully against an intentional tort (Varcarolis, 1990). Intentional torts are not covered by malpractice insurance.

Battery. Battery, in the most general terms, is committed when an intentional contact (touching) is made with the person's body and that person has neither consented to it nor is legally bound to endure it. A successful suit for battery does not require that the plaintiff be physically injured, that the plaintiff suffer financial loss, or that the medical treatment be unsuccessful. Contacts may be offensive to personal dignity, trivial, or insulting in nature (Northrop and Kelly, 1987). The justification for an alleged act of battery to minors may be quite different from to adults, since what may be trivial or insulting may differ.

Based on this definition, which of the following situations represents an action for charges of battery?

- Nurse Walker bathes 14-year-old Robert, even though he protests having a bath.
- Mary, a patient experiencing an epileptic seizure, strikes Nurse Jones.

In the first situation, Nurse Walker acts purposefully in bathing Robert. Although the bath may not be harmful, it is probably offensive in that a forced bath would probably offend an adolescent's sense of dignity. The minor and the parents could bring an action against the nurse. In the second situation, Mary neither committed a voluntary act nor intended to strike Nurse Jones; therefore no battery existed.

Assault. An assault is an act resulting in the plaintiff's apprehension of an immediate harmful or offensive contact (Northrop and Kelly, 1987). In an assault no actual contact needs to occur. The defendant's act must amount to a threat to use force, although threatening words alone are not enough. The defendant also must have the opportunity and ability to carry out the threatened act immediately.

Based on this definition, which of the following situations represents an action for a charge of assault?

- Patient A kisses Patient B on the cheek while Patient B is sleeping.
- While Nurse Rogers is making rounds, Ms. Smith, a patient's parent, picks up a chair to strike the nurse.

No grounds for charges of assault exist in the first situation. Patient B is asleep and therefore has no knowledge or apprehension of an immediate battery. The second situation is an actionable assault because the nurse has an awareness of the patient's ability and opportunity to strike him or her with the chair.

False imprisonment. False imprisonment is an act intended to confine a person to a specific area. The restraint must have been imposed with an appearance of force in the defendant's words, actions, or gestures. The force must have been imposed for some period of time, during which the plaintiff was detained or had to stay somewhere against his or her will (Northrop and Kelly, 1987).

Based on this definition, which of the following situations represents an action for charges of false imprisonment?

- Joe becomes combative, striking out at staff and other patients. Nurse Hawkins restrains him without a physician's order.
- Jane, a voluntarily committed emancipated minor, wants to leave the hospital against medical advice. Nurse Smith prohibits her leaving by assigning an orderly to stand in front of her room.

In the first situation Nurse Hawkins may defeat a charge of false imprisonment because restraining Joe prevented him from doing harm to himself or others. The nurse should obtain a restraint order from the physician as soon as possible after her action and document this in the patient's record. To maintain the patient's right to a safe environment, the nurse may need to use restraints or seclusion. To accord with the standard of the least restrictive environment, body restraints or seclusion may be used only when clinically necessary—never as a form of punishment or for staff convenience (Joint Commission on Accreditation of Hospitals, [JCAH], 1981). The second situation is an action for which a charge of false imprisonment may be brought. Generally, a voluntarily admitted patient may not be detained against his or her will. However, the nurse should be aware of other statutory criteria regarding a psychiatric patient's admission and release status.

NURSING CONSIDERATIONS

Whether the nurse is caring for adults or children, the standard of care is simply what a *reasonable nurse* would provide in similar circumstances. In addition to the duty to provide safe and effective care for adolescents, the nurse has a duty to protect their rights once they are admitted to a mental facility.

Perhaps the single most important step a nurse can take to protect minors' rights is to be familiar with federal and state statutes regarding their admission, treatment, and release. Moreover, nurses should be familiar with their own institution's policies and customs. Other standards, such as those enumerated by the JCAH, as well as those guaranteed by the Constitution of the United States, must be taken into account.

The law is currently in flux. This lack of definitive answers creates an opportunity for nurses to focus on ethical issues. Although few clear answers to legal questions regarding adolescent mental health exist, such ambiguities serve to raise ethical questions concerning professional liability with regard to treatment decisions. In light of this reality, nurses should look to the Professional Code of Ethics (ANA, 1985) and the ANA Standards (1985) for direction. Courts often defer to the judgment or consensus of a hospital ethics committee. This gives nurses the opportunity to be proactive in a legal vacuum regarding the needs of adolescents.

REFERENCES AND SUGGESTED READINGS

Adelman HS, Kaser-Boyd N, and Taylor L (1984) Children's participation in consent for psychotherapy and their subsequent response to treatment, Journal of Clinical Child Psychology 13:170-178.

American Bar Association (1988) Involuntary civil commitment, Washington, DC, Commission on the Mentally Disabled, American Bar Association.

American Nurses Association (1985) Code for nurses, Kansas City, Mo, The Association.

American Nurses Association (1985) Standards of child and adolescent psychiatric and mental health nursing practice, Kansas City, Mo, The Association.

Bartley v Krimins (1975) 402 F Supp 1039 (ED Pa).

Bellotti v Baird (1976) 428 US 132.

Bellotti v Baird (1979) 443 US 622.

Bethel School District No 403 v Fraser (1976) 106 S Ct 3159.

Blackstone W (1765) Commentaries on the laws of England in four books, London, Robert Bell Editory.

Bonham B (1989) The development of a clinical nurse specialist role in an elementary school. Presented at ACPN Conference, White Plains, NY.

Carey v Population Services International (1977) 97 S Ct 2010.

Chally P and Yorker B (1989) Legal parameters of nursing practice, Journal of Neuroscience Nursing 37:8.

Davis S and Schwartz M (1987) Children's rights and the law, Lexington, Mass, Lexington Books.

Gault, In Re: (1967) 387 US 1.

Georgia Department of Human Resources (1989) State Mental Health Plan.

Ginsberg v New York (1968) 390 US 629.

Goss v Lopez (1975) 419 US 565.

Horowitz R and Davidson H (1984) Legal rights of children, Colorado Springs, Colo, McGraw-Hill Book Co.

Ingraham v Wright (1977) 430 US 651.

Joint Commission on Accreditation of Hospitals (1981) Consolidated standards manual for child, adolescent and adult psychiatric, alcoholism and drug abuse facilities, Chicago, The Commission.

Laben J and McLean C (1989) Legal issues and guidelines for nurses who care for the mentally ill, Owings Mills, Md, National Health Publishing.

Lessard v Schmidt (1972) 349 F Supp 1078 (ED Wis); vacated on procedural grounds, 414 US 473 (1974); vacated on procedural grounds, 421 US 957 (1975); reinstated 413 F Supp 1318 (ED Wisc 1976).

Lindsay A, Haimowitz S, and Lockwood R (1988) Involuntary civil commitment. A manual for lawyers and judges. In Commission on the Mentally Disabled, Dooley IA and Parry J, editors, Washington, DC, American Bar Association.

Melton G (1984) Family and mental hospital as myths: civil commitment of minors. In Repucci N, Weithorn L, Mulvey E, and Monaham J, editors, Children, mental health, and the law, Beverly Hills, Calif, Sage Publications, Inc.

Melton G and Schmechel L (1989) Legal issues. In Hsu L and Hersen M, editors, Recent developments in adolescent psychiatry, New York, John Wiley & Sons, Inc.

Meyer v Nebraska (1923) 262 US 390.

Miller R (1987) Involuntary civil commitment of the mentally ill in the post-reform era, Springfield, Ill, Charles C Thomas Publishers, Inc.

Mnookin R (1978) Child, family and state, Boston, Little, Brown & Co.

National Institute of Mental Health (1987) Model plan for a comprehensive community based mental health system, (Technical assistance document) Rockville, Md.

New York v Ferber (1982) 458 US 7474.

Northrop C and Kelly M (1987) Legal issues in nursing practice, St Louis, Mo, The CV Mosby Co.

O'Connor v Donaldson (1975) 422 US 563.

Opton E (1974) Psychiatric violence against prisoners: when therapy is punishment, Mississippi Law Journal 45:605-640.

Parham v J.R. (1979) 442 US 584.

Perr I (1985) Suicide litigation and risk management: a review of 32 cases, Bulletin of the American Academy of Psychiatry and Law 13(3):209-219.

Planned Parenthood of Central Missouri v Danforth (1976) 428 US 52.

Prince v Massachusetts (1944) 321 US 158, 166.

Prosser W (1971) Handbook of the law of torts, ed 4, St. Paul, Minn, West Publishing Co.

Rennie v Klein (1979) 476 F Supp 1294 (DNJ), (1981) 653 F 2d 836 (3rd Cir), (1983) 720 F 2d 266 (3rd Cir)

Rogers v Commissioner of the Department of Mental Health, (1983) 458 (NE 2d 308).

Rogers v Okin (1979), 478 F Supp 1342 (D Mass), (1980) 634 F 2d 650 (1st Cir.)

Rouse v Cameron (1966) 373 F F 2d 451 (DC Cir).

Smith v Seibly (1967) 72 Wash 2d 16, 431 P 2d 719.

Tarasoff v Regents of the University of California (1976) Supp 131 Cal Rptr 14.

Tinker v Des Moines Independent Community School District (1969) 393 US 503.

US Code (1982) Title 29§ 701 et seq.

Varcarolis E (1990) Foundations of psychiatric nursing, Philadelphia, WB Saunders Co.

Wald M (1979) Childrens' rights: a framework for analysis 12 UCDL Rev 255, 260.

Wilson J (1978) The rights of adolescents in the mental health system, Lexington, Mass, Lexington Books.

Wisconsin v Yoder (1972) 406 US 205.

Chapter 5

Disordered Adolescents and Families

Patricia Clunn
Christina R. Hogarth

Diagnostic and Statistical Manual of Mental Disorders (DSM-III-R)

In 1980 a section on mental disorders that first are evident in infancy, childhood, and adolescence was included in the Diagnostic and Statistical Manual of Mental Disorders (DSM-III) of the American Psychiatric Association (1980), and it marked a major milestone in the advancement of adolescent psychiatry. For the first time, mental disorders of the young were part of the official nomenclature, acknowledging their importance and placing them in the mainstream of psychiatry.

The DSM-III (1980) and DSM-III-R (1987) use the term "children" to refer to anyone younger than 18 years of age. No age distinctions are made within the "pediatric" age-group disorders. For symptoms that do not fit the diagnostic criteria in the childhood section, disorders discussed elsewhere in the manual are to be used, making available about four times the number of diagnoses for use with adolescents than previously had been possible (Levy, 1982). When it is appropriate, adults are assigned diagnoses from the child section; those most frequently used for adults are conduct and attention deficit disorders, residual type.

The DSM-III criteria have provided uniform diagnostic criteria that has resulted in profound advances in understanding adolescents' mental disorders during the last decade. The major criticism of the DSM-III child and adolescent section was its failure to cast the diagnostic criteria within a developmental framework (Quay, 1986).

Although there was some resistance in the beginning, the DSM-III and DSM-III-R diagnoses were quickly adopted by the psychiatric community. They have provided the framework for the teaching psychiatry in most educational programs and are used in most treatment settings (Klerman, 1986).

PREVALENCE OF ADOLESCENT DSM-III DISORDERS

Epidemiological studies completed since 1980 have shifted the focus from overall incidence to the incidence of specific diagnostic diseases. They describe the DSM-III and DSM-III-R categories and analyze the reliability and validity of the commonly used diagnoses for adolescents (Cantwell and Baker, 1989; McGee and others, 1990). This chapter reviews those DSM-III-R disorders that occur most commonly among adolescents.

In most current follow-up studies, agreement among several sources (such as parents and teachers) is required to label an adolescent's problem a "disorder" (Anderson and others, 1987). As with younger children, the dependence of adolescents on adults and the adult's observations are critical factors in substantiating the clinician's assessment data and diagnostic formulation.

Although studies differ in terms of geographical location, age-range of the samples, and methodology, there is significant agreement that about one in five adolescents has some type of mental disorder (McGee and others, 1990). Using DSM-III-R criteria and a sample population of adolescents between the ages of 13 and 18 years, McGee and others found oppositional disorders to be the most prevalent diagnosis and separation anxiety the least frequently used diagnosis. Sex difference was pronounced in the prevalence of conduct disorder diagnoses; three times more male adolescents were diagnosed with conduct disorders than females, whereas overanxious disorders were five times more prevalent in female adolescents.

Anxiety and overanxious disorders were found to be the most frequent diagnosis in adolescents in a recent survey, and most had concurrent (comorbid) depressive disorders (McGee and others, 1990). Conduct and oppositional disorders were the second most prevalent disorder. Most disorders in males were diagnosed as aggressive subtypes; most females as nonaggressive subtypes. Findings showed significant changes over time in truancy, underage drinking, and petty theft among adolescent girls. Depressive disorders had the greatest degree of comorbidity: about two thirds of the adolescents had depressive disorder and coexisting conduct or anxiety disorders.

It was found that more than half the adolescents had been referred for treatment by school counselors, confirming findings of other recent surveys that, at this time, most adolescents have access to psychiatric services; however, these services do not appear to be used to any extent. Most adolescents who participated in these studies had poor or inappropriate coping skills, poor social competency, and low levels of social support, all of which are areas of psychiatric nursing concern. The persistence of this finding strongly suggests that these areas require careful attention in nursing assessments and that related nursing diagnoses be included in all nursing care plans, which should be adapted to the DSM-III-R diagnoses of adolescents. Self-care deficits also were pronounced; although very few adolescents were receiving prescription medications for their mental health problems, many, especially females, were self-medicating with alcohol and drugs to help themselves feel better (McGee and others, 1990).

In this chapter, DSM-III-R diagnoses for mental disorders in adolescence are discussed in terms of psychiatric mental health (PMH) nursing diagnoses typically used with the DSM-III-R categories. Diagnostic formulations are based on a thorough assessment of the adolescent, as discussed in Chapter 6. The development of a diagnosis is the initial step leading to the formulation of a treatment plan, providing the rationale for interventions in specific psychopathological conditions broadly covered in this chapter and presented in detail in Chapter 14. Prevention, crisis, and therapeutic milieu interventions and somatic therapies are discussed in Chapters 9, 10, and 11, respectively.

The Concept of Acting Out

The concept of acting out was first used by Freud (1953) to denote manifestations of resistance to psychoanalytical therapy. The use of the term was expanded to describe the tendency of some patients to communicate aspects of their past experiences in nonverbal forms. Freud's concept of the need to put past repressed experiences into action—the compulsion to repeat—later became known as "acting on impulse." Since Freud the psychoanalytic concept of acting out has broadened to include impulsive, conduct-disordered, and other antisocial behaviors.

In contemporary literature, some theorists have defined acting out as having both positive and negative connotations, which has resulted in an emphasis on the adaptive and creative nature of acting out. A humanistic position is that much of what is called acting out is an attempt at "working through" conflict. True acting out is used to maintain repression, whereas working through involves expression. For example, acting out for mastery reflects actions that are essential for development of ego strength and change (Robertiello, 1987).

Normally, people react to certain common situations in stereotypical ways, in contrast to reactions to isolated incidents; some develop a "life-style" of acting out. On the other hand, another kind of acting out is sporadic and related to poor impulse control, which frequently is seen in adolescents. These youngsters have low frustration tolerance that often is related to developmental interferences, parental inconsistency, overindulgence, insufficient discipline, and general overcharging of sexual impulses because of biological changes, that is, biological "activation" explanations (Offer and Offer, 1975).

Clinically, acting out has come to mean any behavior that is typical or characteristic of an individual under stressful conditions that would be minimal for others in the same situation. In its strictest definition, acting out is characterized by uncontrolled and aggressive actions. To qualify for classification in the category of acting out, the behavior must be detrimental either to the person or to the society in which he or she lives (Brown, 1987).

According to Miller (1980, 1983) the psychodynamic origins of action communications occur in early adolescence as children enter puberty and begin to detach themselves emotionally from their parents. At that time, they experience a simultaneous self-preoccupation as a result of the many physical changes that are occurring and a lack of replacement love objects. They have difficulty understanding their feelings and feeling emotionally supported by involved with others.

The adolescent's need for action is due, in part, to the need to discharge tensions resulting from the heightening of sexual and aggressive drives. Like younger children, those in the early years of adolescence often have limited verbal skills and rely on actions to communicate with others. They tend to be bored and depressed because they are severing ties with parents and expecting to move into more independent social roles (Rutter and others, 1976).

Acting out is an attempt to resolve conflict by manipulating oneself and one's environment, often to recreate earlier experiences of being loved. In contrast, *acting up* is defined as the behavior that children and early adolescents engage in to obtain responses from adults when, for example, they seek external controls, and this behavior is developmentally appropriate (Miller, 1986). Rosen (1987) has added the concept of *acting in*, which is the turning inward of destructive drives and energies, resulting in self-destructive behaviors, often of a somatic nature, such as eating disorders and other psychophysiological manifestations, such as tension headaches, or "nervous" stomach. The continued arousal of this neuropsychological system is said to result in chronic illnesses and learning disorders (Rodriguez and Routh, 1989).

Blos (1962), in contrast, claims that the adolescent's tendency is toward action; thus "acting out" is as normal for adolescents as nursing is for infants. Much of adolescent acting out has a theatrical component that is similar to the dramatic play of young children. Adolescents often choose a stereotypical hero and act "as if" they were that person. Other experts agree that acting out provides the adolescent the vehicle for "blowing off steam" and reducing tension and claim that the function of acting out is denial through action that usually is unconscious (Freud 1965, 1969).

Other experts attribute acting out to the family dynamics and family style of dealing with tensions. Young persons learn how to respond to stress through parental examples and family circumstances, such as covert and overt attitudes toward society and authority. It is suggested that many parents are able to gratify their own poorly integrated impulses through their adolescent's acting out, which they unconsciously encourage and condone (Josselyn, 1987; Calabrese, 1987).

Similarly, inpatient staff dynamics may unwittingly stimulate adolescents to act out (Offer, Ostrov and Howard, 1981). Stanton and Schwartz (1949) were the first clinicians to identify that patients' "act out" the conscious and unconscious conflicts among the staff. Rashkis and Wallace (1959) expanded this notion and identified the reciprocal effects of patient disturbance; that is, staff attitudes affect and are affected by patient behavior. This reciprocal relationship, frequently referred to as the "Stanton-Schwartz syndrome," is named for the researchers whose study found that in cases of interstaff conflict, an increase in regressive behavior, such as incontinence, occurs among the patients (Poal and Weisz, 1990).

CLINICAL MANIFESTATIONS

Acting out is defined as a faulty reaction to normal life; *pathological acting out* involves various degrees of a variety of behaviors, as well as certain mental disorders in which acting out occurs in an extreme form. Typically this behavior involves overt aggression or self-destructive behaviors; however, acting out involves any behavior that translates an unconscious statement into an overt act. Not all such behaviors — suicide, for example — are included as DSM-III diagnoses, even though they harm the individual. Although aggression and violence are not DSM-III diagnoses in themselves, they are frequently used nursing diagnoses. Severe forms of acting out, such as suicide and violence, occur in many DSM-III-R psychiatric disorders, but as specific entities, they are diagnostical. In contrast, many possible nursing diagnoses relate to these behaviors.

Acting out is a term that often is used in describing psychotic behaviors. Critical assessment issues are involved in determining whether a psychotic adolescent will act out, that is, attempt suicide or attack others. The potential for acting out unrealistic perceptions or ideations needs to be carefully noted. Among the most difficult conditions to evaluate are dissociated personality disorders, in which clients split off part of their personality so they can "act out" things that under ordinary circumstances would be unacceptable.

Psychopathic and delinquent adolescent behaviors are additional examples of acting out, in which persons translate their conflicts and drives into behavior such as drug abuse and addiction. Adolescents with character disorders also act out, and this acting out is described as the tendency to persist in masochistic or sadistic behaviors.

When anxiety disorders are "acted out," these behaviors are intervention. Anxiety is related to the adolescent's capacity to identify with society and its controlling aspects, which illuminates the adolescent's awareness and thus potential for eventual internalization of social values and controls. The lack of anxiety, often seen in more severe forms of sociopathic acting out, suggests that the behavior effectively contains the anxiety and makes intervention more difficult.

Many forms of acting out are culturally, socially, and environmentally prescribed. For example, in some forms of mental illness, acting out occurs more frequently in less verbally oriented cultures. Cross-cultural studies indicate that the more primitive the society, the more motor manifestations of mental disorders. Catatonic motor-type schizophrenia is more frequently found among adolescents in underdeveloped societies, where there is a tendency toward action (Nichtern, 1982).

INTERVENTIONS

Acting out behaviors are usually opportunities for intervention and corrective experiences. While some inexperienced adolescent psychiatric nurses may think that a quiet, compliant adolescent or milieu is a goal of treatment, acting out behavior is often therapeutic, can be described in nursing diagnosis terms, and appropriate treatment plans can be developed for helping the adolescent.

An important aspect of clinical treatment for adolescents who act out, regardless of underlying psychopathology, is providing a structured environment to assist adolescents in understanding their role in society, as well as the roles of others. Socializing adolescents with conduct disorders or antisocial behavioral patterns consists mainly of showing them, interpreting for them, and helping them understand, accept, and respect the role and function of others through social skills training. In the inpatient setting, a variety of milieu and group techniques are used, including limit setting, self-government, and recreational, work, and school (educational) opportunities (Rome and Barry, 1987).

Interventions that have proven successful with adolescents who act out are psychodrama or sociodrama and role playing, in which the reenactment by various people shows the adolescent alternative solutions and problem solving in a more relaxed, constructive way. In reenactment, the actors can take roles of persons with whom they are in conflict, and through role playing and role reversals, they are better able to understand the motivation of the persons they oppose. In this kind of learning, adolescents can redo or "replay" their actions and change the behaviors and responses they believe were ineffective (Papanek, 1987).

Defiant, Conduct, and Attention Deficit Disorders

Defiant, conduct, and attention deficit hyperactivity disorders are categorized under disruptive behavior disorders in the DSM-III-R category and, as noted earlier, are the most prevalent acting out disorders of adolescence (see box).

Oppositional defiant disorders are included in the conduct disorder classification. Adolescents with this diagnosis exhibit socially disruptive behaviors that usually are more distressing to others than to themselves. In contrast to parent and teacher reports and concerns, these adolescents see themselves as victims of circumstances and do not understand what it is they do that causes adults to describe them as oppositional, defiant, or noncompliant. Some experts claim that disruptive behavior disorders are as much a social and political issue as a biomedical indexing and categorization (Adams and Fras, 1988), since the appraisals and diagnoses are based, for the most part, on moral evaluations by parents and teachers.

Medical and Nursing Diagnoses Related to Conduct Disorders and Oppositional Disorders

Medical Diagnoses (DSM-III-R)

312   Conduct disorder
313.8.1   Oppositional defiant disorder

Nursing diagnoses (PMH)

4.1.2.1   Anger
5.3.1.1   Potential for violence
5.3.2.2   Aggressive/violent behavior toward environment
5.3.2.3   Delinquency
5.3.2.4   Lying
5.3.2.5   Physical aggression toward others
5.3.2.7   Promiscuity
5.3.2.8   Running away
5.3.2.9   Substance abuse
5.3.2.10   Truancy
5.3.2.11   Vandalism
5.3.2.12   Verbal aggression toward others
6.3.2.3.1   Chronic low self esteem
2.2.2   Altered judgment
1.1.99   Motor behavior (NOS): poor impulse control

From American Psychiatric Association (1987) Diagnostic and statistical manual of mental disorders III-R, Washington, DC, The Association.

Attention deficit disorders are more oppositional, defiant, and pervasive, and the life-style of adolescents with these problems seriously influences their cognition, feelings, learning, and social functioning. Estimates are that 75% of the youth diagnosed with attention deficit hyperactivity disorder also have conduct disorder problems (Safer and Allen, 1976). The concurrence of these disorders has led some experts (McMahon and Forehand, 1988) to suggest that hyperactivity is the "driving force" in conduct disorders, that is, the necessary element in severe conduct disorders. Estimates are that more than 50% of the youngsters seen in mental health care settings have disruptive behavior disorders, which emphasizes the clinical importance of these problems.

Disruptive adolescents usually are referred because their acting out behaviors are "out of control" of their parents and/or significant others. It is estimated that boys more often than girls have disruptive behavior problems, ranging from 4:1 to 12:1 (DSM-III-R, 1987). Developmental studies that compare both sexes whose behaviors are not a problem for adults (nonreferred) and those referred because of their disruptive behaviors show that most adolescents, referred and nonreferred, exhibit disruptive behavior at some point earlier in their childhood (Patterson, 1982).

The usual age of onset is during the early latency stage, when diagnoses of disruptive disorders are first used. The older the child is when they are first seen for conduct disorders, the greater the likelihood of their engaging in delinquent and criminal behaviors as adults. They are at increased risk for adult psychiatric impairments, such as antisocial personality disorders, poor occupational adjustment, low educational attainment, marital disruptions, and poor physical health (Kazdin, 1985; Kay and Kay, 1986).

The overwhelming number of referrals for professional help for adolescents with conduct disorder taxes the educational, treatment, and legal systems. Because these problems are so commonly encountered and span a continuum from minimal to severe, nurse clinicians who work with children and adolescents need to assume a positive attitude toward treatment, and be able to evaluate the degree of severity of the behavior and the appropriate interventions. They need to instruct and enlist parents and teachers in planning and management, to therapeutically intervene in direct care when appropriate, and to know when more sophisticated interventions and medications are indicated (Patterson, 1976, 1974).

CONDUCT DISORDER: DEFINITIONS AND CONCEPTS

An age limit of 18 years is a criterion for antisocial personality disorders in the DSM-III-R classification. A diagnosis of antisocial personality disorder in adolescents or adults includes a history of childhood conduct disorder that indicates the client has a life-long pattern of acting out in socially unacceptable ways. Historically, classification systems for conduct disorders were combined with problems of crime and antisocial behaviors (see box on p. 76). This lumping of legal and psychological perspectives has resulted in diverse explanations and management techniques, disputed among scholars in juvenile delinquency and child psychology. Despite disagreements, there is a strong consensus among all disciplines that conduct disorders during childhood are the precursors to adolescent delinquency, which in turn leads to adult crime (Farrington, 1986; Lewis and others, 1985).

Conduct Disorder

NOTE: The following items are listed in descending order of discriminating power on the basis of data from a national field trial of the DSM-III-R criteria for disruptive behavior disorders. Conduct disorder is defined as a disturbance of conduct lasting at least 6 months, during which at least three of the following events have occurred:

1. Has stolen without confrontation by a victim on more than one occasion (including forgery)
2. Has run away from home overnight at least twice while living in parental or parent-surrogate home (or once without returning)
3. Often lies (other than to avoid physical or sexual abuse)
4. Has deliberately engaged in fire setting
5. Is often truant from school (for adult, absent from work)
6. Has broken into someone else's house, building, or car
7. Has deliberately destroyed others' property (other than by fire setting)
8. Has been physically cruel to animals
9. Has forced someone into sexual activity
10. Has used a weapon in more than one fight
11. Often initiates physical fights
12. Has stolen with confrontation by a victim (mugging, purse snatching, extortion, armed robbery)
13. Has been physically cruel to people

From American Psychiatric Association (1987) Diagnostic and statistical manual of mental disorders III-R, Washington, DC, The Association.

The lack of consensus among theorists is reflected in the dilemmas clinicians encounter in the use of the DSM-III-R classification systems. Acting out behaviors do not neatly fit into one distinct pattern or cluster of behaviors. Because acting out behaviors are associated with chemical dependency and substance abuse, depression, bipolar affective disorder, and manic and borderline personality disorder, diagnosis is difficult and often incorrectly made.

Etiological explanations for these disorders vary and are similar to the explanations for adult personality disorders, which stress biological and genetic factors. Psychoanalytical interpretations stress separation-individuation, trait, and temperament. According to this perspective the first signs of oppositional behaviors appear between the ages of 18 to 36 months.

Most authorities agree that certain biological and genetic influences predispose children to these behavioral problems as a result of temperament (Thomas and Chess, 1981; Chess and Thomas, 1986). Of special interest is the temperamentally difficult child, who, from birth, exhibits intense, irregular, negative, and nonadaptive behavior, which some view as predisposing the child to maladaptive parent-child interactions. The parents' role in this interaction has been described as one of negative reinforcement that escalates and maintains coercive behaviors.

Social bonding theorists emphasize that the ability to form intimate and enduring relationships that are mutually enjoyable and satisfying is established during early infant-mother interactions (Reid and others, 1981). Failure to establish affection, empathy, and bonding with others is a criterion for conduct disorders. Signs of bonding include the following:

1. Has one or more peer group friends of at least 6 months' duration
2. Extends self to others when no immediate advantage is likely
3. Apparently feels guilt or remorse if a reaction is inappropriate
4. Avoids blaming or informing on companions
5. Shows concern for the welfare of friends

Table 5-1 presents a developmental model based on the empirically derived conduct disorder dimension discussed earlier. This model identifies a hierarchical progression of conduct disorders through four developmental stages: oppositional, offensive, aggressive, and delinquent and from overt to covert behaviors, from minor to more serious disruptive behaviors, and from parents and home to school and community. Earlier behaviors do not disappear but continue as the hierarchy of more complex patterns develops. The model is incremental, with initial behavior patterns continuing and existing simultaneously with later patterns.

Family characteristics and parenting behaviors are also frequently cited causative factors. Epidemiological studies show that children with conduct disorders are from families in which more marital and personal problems occur, and have parents with antisocial personalities who are more alcohol dependent more often than are families of children in the general population (Wicks-Nelson and Israil, 1984).

Parenting behaviors, especially those of mothers, have been studied extensively and are considered by experts (Brody and Forehand, 1986) the basis for many conduct disorders. Dysfunctional parenting and parenting variables that have been related specifically to the development and maintenance of the child's noncompliance, are considered a key concept in conduct disorder diagnoses. Rey and Plapp (1990) propose that if oppositional defiant and conduct disorders are different diagnostic conditions, the distinctions are due to differences in parenting styles.

Table 5-1   Developmental Progression of Conduct-Disordered Behaviors

Oppositional	Impulsive	Aggressive	Delinquent
Argues	Offensive	Destroys	Sets fires
Bragging	Cruelty	Threatens	Steals outside
Demands atten-	Disobeys at school	Attacks	Alcohol/drug use
tion	Screams	Bad friends	Truancy
Disobeys at home	Poor peer rela-	Steals at home	Runs away
Temper tantrums	tionships		Vandalism
Stubborn	Fights		
Teases	Sulks		
Loud	Swears		
	Lying/cheating		

From Edelbrook E (1985) Conduct problems in childhood and adolescence: developmental patterns and progressions, Unpublished manuscript. Reprinted by permission of the author.

DSM-III-R criteria. Suggestions for unifying oppositional defiant and conduct disorders on a continuum within a single diagnosis, presented earlier, illustrate overlapping and the need for extreme care in diagnostic formulations. Recent behavioral research reflects the continuing efforts of scientists toward finding more precise definitions and the notable strides that have been made in this area during the last few decades. The revised DSM-III-R category for conduct disorders represents a major effort to correct the past problem of clinicians' use of conduct disorders as a catchall label. Instead it is an important and clinically useful category. This is especially true in child inpatient settings, where interdisciplinary team function is customary, and the nurse clinician's work milieu includes coordinating interventions of special educators, psychologists, psychiatrists, and parents. The revised criteria and descriptions separate the more serious juvenile delinquent behaviors from conduct disorders and provide more socially acceptable and useful diagnoses.

Isolated acts of conduct disorder are not sufficient for the diagnosis of conduct disorder and are to be coded as antisocial behavior. Behaviors must continue over time in a pattern, with impairment in social and school functioning. The DSM-III-R definition stresses that the repetitive, persistent patterns of behavior be of at least 6 months' duration, with signs of violating the basic rights of others and major age-appropriate societal roles.

Two elements combine the components of aggression and socialization found in conduct disorders: lack of empathy, which varies in amount or degree, and the inability to fit in with rest of society and its demands for inner values and outward conduct. These children, who seem to have no concern for the feelings, wishes, or well-being of others, exhibit callous behavior. They readily inform on their companions and blame others for their misdeeds. They initiate physical aggression, are physically cruel to other persons and to animals, and deliberately destroy the property of others. Stealing is common, ranging from taking possession, shoplifting, and forgery to breaking into homes and cars. Lying and cheating in games and schoolwork are common occurrences. Aggressive behaviors include direct confrontation with victims and extreme behaviors, such as vandalism, fire setting, rape, and murder. Nonaggressive behaviors include disobedience, violations of home and school rules, truancy, substance abuse, running away, thefts not involving victim confrontations, and persistent lying and stealing.

Indicators of the absence of adequate social empathy (undersocialization), bonding, and attachment include superficial peer relations, egocentricity, manipulation, lack of concern for others, and lack of guilt and remorse. Attachment bonds are judged by peer-group friendships, the ability to extend the self for others through helping, the degree of guilt feelings, loyalty for companions, and concern for the welfare of others. If only one of these characteristics is present, the undersocialized subtype diagnosis is appropriate. Associated features include the regular use of tobacco, liquor, and other drugs. Sexual activities usually begin earlier in these children than in other children in their peer group (Harnet, 1989).

Conduct disorders are present in 9% of the males and 2% of the females in the general population (DSM-III-R). The age of onset for conduct disorders varies; onset usually occurs at prepuberty, especially in girls, who usually are assigned in the solitary aggressive group type.

The outcome and course varies. Early onset is a poor prognostic indicator, with high prediction for antisocial personality disorders during adulthood. Although milder forms of these disorders may dissolve with maturity, when children with more severe forms remain untreated, their condition tends to become chronic. The solitary aggressive group type has the best prognosis; however, the child's antisocial behaviors usually persist into adulthood, with illegal activity. Complications of conduct disorders noted in the DSM-III-R include school suspension, legal difficulties, substance abuse, venereal diseases, and high rates of physical injury from accidents, fights, and suicidal behavior.

Oppositional defiant disorder. Oppositional defiant disorder (ODD) and conduct disorders both feature disobedience and opposition to authority figures. The important distinction, however, is that clients with conduct disorders violate the rights of others, whereas clients with ODD do not (see box on p. 80). The latter are disobedient, defiant, negative, angry, and aggressive in their opposition to adults (Allen and Fras, 1988).

Typically, ODD becomes a diagnostic entity when the child is about 8 years of age. The course of the disorder is unknown. Usually when it appears before puberty, it is more common in boys than in girls.

The major symptoms and behaviors include irritability, hypomania, and antisocial behaviors which are also seen in bipolar disorders. These behaviors may also be early signs of schizophrenia. Attention deficit with hyperactivity and specific developmental disorders are problems also commonly associated with ODD. These problems may progress from conduct disorder (Axis I) to adult passive-aggressive or antisocial disorder (Axis II).

Interventions. The clinical management of care of adolescents with oppositional defiant, conduct disorder and attention deficit disorder with hyperactivity include many similar techniques. With regard to conduct disorders, variations in planning are based on the symptoms and predominating behaviors. Most interventions include a combination of behavioral, emotional, cognitive, and family group therapies. The success of these interventions hinge on including the family, teachers, and other adults who are involved with the child and on gaining their support and assistance in treatment plans.

Discipline and consistent external parental controls are the most important aspects of working with adolescents with conduct disorders. Fostering self-control is vital, and changes and growth can be measured against the context of adult/parental authority. These adolescents, especially during the early adolescent period, are disobedient, negativistic, confronting, resistive, provocative, dawdling, foot-dragging, and defiant. Helping parents or staff members in inpatient settings to master successful disciplinary techniques in working with these youngsters has been called the "triumph of helping empathy over the distortions of projective identification, narcissistic identification, splitting, role reversals and identification with the aggressor" (Adams and Fras, 1988).

Adolescents with undersocialized and aggressive conduct disorders respond best to long-term, high-quality residential treatment settings that provide structure, support, and identification. In these settings, affective and cognitive deficiencies can be addressed by an interdisciplinary team. The traditional uncovering or analyzing techniques should be avoided because they usually cause acting out and may make

---

Oppositional Defiant Disorder

Note: Consider a criterion met only if the behavior is considerably more frequent than that of most people of the same mental age.

A. A disturbance of at least six months during which at least five of the following are present:

   (1) often loses temper
   (2) often argues with adults
   (3) often actively defies or refuses adult requests or rules, e.g., refuses to do chores at home
   (4) often deliberately does things that annoy other people, e.g., grabs other children's hats
   (5) often blames others for his or her own mistakes
   (6) is often touchy or easily annoyed by others
   (7) is often angry or resentful
   (8) is often spiteful or vindictive
   (9) often swears or uses obscene language

From American Psychiatric Association (1987) Diagnostic and statistical manual of mental disorders III-R, Washington, DC, The Association.

---

the adolescent's problems worse. However, adolescents with undersocialized, nonaggressive conduct disorder often exhibit sneaky, devious behaviors that frustrate the unseasoned therapist. These passive-aggressive, shy personality types frequently are exploited by others; thus their family and peer relationships need be carefully monitored. As a group they have been found to be less physically robust, and it has been suggested they may feel weak and consequently resort to handling their anger by devious methods of revenge (Adams and Fras, 1988).

Adolescents with socialized, nonaggressive diagnoses are more socially aware, responsive, have better prognoses and are easier to treat. They are less self-centered, and their ability to relate to others provides them a high degree of rehabilitation potential. With long-term psychotherapy they can be helped to outgrow antisocial relationships and to change and grow in different, constructive, new relationships. Their identification with stable adults is a strength to be fostered. They are more amenable to traditional psychotherapies and educational help than are clients with aggressive conduct disorders (Loeber, 1988; Loeber and Schmaling, 1988).

Clinical specialists and nurses who are imaginative and patient are best suited to work with adolescents with conduct disorders. The time required for them to show change may cause even the most seasoned clinician frustrations and fears that these clients will continue in their nonfunctional patterns. Thus, mentor and peer supervisory support for clinicians working in long-term relationships with adolescents with these disorders is highly recommended.

The short-term goals of care are to alleviate the immediate difficulties and, long-range, to prevent juvenile and adolescent delinquency and adult adjustment problems through redirection and reeducation of the parents and adolescent.

ATTENTION DEFICIT HYPERACTIVITY DISORDER

During the last decades, valuable research has provided remarkable expansions in the understanding and treatment of hyperactive children and adolescents, a condition now referred to as attention deficit hyperactivity disorder (ADHD). This disorder is the most frequently seen disorder in child and adolescent guidance and mental health clinics (see box below).

At this time there is more information on the prevention, etiology, developmental course, and prognosis of ADHD than has ever before been available. In addition, many reliable and valid tools and techniques have been developed that assess, as well as measure treatment intervention outcomes.

Some authorities claim that one of the greatest successes in the area of child and adolescent psychiatry, which has placed the treatment of clients with ADHD in the mainstream of medicine, has occurred through the use of pharmacology to reach definable and measurable treatment goals (Adams and Fras, 1988). Pharmacotherapy and brief parental guidance is now available, with down-to-earth, economical, and accessible services for youngsters needing treatment for ADHD.

Definitions and concepts. The most basic definition of ADHD is that it is a syndrome whose essential traits are distractibility and inability to contain stimuli. This results in excessive and random movements and short attention span (Adams and Fras, 1988). ADHD is characterized by developmentally inappropriate degrees of inattention, with the specific features of gross motor activity, impulsive, careless performance, and excessive running or climbing. These clients are described as "always having their motors running" (DSM-III-R, 1987, p. 50). Associated features include low self-esteem, mood lability, low frustration tolerance, and temper outbursts. ADHD cannot be viewed in terms of a uniform concept and requires the same care and multiple assessment measures used for screening children and adolescents with conduct disorders.

The lack of etiological explanations for this disorder has resulted in an emphasis on descriptions stated in behavioral terms. In the vast literature on hyperactivity, most definitions emphasize the triad of developmentally inappropriate behaviors: inattention, impulsiveness, and hyperactivity. The concept of immaturity is inherent

---

Medical and Nursing Diagnoses Related to Attention Deficit Disorder

Medical diagnoses (DSM-III-R)

314.01   Attention deficit hyperactivity disorder

Nursing diagnoses (PMH)

1.1.2   Altered motor behavior
    1.1.2.6   Hyperactivity
    2.6.2.1   Altered abstract thinking
    2.6.2.2   Altered concentration
    2.6.2.3   Altered problem solving

in this diagnosis. Signs and symptoms cannot be uncovered in laboratory tests; thus, like conduct disorders, the diagnosis is made from the reports of significant adults such as parents and teachers.

Terms used in the past for ADHD reflect the changing schools of thought on its causes, symptoms, and treatment contributing to its continued negative connotation. ADHD first was described in 1902 as "volitional inhibition," that is, defects in moral control. During the past 80 years, hyperactivity has been renamed more than 20 times (Barkley, 1988).

The most recent DSM-III-R term reflects the general consensus of scientists at this time — that the major deficiency in hyperactive clients is their attention problems and these problems are because of organic or physiological-based factors. Terms in the earlier literature such as hyperactive, hyperkinesis syndrome, and minimal brain damage are confusing and imprecise. In most contemporary writings, hyperactivity, hyperkinesis, and attention deficit disorder are terms that continue to be used interchangeably; however, some scientists precisely distinguish among these terms and use "hyperactivity" to describe activity level problems and the latter two terms to describe symptoms that appear in addition to the hyperactivity.

Theoretical explanations. Hyperactivity has a long history in clinical literature and practice. Although many theoretical explanations have been considered etiologically important, few specific causes have been identified. Hyperactivity is the result of not one but of many etiological factors.

Since the first writings describing hyperactivity in the 1900s, neurological factors have been postulated as a cause for hyperactivity. The similarity between the behaviors of clients with ADHD and those with brain injuries has been attributed to the same organic factors. Youngsters who were overactive, distractible, and inattentive and who had poor impulse control were diagnosed as having brain injury, even in the absence of laboratory evidence or history of brain injury. The popular diagnoses of minimal brain damage (MBD) and minimal brain dysfunction implied an underlying brain impairment that was not organically visible by means of diagnostic laboratory tests until recently.

The terminology for primary behavior symptoms that appeared in the literature during the 1970s and the diagnostic term in DSM-II (1952), "hyperkinetic reaction of childhood," were later changed to "attention deficit disorders." Many genetic explanations for hyperactivity continued popular as interest in other possible biological and genetic explanations replaced the earlier notion of minimal brain dysfunction. For example, research on the personality and temperament traits of parents of hyperactive youths showed that impulsiveness, poor judgment, and sociopathy occur more commonly than they do in the parents of youngsters who do not have ADHD. Ongoing twin and adoption studies continue to strongly support these genotype factor influences (Zametkin and Rapoport, 1987).

Maturation or developmental lags also have been studied as etiological factors that contribute to hyperactivity. In these research studies, "lag" refers to the fact that the youngster's nervous system has not developed according to the expected norm. This biological dysmaturation is neither global nor found in all areas; it affects some areas more than others. For example, gross motor development may occur on schedule whereas fine motor coordination and perception do not. When these youngsters are tested, there is a "scattering" of results, and this scattering also appears when the client is tested for perceptual motor functioning.

Other biological factors suspected as causative of ADHD are associated with the mother's environment during pregnancy. Intrauterine damage includes congenital anomalies, intrauterine subclinical lead poisoning, and effects of maternal cigarette smoking, alcoholism, and drug abuse.

Allergies and intolerance to dyes and carbohydrates are other physical responses that have been viewed as causative factors for hyperactivity, and they have received considerable popular press. To date, no systematic studies in the area of foods and dyes have been conducted that definitively support these food dye hypotheses.

The following factors in the adolescent's developmental history may contribute to the diagnosis of ADHD:

- Prematurity
- Signs of fetal distress
- Precipitated or prolonged labor
- Perinatal asphyxia and low Apgar scores
- Feeding and sleeping difficulties during first few weeks of life
- Three-month colic, that is, sleeps all day, cries all night
- History of brain damage or injury to the central nervous system as a result of trauma or infections, cerebral palsy, and neurological disorders

Family history is an additional factor. It includes family members with the triad of alcoholism, hysteria, and sociopathy; parents who report a childhood history of hyperactivity; family members with learning disabilities, such as a father with reading problems; and family members with developmental learning disorders and/or impulse control problems, such as violent behaviors and uncontrollable rages, child abuse, and neglect.

Most psychological explanations for hyperactivity focus on a social-learning framework. Some attribute hyperactivity of childhood to a syndrome of "conditioned life-style hyperactivity," a theory positing that the young person's interaction patterns with significant adults produce short attention spans, hyperactivity, and impulsiveness. Direct imitation of parental actions and reactions, plus conditioning by parental rewards for styles of excessive activity, are contributing factors.

Clinical description. Hyperactivity disorder includes all the symptoms of oppositional defiant disorder, conduct disorder, and other specific developmental disorders (see box on p. 84). Nonlocalized neurological soft signs and motor perceptual dysfunctions, such as poor eye-hand coordination, may be present.

According to the current DSM-III-R criteria, hyperactivity occurs in about 3% of the general population younger than 18 years of age, and it is seen nine times more often in males than in females. Although onset is before the age of 7 years, ADHD is diagnosed at 3 or 4 years of age, when the child enters kindergarten or preschool. The behaviors must be present for at least 6 months for verification of the diagnosis. Symptoms reported by significant adults include distractibility, inability to contain stimuli, random movements, short attention span, developmentally inappropriate inattention, impulsiveness, hyperactivity, and immaturity.

Hyperactivity is exhibited differently at various developmental stages, and characteristic signs and symptoms alert the clinician to the problem during the

---

Attention Deficit Hyperactivity Disorder

NOTE: A criterion is considered to be met only if the behavior occurs considerably more frequently than in most persons of the same mental age.

Attention deficit hyperactivity disorder (ADHD) is a disturbance of at least 6 months during which at least eight of the following signs are present:
1. Often fidgets with hands or feet or squirms in seat (in adolescents, may be limited to subjective feelings of restlessness)
2. Has difficulty remaining seated when required to do so
3. Is easily distracted by extraneous stimuli
4. Has difficulty waiting for turn in games or group situations
5. Often blurts out answers to questions before they have been completed
6. Has difficulty following through on instructions from others (not because of oppositional behavior or failure of comprehension), for example, fails to finish chores
7. Has difficulty sustaining attention in tasks or play activities
8. Often shifts from one uncompleted activity to another
9. Has difficulty playing quietly
10. Often talks excessively
11. Often interrupts or intrudes on others, for example, may break into other children's games

From American Psychiatric Association (1987) Diagnostic and statistical manual of mental disorders III-R, Washington, DC, The Association.

---

collection of the child's developmental history from parents. During infancy these children have higher activity levels than do other children and reject the usual comforting measures. Parents report the need for extraordinary measures to restrain these children in their cribs and ensure their safety. As the child becomes mobile and is able to crawl and climb, the child seems "fearless," and safety becomes a preoccupation.

By the early adolescent phase, the hyperactive youth show signs of depression and low self-esteem. Success at school, at home, and in social relations is rare, and acting out behavior increases as a result of chronic failure. These youngsters brag about false accomplishments, lie and cheat in school, and try anything to be accepted. Truancy begins as they learn to avoid school and failure experiences, and they often run away from home when tensions peak. Many hyperactive children have their first contacts with juvenile authorities during this time (Ross and Ross, 1982).

During adolescence, impulsive, angry outbursts usually interfere with interpersonal relationships and may result in guilt, self-hate, helplessness, inadequacy, and low self-esteem. Antisocial acts that defy authority are frequent. Given the need to belong to a group and the multiple rejections they experience, hyperactive adolescents are easily led to membership in gangs. Here they find the structure they need, as well as the acceptance and spirit of adventure. Stealing, fighting, truancy, and drug and alcohol abuse occur more often in adolescents with ADHD than among this age-group in the general population. Often these adolescents find acceptance in socially questionable cultures and cults, such as the Unification Church or the Divine Light Missions (Galanter, 1989, 1990).

When childish traits of immaturity, such as superficiality, poor judgment based on concreteness, immediate gratification, and poor impulse control, continue into adolescence, both sexes are at greater risk for alcoholism and drug abuse as adults. The prognosis depends on psychosocial conditions, such as the family and school providing the appropriate structure and support and encouraging strengths. Adolescents from stormy environments have poorer prognoses. Considerable overlap with conduct disorder problems make this diagnosis a serious concern. Physical violence, repeated fire setting, and cruelty to animals are often reported.

There is controversy as to whether the incidence of hyperactivity is increasing. Some experts claim that the incidence is not increasing but that hyperactivity is being detected more frequently because of more preschool screening programs, greater dissemination of information about hyperactivity to professionals and parents, and an increased awareness in adults in the general population about developmental and psychiatric conditions in general. Others claim there is an alarming growth in the incidence in hyperactivity as a result of the increase of divorced and dysfunctional families, increased environmental pollutants, permissive child-rearing practices, and poor nutritional habits. Other experts say that increased incidence is due to sophisticated medical neonatal technology and more effective lifesaving techniques for endangered infants. Residual deficits of these surviving infants increases the incidence of psychiatric and developmental disorders. However, it should be kept in mind that the life histories of many highly successful, intelligent, and creative individuals indicate that they had hyperactivity problems when young. Part of what enhances their outstanding contributions is keeping that "childlike" inquisitiveness, activity, and involvement for the rest of their lives.

Interventions.   Behavioral modification interventions and operant conditioning that rewards self-control and the delay of gratification are among the most widely and successfully used interventions, combined with parental guidance and educational and psychopharmacological measures (Barkley, 1987).

Parental counseling and guidance need to be directed toward helping parents clarify their perceptions of the adolescent and provide them a framework for understanding normal adolescent development, as well as ADHD. The gradual building of new parenting skills helps adults cope with their adolescent. Prevention is emphasized, for example, keeping a step or two ahead of the adolescent, thinking ahead, and planning toward situations that will minimize disruption and overstim-ulation. Social interactions need be monitored because controlled children and adolescents with ADHD are highly susceptible to the influences of peers with impulse control difficulties, and these peers stimulate the adolescent's quest for quick stimulation and immediate gratification.

Individual psychotherapy usually follows psychodynamic principles adapted to the adolescent's concrete, short-term perspective, with shorter sessions and longer intervals between them. Nurse clinicians who embark on a career in this area need supervision to ensure the use of sound psychodynamic principles and to tailor therapy to the special needs of the adolescent with ADHD (Brunstetter and Silver, 1985). The successful use of psychopharmacology does not exclude the need for individual therapy nor the parents' need for guidance. Indeed, psychopharmacology is most successful when administered concurrently with supportive, educational therapy. All too often parents and teachers hold a simplistic views that pharmacological treatment and/or strict discipline will solve the problem.

ADHD and developmental learning disabilities often coexist. Thus the nurse needs to work with school personnel and offer teachers support and counseling. Teachers, like nurses, often experience considerable stress in their jobs; children with conduct disorders and hyperactivity frequently manifest behaviors that add to the stress teachers experience in inpatient and community settings (Satterfield, Satterfield, and Cantwell, 1981).

Depression and Bipolar Affective and Mood Disorders

The behavioral disorders discussed thus far, requiring psychiatric care, involve overt disturbances in action behaviors. Emotional disorders that need psychiatric attention, in contrast, involve disturbances of mood or feelings. They fall into two major categories: (1) anxiety disorders, including separation anxiety, avoidance, and overanxious disorders and (2) affective disorders, such as major depression, dysthymic and cyclothymic, and bipolar disorders, often referred to as the pure emotional disorders.

Mood refers to a prolonged, pervasive emotional state that colors people's perceptions of themselves and their world. Mood disorders have in common a disturbance of mood and symptoms of manic or depressive behaviors. The DSM-III-R divides mood disorders into two groups, depressive and bipolar disorders. The criteria indicate that these disorders are not caused by organic or physical factors or by prescribed or self-medications, such as in substance abuse disorders.

An understanding of the definitions of and distinctions between depressive and bipolar disorders requires knowledge of the concept of episodes and the distinctions among manic, hypomanic, and depressive episodes as they are used in the adult DSM-III-R diagnostic categories (Table 5-2). Although shifting episodic mood states require constant adaptations of nursing diagnoses and interventions, insidious and ongoing episodes of depression are of the greatest concern, because suicide is a potential danger (see boxes on pp. 89-91). Adolescents often become depressed after admission to an inpatient treatment setting; however, staff nurses need be alert to the observable behaviors that are signs and symptoms of depression at all times during hospitalization (Khouri and Akiskal, 1986).

Adolescent behaviors that suggest the development of a depression episode include diminished social activity, such as changes in talking and participating in group activities; failure to initiate social contacts and interactions with staff members; solitary behaviors, such as the inability to work on tasks and engage in activities and games; changes in grooming; and affect expressions, such as smiling, frowning, arguing, and complaining (Kazdin and others, 1985). Most adolescents who are depressed, however, exhibit acting-out behaviors. Once the adolescent can make the connection between acting out behaviors and a depressed mood, clinicians will observe signs associated with depressed mood, such as crying, hopelessness, and suicidal ideas (Robbins and Alessi, 1985; Kutscher and others, 1990).

Table 5-2   Comparison of Manic, Hypomanic, and Major depressive episodes

Manic	Hypomanic	Major depressive

A. A distinct period of abnormal, persistently elevated, expansive, or irritable mood
B. During mood disturbance, at least three (four if irritable mood) of the following symptoms have persisted and have been present to a significant degree:
  1. Inflated self-esteem or grandiosity
  2. Decreased need for sleep
  3. More talkative than usual
  4. Flight of ideas or subjective experience that thoughts are racing
  5. Distractability
  6. Increase in activity (socially, sexually, vocationally) or psychomotor agitation
  7. Excessive involvement in potential risk, such as buying sprees, driving at high speeds)
C. Mood disturbance is severe enough to cause marked impairment in occupation function, social activities, or relationships, or severe enough to necessitate hospitalization to prevent harm to self or others
	A. The predominant mood is elevated, expansive, or irritable with similar symptoms associated with manic episodes. However, disturbance is not severe enough to cause marked impairment in job, social activities, and relationships or to require hospitalization. Delusions or hallucinations are never present.
	B. On the basis of manic episode criteria, a hypomanic episode includes items *A* and *B* but not *C* (marked impairment) or *D* (delusions or hallucinations)
		A. At least five of the following symptoms must be present simultaneously for a 2-week period or more, representing a change from previous levels of functioning. One sign must be depressed mood or anhedonia:
		  1. Depressed mood; in adolescents, an irritable mood
		  2. Anhedonia (inability to express pleasure)
		  3. Significant weight loss not by dieting, chronic disease, increase in appetite
		  4. Insomnia/hypersomnia nearly every day
		  5. Notable psychomotor agitation/retardation almost every day
		  6. Loss of energy or presence of fatigue almost daily
		  7. Feels worthless, excessive and inappropriate guilt almost daily
		  8. Decreased ability to concentrate or experience indecisiveness almost daily
		  9. Recurrent thoughts of death or recurrent suicidal ideation

Modified from Reid WH and Wise MG (1989) DSM-III-R training guide, New York, Brunner/Mazel, Inc.

Continued.

Table 5-2   Comparison of Manic, Hypomanic, and Major depressive
episodes—cont'd

Manic	Hypomanic	Major depressive
D. At no time have delusions or hallucinations been present for 2 weeks in the absence of prominent mood symptoms. E. Not superimposed on schizophrenia, schizophreniform disorder, delusional disorder, or psychotic disorders not otherwise specified F. No organic factor is known to have initiated or maintained the disturbance. Somatic conditions such as postpartum depression that apparently precipitate a mood disturbance requiring antidepressant medications are not considered organic factors.		B. Not caused or maintained by an organic factor or uncomplicated bereavement C. At no time have delusions or hallucinations been present for 2 weeks; no prominent mood symptoms D. Not superimposed on schizophreniform, delusions, or psychotic disorders not otherwise specified

MAJOR DEPRESSION

Concepts and theories. Depressive symptoms include dysphoric mood, irritability and weeping, low self-esteem, self-deprecation, hopelessness, recent poor academic performance, disturbed concentration, diminished psychomotor behavior, withdrawal, sleep problems, weight loss or gain, and somatic complaints (DSM-III-R). Other interpersonal difficulties may be present, such as conflicts with parents, fighting with peers and siblings, drug abuse, antisocial behaviors resulting in involvement with the law, and sexual acting out. In contrast to adult clients, most adolescents acknowledge that they are, or have been, depressed, and they give explanations for their depression, such as academic failure and problems with the opposite sex.

Explanations based on genetic studies have dominated the recent theoretical literature because of the revolutionary advances in the field of molecular genetics and the ability to localize and characterize abnormal genes. Recombinant DNA

DSM-III-R and Nursing Diagnoses Related to Mood (Affective) Disorders

Medical diagnoses (DSM-III-R)

296.2x	Major depression, single episode
296.3x	Major depression, recurrent
296.4x	Bipolar disorder, manic
296.5x	Bipolar disorder, depressed
296.6x	Bipolar disorder, mixed
300.40	Disrhythmic disorder
301.13	Cyclothymia

PMH nursing diagnoses related to mood (affective) disorders

1.1   Motor behavior

   1.1.2   Altered motor behavior
      1.1.2.1   Activity intolerance
      1.1.2.5   Fatigue
      1.1.2.6   Hyperactivity
      1.1.2.7   Hypoactivity
      1.1.1.8   Psychomotor agitation
      1.1.1.9   Psychomotor retardation
      1.1.1.10   Restlessness

1.3   Self-care

   1.3.3   Altered self-care
      1.3.3.3   Altered grooming
      1.3.3.4   Altered health maintenance
      1.3.3.6   Altered participation in health care

1.4   Sleep/arousal patterns

   1.4.2   Altered sleep/arousal patterns
      1.4.2.1   Decreased need for sleep
      1.4.2.2   Hypersomnia
      1.4.2.3   Insomnia
      1.4.2.4   Nightmare/terrors
      1.4.2.5   Somnolence

2.2   Judgment

   2.2.2   Altered judgment

Continued.

---

biological research findings also strongly support theories that biological and genetic vulnerability is associated with affective disorders. Although the findings of these studies are tentative because of the newness of this area, family studies that focus on genetic linkage of large extended families have localized some of the genes responsible for bipolar affective disorder. Research studies (Orvaschel, 1990; Orvaschel and others, 1982) focusing on children at risk for the development of

(Text continued on p. 92).

DSM-III-R and Nursing Diagnoses Related to Mood (Affective) Disorders — cont'd

2.6   Thought processes

2.6.2   Altered thought processes
       2.6.2.2   Altered abstract thinking
       2.6.2.3   Altered problem solving
       2.6.2.4   Confusion/disorientation
       2.2.2.6   Delusions
       2.2.2.7   Ideas of reference
       2.2.2.8   Magical thinking
       2.2.2.9   Obsessions
       2.2.2.10   Suspiciousness
       2.2.2.11   Thought insertion

4.1   Feeling states

4.1.2   Altered feeling state
       4.1.2.2   Anxiety
       4.1.2.3   Elation
       4.1.2.6   Grief
       4.1.2.7   Guilt
       4.1.2.8   Sadness

4.2   Feeling processes

4.2.2   Altered feeling processes
       4.2.2.1   Lability
       4.2.2.2   Mood swings

5.3   Conduct/impulse processes

       5.3.1.1   Potential for violence
       5.3.1.2   Suicidal ideation
5.3.2   Altered conduct/impulse processes
       5.3.2.1   Accident prone
       5.3.2.2   Aggressive/violent behavior toward environment
       5.3.2.6   Physical aggression toward self
               5.3.2.6.1   Suicide attempt(s)
       5.3.2.12   Verbal aggression toward others

5.4   Family process

5.4.1   Altered family processes
       5.4.1.1   Ineffective family coping
               5.5.2.1.2   Disabled
5.5.3   Altered role performance
       5.5.2.3   Altered student role
5.5.3   Ineffective individual coping
       5.5.3.1   Defensive coping
       5.5.3.2   Ineffective denial

Continued.

DSM-III-R and Nursing Diagnoses Related to Mood (Affective)
Disorders — cont'd

5.7 Social interaction

5.7.2   Altered social interaction
     5.7.2.2   Compulsive behaviors
     5.7.2.3   Disorganized social behaviors
     5.7.2.5   Social isolation/withdrawal
     5.7.2.6   Unpredictable behaviors

6.1 Attention

     6.1.2.1   Hyperalertness
     6.1.2.2   Inattention
     6.1.2.3   Selective attention

6.3 Self-concept

6.3.2   Altered self-concept
     6.3.3.2   Altered personal identity
     6.6.6.3   Altered self esteem
          6.3.2.3.1   Chronic low self-esteem
          6.3.2.3.2   Situational low self-esteem

6.4 Sensory perception

6.4.2   Altered sensory perception
     6.4.2.1   Hallucinations

7.6 Neuro/sensory processes

7.6.2   Altered neuro/sensory process
     7.6.2.2   Altered sensory acuity

8.1 Meaningfulness

8.1.2   Altered meaningfulness
     8.1.2.1   Helplessness
     8.1.2.2   Hopelessness
     8.1.2.3   Loneliness
     8.1.2.4   Powerlessness

8.3 Values

8.3.2   Altered values
     8.3.2.1   Conflict with social order
     8.3.2.3   Unclear values

affective disorders have found that an etiological heterogeneousness underlies all mood disorders. Other genetic and DNA studies stress the mixture or comorbidity of anxiety and depression (Leckman and others, 1983; 1990).

Although statistics vary, it generally is held that the presence of a major depression in first-degree relatives predisposes a person to this diagnosis. In one family study it was reported that of subjects diagnosed with mood disturbances, 20% to 37% had relatives with similar difficulties, whereas only 7% of the normal subjects participating in the study had relatives with diagnoses of depression (Gershon and others, 1982). Some studies hold that as many as 30% of adolescents are mildly or clinically depressed. There is a preponderance of depression in females, which increases with age (Cantwell and Carlson, 1983).

There is a strong relationship between depression and suicide, and the escalating adolescent suicide rate suggests that adolescent depression is seriously under-diagnosed. Thus, diagnosis of depression and suicide potential has become the major clinical and research concern, as well as the most explored and rapidly changing area in adolescent psychopathology (Kovacs and others, 1984).

Although the DSM-III-R holds that the adult criteria for depression apply to children and adolescents, it appears that adolescent depression is more difficult to recognize than is the adult equivalent. The applicability of the adult taxonomy for adolescents has been questioned, and considerable evidence supports the theory that there are several types of depression in adolescents. Failure to recognize them contributes to the underdiagnosis of adolescent suicide, which is highly related to depressive disorders.

Adolescent depression has been referred to as "masked depression." According to this theory some adolescents do not express their depressed mood directly but "mask" it in symptoms such as somatic complaints, conduct disorders, aggressive behavior, delinquency, school phobias, and academic underachievement. Studies of masked depression support suggestions that the symptoms of adult and adolescent depression differ. Masked depression symptoms have been found to be strongly related to substance abuse in adolescents but not in adult substance abuse. A strong relationship between major depressive disorders and antisocial behavior also has been found in youths but not in adults (Carlson and Cantwell, 1980). Depression in these adolescents usually is characterized by irritable moods and acting out behaviors, in contrast to the classic "depressed mood" and "loss of interest" or pleasure symptoms characteristic of depressed adults (American Psychiatric Association, 1987) (see case study).

Case Study: Major Depression

John, a 15-year-old middle-class male, was assessed in the juvenile detention facility of a rural county. He was being held in detention after an incident in which he attacked his father. He was on probation for curfew violations. The adolescent was assessed while wearing prison garb and handcuffs.

John had a depressed affect, poor eye contact, suicidal ideas, and a sense of hopelessness. He said his grades had fallen during the past year. He gave a history of being beaten by his father since he was 5 or 6 years old. He reported that after a particularly severe beating about 8 months ago, he called the children's protective services in his county. The worker came to the home but was persuaded there was no abuse. John then learned that if he got into trouble with the police, the juvenile court would send his parents to a parenting class. He subsequently stayed out past the town curfew for teenagers and was processed through juvenile court, and his parents attended the class as he had hoped. His father stopped hitting him, but John discovered that he was still angry with his father and became physically aggressive, including getting his father's gun out of the gun cabinet during an argument. He was feeling angry, tearfully depressed, and afraid of his own aggressiveness. Because of his potential for suicide and aggression along with significant depression, John was referred for inpatient treatment. The evaluation there validated the presence of a major depression, as well as evidence of posttraumatic stress disorder. Shortly after treatment was initiated, John began experiencing episodes of violent behavior toward the environment and toward himself, including tying a shoelace tightly around his neck. John was placed on an antidepressant regimen and was assisted by the nursing staff to redirect his rage into physical activity (punching bag) and verbal expression. Family therapy was aimed at healing the relationship between John and his parents, who were seeking his forgiveness and sincerely wanted to change.

BIPOLAR AND UNIPOLAR AFFECTIVE DISORDERS

Persons with bipolar affective disorders have episodes of depression and mania, whereas those with unipolar disorders have depressive episodes only. Estimates of the prevalence of bipolar disorders are that approximately 1% of the population is affected (Klerman, 1986); approximately 1 to 3 million men and women in the United States suffer from bipolar mood disorder (McEnany, 1990; Klerman, 1978).

The onset of bipolar disorders usually occurs before the age of 30 years (Cancro, 1985). There is an increased incidence of bipolar disorder among first-degree relatives with bipolar or unipolar disorders or alcoholism (Andreasen and others, 1987). Because bipolar disorders are chronic, lifelong medication maintenance usually is required. In a summary of recent research on the biological indices of bipolar mood disorders, McEnany (1990) organized the current understandings of bipolar disorders into four major areas: (1) biological rhythms, (2) biochemical brain function and bipolar states, (3) related biological influences of bipolar mood states, and (4) genetics and bipolar mood disorders.

Although biochemical theories and investigations have focused predominantly on major depression, these studies have provided the basis for postulates concerning bipolar disorders. Neurotransmitters such as norepinephrine, serotonin, and dopamine reabsorb, release, or break down in the central nervous system (Bunney and others, 1979; Goldstein and others, 1980). On the basis of these findings, it has been suggested that depression is associated with insufficient activity of neurotransmitters. Mania, in contrast, is due to excessive activity of these neurochemicals (Schildkraut and others, 1985). With the use of antidepressants or lithium, a balance is reestablished at these neurotransmitter sites, further supporting this explanation (Levy, 1982). Additional studies are needed to develop the classification and clinical laboratory tests necessary to determine the type of affective disorder and the most effective treatment. Current biochemical research is focusing on investigations of the relationship of hormones to mood disorders, and endocrine research studies are focusing on the hypothalamic-pituitary-adrenal link, the hypothalymic-pituitary-growth hormone link, and the hypothalymic-pituitary-gonadal link, as well as the interactions of chemical imbalances in affective disorders (Schildkraut and others, 1985).

The clinical picture of persons with bipolar disorder is based on the client's and family's historical accounts of mood swings or descriptions of feelings such as high or low, euphoric or flat. Many older adolescents have mixed bipolar disorders, which are characterized by symptoms of simultaneous depression and mania, intermixed or alternating rapidly every few days (Puig-Antich, 1985). The onset and duration of these episodes are unpredictable and may last a few days to several weeks (Goldstein and others, 1980).

Hypomanic behaviors may occur without a preceding depressive episode. Hypomanic adolescent behaviors include impulsiveness; uninhibited, loud, theatrical actions; rapid, pressured speech; an overly self-confident manner; difficulty completing tasks or sitting still; decreased eating and sleeping requirements; low frustration level; risky, delinquent behaviors; and sexual promiscuity.

The adolescent with manic behavior exhibits many of the same symptoms but at an increased level of intensity and rapidity. In addition, the manic stage includes symptoms of delusions, hallucinations, disorientation to time and place, and bizarre psychomotor behaviors (Goldstein and others, 1980). These adolescents often self-medicate with alcohol or other drugs to calm or energize themselves and frequently have a dual diagnosis of chemical dependency.

SUICIDE

Statistical reports of suicide vary. Some reports (Spirito and others, 1987), however, claim that suicide is the third leading cause of death in the United States among persons younger than 20 years of age. Suicides occurring in children younger than 10 years of age have been reported and are especially disturbing, as are reports that during the last three decades, adolescent suicide rates have been escalating throughout the world (Izard and Schwartz, 1986). These increases vary considerably from one country to another, with the United States among the highest rates reported. These variations reflect cultural differences in acting out.

While suicide has historically fallen within the domain of psychiatry and mental health, in 1987, concerns that the incidence of suicide had reached epidemic proportions caused the Centers for Disease Control to make it a priority concern. Most experts (Miller, 1986) agree that the statistics for this age-group are misleading and that there are at least five times as many adolescent suicides as reported. Accidental deaths related to automobiles and firearms often are unrecognized suicides.

The alarming increase in suicide in the young has been attributed to social changes, such as divorce and separating parents, destruction of the nuclear family, and the emotional divorce of a parent from a child (Miller, 1986). The emotional susceptibility of adolescents, coupled with parental shifting, confusing societal norms, and a lack of parental and peer support also are stressed as factors that set the stage for self-destructive acts (Steer and others, 1988).

The incidence of suicide is associated with psychopathology, including affective disorders, antisocial problems, and substance abuse (Brent and Kolko, 1990). Risks of suicide, suicide ideation, and suicide attempts among adolescents with affective disorders are particularly high; thus adolescent depression is a major clinical concern (Peck and others, 1985).

Suicides, suicide threats and gestures, and suicide attempts are severe forms of acting out that are directed against the self. The act has a symbolic importance in that it often is intended to hurt or destroy others. These acts present a danger to life and possible permanent crippling; thus self-destruction acts constitute psychiatric emergencies that require special therapeutic approaches (Glaser, 1987).

A number of categories of suicidal behavior, that is, forms of expressing suicidal intent, have appeared in the literature. Although grouping by severity has been attempted, the mode of expression is not a reliable indicator of the conflict or the likelihood of repetition (Glaser, 1987).

Casual statements and suicidal gestures may constitute attempts to indicate verbally or nonverbally a desire for self-destruction. Although these threats may reflect attention-seeking behavior, they should not be discounted or minimized. The threat may be better understood as a hope that someone will recognize the danger and rescue the adolescent from self-destructive behaviors.

A suicide attempt is any action taken by the individual toward the self that will lead to death if not interrupted. A successful suicide is one that results in death (Stuart and Sundeen, 1991).

To date most research on youth suicide has been based on models developed from research on adult populations. Thus it is difficult to apply these findings to clinical situations with adolescents. Depression has been the most frequently explored factor in studies of adolescent suicidal behavior, and the link between depression, suicidal ideation, and acting out has been emphasized. The lack of social support and interpersonal relationships are factors strongly indicated as contributing to suicide, although research is limited in this area. Family, girlfriend/boyfriend, or school problems usually are present at the time of death. Hopelessness is a factor as suicidal ideation moves from nonspecific ideas to specific intent. Attention deficit, conduct disorder, and anxiety also are correlated with adolescent suicide attempts, suggesting that other factors, such as poor social skills, may contribute to adolescent suicide (Klorman, 1986; McClennan and others, 1990) (see box).

Risk Factors For Adolescent Suicide

Family constellation
Psychiatric history
Family history of substance abuse
Individual substance abuse
Frequent moves
Physical abuse
Sexual abuse
Anger
Hostility

Schizophrenia

Schizophrenia is one of the most challenging clinical problems that clinicians who work in adolescent psychiatry encounter (see boxes on pp. 97-98). The changing, unpredictable, up-and-down, sporadic behaviors of these clients are of major concern. Schizophrenia is characterized by various psychotic symptoms of delusions, hallucinations, incoherence, loose associations, catatonic behavior, or grossly inappropriate affect (see box on p. 99). The disorder is classified into catatonic type, disorganized type, paranoid type, and undifferentiated and residual type. The symptoms quickly lead to dysfunctions in relationships, work, and self-care. Behaviors that family members or caregivers may notice before or after the actual phase of the illness include social withdrawal, poor hygiene or grooming, talking to self, hoarding food, odd beliefs such as unusual superstitiousness, telepathy, and vague, overelaborate, or circumstantial speech, a marked lack of initiative, interests, or energy are also noted.

The symptoms of schizophrenia are classified as either positive (hallucinations, delusions, disordered thinking) or negative (emotional withdrawal, apathy, inattentiveness, poor social function). These groups of symptoms are associated with the client's other characteristics. It appears that the number of positive symptoms decrease as negative symptoms increase and that negative symptoms increase as the illness continues.

Historically, about 1% of the population is diagnosed as having schizophrenia, and in most cases the condition eventually becomes chronic (Cancro, 1985). Recently it was estimated that 1.2 to 6 million Americans suffer from schizophrenia (Babigian, 1985) and that the cost of this illness is between $10 and $20 billion dollars a year (Cancro, 1985). During the last few years, scientific advances in understanding mental disorders have changed profoundly as technological advances rapidly alter previous conceptions of the etiologic factors in many of these conditions. As a result of advances in the biological sciences, the present "biological revolution" in psychiatry has provided new insights in the areas of brain structure, functioning, and chemistry. Historically these disorders have been a major concern of clinicians who work in child and adolescent psychiatry. The new psychobiological findings require a reframing, reevaluation, and expansion of many nursing assessment and intervention techniques. The field of adolescent psychiatric nursing will change remarkably in the coming decade as nurses integrate and implement recent psychobiological discoveries in clinical adolescent care.

One of the most important questions to be answered in the treatment of schizophrenic adolescents is the role of biology and the brain function in schizophrenia. Some 50 years ago results of the first studies of twins provided evidence of important biological factors and supported the role genetics play in the disorder. Findings showed that monozygotic twins have three to four times higher concordance rates than do dizygotic twins. Studies of adopted offspring also show that schizophrenia in the biological father increases probability of schizophrenia in the offspring; however, conclusive gene identification is yet to be found. Ongoing concordant twin studies stress interaction of gene vulnerability and environmental stress (Zubin, 1983; Kallman and Roth, 1956).

Medical and Nursing Diagnoses Related to Psychosis and Schizophrenia

Medical diagnoses (DSM-III-R) *Schizophrenia*

295.2x	Catatonic
295.1x	Disorganized
295.3x	Paranoid
295.9x	Undifferentiated
205.6x	Residual
310.10	Organic personality disorder (etiology noted on Axis III or is unknown)

Nursing diagnoses (PMH)

2.6   Thought processes
    2.6.1   Potential for alteration
    2.6.2   Altered thought processes
        2.6.2.1   Altered abstract thinking
        2.6.2.2   Altered concentration
        2.6.2.3   Altered problem solving
        2.6.2.4   Confusion/disorientation
        2.6.2.5   Delirium
        2.6.2.6   Delusions
        2.6.2.7   Ideas of reference
        2.6.2.8   Magical thinking
        2.6.2.9   Obsessions
        2.6.2.10   Suspicions
        2.6.2.11   Thought insertion
5.2   Communication processes
    5.2.2   Altered communication processes
        5.2.2.1   Altered nonverbal communication
        5.2.2.2   Altered verbal communication
            5.2.2.2.1   Aphasia
            5.2.2.2.2   Bizarre content
            5.2.2.2.3   Confabulation
            5.2.2.2.4   Ecolalia
            5.2.2.2.5   Incoherent
            5.2.2.2.6   Mute
            5.2.2.2.7   Neologisms
            5.2.2.2.8   Nonsense/word salad

Continued.

Another focus of research in schizophrenia is the use of radiological and nonradiological techniques computed tomographical scans or magnetic resonance imaging to study the structural pathology in the brain of patients with schizophrenia. Studies demonstrate that the brains of persons with this diagnosis are not structurally normal, and there is evidence of quantitatively determined decreased tissue mass in this population. Further, data about the brain's structural pathology are similar to data about neurodevelopmental disability. There are signs that patients with schizophrenia have some disorder in normal brain development, such as delayed

Medical and Nursing Diagnoses Related to Psychosis and Schizophrenia — cont'd

1.4 Sleep/arousal patterns
    1.4.2 Altered sleep/arousal patterns
        1.4.2.1 Decreased need for sleep
        1.4.2.2 Hypersomnia
    1.1.2 Altered motor behavior
        1.1.2.1 Activity intolerance
        1.1.2.2 Bizarre motor behavior
        1.1.2.3 Catatonia
        1.1.2.4 Disorganized motor behavior
        1.1.2.6 Hyperactivity
        1.1.2.7 Hypoactivity
        1.1.2.8 Psychomotor agitation
        1.1.2.9 Psychomotor retardation
        1.1.2.10 Restlessness
6.4 Sensory perception
    6.4.2 Altered sensory perception
        6.4.2.1 Hallucinations
            6.4.2.1.1 Auditory

motor disabilities, performance IQ higher than verbal IQ, and conduct difficulties (Hendren and others, 1990). By means of positron emission tomography and blood flow scanning in living persons, regional functional dissimilarities between clients with schizophrenia and normal individuals have been found in the frontal lobe, particularly the prefrontal cortex (Hendren and others, 1990).

Traditionally, schizophrenia that has its clinical onset around 14 or 15 years of age can be related to an insult that happened many years earlier, such as a brain deficit at birth. For example, the frontal lobe, which controls reasoning, is the last part of the brain to develop, and Piaget's theory of formal operations and development of cognitive strategies, which depend on the prefrontal cortex, gives support to this. At adolescence, greater demands for autonomous independent cognitive and psychological functions, including stress management, are related to prefrontal integrity. Thus organic deficits in the prefrontal cortex may be related to the onset of schizophrenia in adolescents.

Other theoretical areas of current research involve dopamine, which reaches its peak of activity in adolescence and diminishes around the age of 20 years. Chemical dopamine is altered in the brain of some persons with schizophrenia, a finding confirmed by the effectiveness in schizophrenia of drugs that block dopamine receptors in the brain. Biochemical research proposes two explanations. One possibility may be an inborn error of metabolism, and the second proposes that there is an imbalance in the neurochemical system of the brain. The reaction in the chemical neurotransmitter may be unstable at the presynaptic or postsynaptic receptor sites (Meltzer, 1979). Persons whose illness is characterized by positive symptoms are most likely to have dopaminergic hyperactivity, whereas those with

---

Schizophrenia

A. Presence of characteristic psychotic symptoms in the active phase: either *1*, *2*, or *3* for at least 1 week (unless the symptoms are successfully treated):
   1. Two of the following:
      a. Delusions
      b. Prominent hallucinations (throughout the day for several days or several times a week for several weeks, with each hallucinatory experience lasting longer than a few brief moments)
      c. Incoherence or obvious loosening of associations
      d. Catatonic behavior
      e. Flat or grossly inappropriate affect
   2. Bizarre delusions (involving a phenomenon that the person's culture would regard as totally implausible, such as thought broadcasting or being controlled by a dead person)
   3. Prominent hallucinations (as defined in [1*b*] above) of a voice with content having no apparent relation to depression or elation, a voice keeping up a running commentary on the person's behavior or thoughts, or two or more voices conversing with each other
B. During the course of the disturbance, functioning in such areas as work, social relations, and self-care clearly below the highest level achieved before onset of the disturbance (or, if the onset is in childhood or adolescence, failure to achieve expected level of social development)
C. Prodromal or residual symptoms:
   1. Marked social isolation or withdrawal
   2. Noticeable impairment in role functioning as a wage-earner, student, or homemaker
   3. Markedly peculiar behavior (collecting garbage, talking to self in public, hoarding food)
   4. Obvious impairment in personal hygiene and grooming
   5. Blunted or inappropriate affect
   6. Digressive, vague, overelaborate, or circumstantial speech, poverty of speech, or poverty of speech content
   7. Odd beliefs or magical thinking that influences behavior and is inconsistent with cultural norms (superstitiousness, belief in clairvoyance, telepathy, "sixth sense," idea that "others can feel my feelings," overvalued ideas, ideas of reference)
   8. Unusual perceptual experiences such as recurrent illusions or sensing the presence of a force or person not actually present
   9. Lack of initiative, interests, or energy

From American Psychiatric Association (1987) Diagnostic and statistical manual of mental disorders III-R, Washington, DC, The Association.

---

social and intellectual deterioration (negative symptoms) as prominent clinical problems may not have dopaminergic hyperactivity. Current research findings suggest that persons with negative symptoms may have structural brain abnormalities, which raises further questions regarding the cause these structural changes, such as viral infections. Also, persons with Parkinson's disease, which causes a hypodopaminergic state, exhibit these negative symptoms (Andreasen and Olsen, 1982; Karson, Kleinman, and Wyatt, 1986).

Interventions for adolescents with schizophrenia include nursing and medical management of acute symptoms, education of the adolescent and the family regarding the illness and its management, and family therapy for family dysfunctions coexisting with the disorder. Nurses who care for adolescents with schizophrenia should be aware of support groups in the community for families of the mentally ill, including the National Alliance for the Mentally Ill. A working relationship with these groups is essential to developing trust with families and for staying abreast of events taking place in these organizations.

Adolescents with schizophrenia often are treated initially in inpatient settings. Planning for school and aftercare sometimes presents difficulties because of lack of resources in the community. In many cases an adolescent would benefit from a partial hospitalization program that provides treatment and school instead of home tutoring and once-a-week outpatient therapy.

Anxiety Disorders

CONCEPTS

Anxiety symptoms in childhood and adolescence are common (see box on p. 101). Children experience anxiety as a part of normal development in the process of individuation from their mothers. Mahler (1968) indicated that anxiety results from a psychological fear of loss, or separation anxiety. Bowlby (1973) described anxiety as a response to the disruption in attachment behavior. Sullivan (1953) believed that the child learns anxiety from anxious parents. More recently, genetic transmission studies indicate a higher incidence of anxiety disorders in the relatives of children and adults who experience anxiety disorders compared with control groups (Bernstein and Garfinkel, 1988). Anxiety disorders in adolescents frequently are associated with depression (Bernstein and others, 1989); panic disorders are especially associated with an abnormality in lactate levels (Pitts and McClure, 1967) and mitral valve prolapse (Crowe and others, 1982).

SEPARATION ANXIETY DISORDER

Separation anxiety disorder in adolescents usually is seen as school refusal, or school phobia. It usually occurs at the transition to junior high school around the age of 12 to 14 years. Half these adolescents meet the criteria for a major depressive episode (Bernstein and Garfinkel, 1986). Many come from chaotic homes where the mother figure is unavailable physically and emotionally, with a history of difficult separations, such as the parents' divorce, placement outside the home, or repeated separations because of hospitalization of a parent. Because these adolescents often have somatic complaints, the parents permit them to stay home.

Interventions. Interventions for school-refusal behavior include behavioral therapy, family therapy, and chemotherapy. Behavior therapies are aimed at reducing the adolescent's anxiety about various aspects of attending school. Contingency contracting often is used to support school attendance. Family therapy is employed to encourage separation from parents and to develop appropriate bonding if it is

---

Medical and Nursing Diagnoses Related to Anxiety

Medical diagnoses (DSM-III-R)

309.21   Separation anxiety disorder
313.21   Avoidant disorder
313.00   Overanxious disorder
300   Panic disorder
300.30   Obsessive-compulsive disorder

Nursing diagnoses (PMH)

4.1.2.2   Anxiety
1.1.2.10   Restlessness
1.4.2.3   Insomnia
5.3.2.10   Truancy
5.5.2.3   Altered student role, guilt
5.5.3.1   Defensive coping, social isolation/withdrawal
2.6.2.9   Obsessive/compulsive behaviors
2.6.2.2   Altered concentration
6.1.2.1   Hyperalertness
7.2.2.1.2   Diarrhea
7.2.2.1.1   Constipation
2.6.2.2   Altered concentration
1.2.2.1   Diversional activity deficit

---

inadequate. The therapist works with the school, often the school nurse or counselor, to develop plans for the return to school. Imipramine and alprazolam, a new benzodiazepine, are useful in the treatment of school refusal. If the adolescent has a concurrent depression, the dosage of imipramine should be adjusted accordingly.

OBSESSIVE-COMPULSIVE DISORDER

Obsessive-compulsive disorder (OCD) is characterized by "recurrent; and persistent ideas, thoughts, or images that are experienced as intrusive and senseless" with "repetitive, purposeful behaviors that are performed in response to the obsession" (American Psychiatric Association, 1987). The rituals are designed to provide relief from the anxiety or the fear regarding the obsessional ideas. The rituals interfere with normal functioning, although adolescents try to hide the problem from others. The disorder often starts in childhood and may be full-blown by the age of 15 years. Although some adolescents have had a severe conscience since childhood, often in a rigid, strict family (Rasmussen, 1986), in other adolescents a sudden onset of symptoms occurs (Rapoport, 1986), leading to the theory that OCD is an organic disorder. Positron emission tomographic findings demonstrated significantly higher glucose metabolism in the left orbital gyrus. Furthermore, patients with OCD had abnormal activity in the subcortical areas of the hemisphere (Baxter and others, 1987). In addition, research has indicated the presence of neurotransmitter dysfunctions, especially in serotonin and norepinephrine regulation. The effectiveness of clomipramine in the treatment of OCD has led to new information in this area.

There is evidence that OCD and Tourette's syndrome are related illnesses (Pauls and others, 1986). It is well-known that children with Tourette's syndrome have significantly more obsessional symptoms than do adults with Tourette's syndrome (Jensen, 1990). Studies of twins indicate a genetic predisposition to OCD (Lieberman, 1984).

Interventions for OCD include behavior therapy, family therapy, and clomipramine.

Other Disorders of Adolescence

BORDERLINE PERSONALITY DISORDER

Although borderline personality disorder (see upper box on p. 103) is not listed in the DSM-III-R for persons younger than 18 years of age, the prevalence of the disorder in adolescents is well documented. Masterson (1985) described the basis of the disorder as a failure of the developmental task of separation and individuation of a toddler from the mother. He proposed that this failure stems from the mother's need to keep the child in the infantile symbiotic state. When the child makes a bid for independence, the mother withdraws nurturance. The child fears the withdrawal or abandonment and clings to the mother. The child also experiences rage toward the mother for frustrating the child's needs. As a result, the child fails to learn to accept the mother as a whole person and splits her into good mother and bad mother. Furthermore, the mother's negative view of the child is internalized (introjected) into the child's own confused self-image. The relationship between the mother and the adolescent resembles the described childhood pattern, with a distant father. Often the mother precipitates the adolescent's anger and anxiety by dealing with the adolescent from a narcissistic point of view. Another result of this scenario is that the small child and later the adolescent, develops a confused self-identity.

The behavior of the adolescent with borderline personality disorder matches the DSM-III-R criteria for the borderline personality in adults (see lower box on p. 103).
The major characteristics include the following:
1. Intense clinging relationships
2. Splitting self and others into "all bad" or "all good"
3. Feelings of emptiness
4. Intense anger and acting out behavior such as temper tantrums and violence
5. Impulsiveness in sex, spending money, and other behaviors, sometimes substance abuse and bulimia
6. Repeated suicide gestures, threats, and self-mutilation
7. Intense fear of abandonment

The adolescent with borderline personality disorder manipulates caregivers and parents through the splitting mechanism, relating to others as if they are "all bad" or "all good" and rages against the "bad" persons in his or her life. Any minor abandonment by significant others (for example, refusing requests, going on vacation, leaving the unit for the day) precipitates high anxiety. This anxiety is often relieved by acting out behaviors, most notably self-mutilation, but also temper tantrums, substance abuse, and sexual activity.

Medical and Nursing Diagnoses Related to Borderline Personality Disorder

Medical diagnoses (DSM-III-R)

Not available for adolescents

Nursing diagnoses (PMH)

5.5.3   Ineffective individual coping
  5.5.3.1   Defensive coping: splitting
  4.1.2.1   Anger
  4.1.2.2   Anxiety
  4.1.2.5   Fear
  4.2.2.1   Lability
  5.3.2.5   Physical aggression toward others
  5.3.2.6   Physical aggression toward self

Borderline Personality Disorder

NOTE: Diagnosis is based on a pervasive pattern of instability of mood, interpersonal relationships, and self-image, beginning by early adulthood and present in a variety of contexts, as indicated by at least five of the following:

1. A pattern of unstable and intense interpersonal relationships characterized by alternating between extremes of overidealization and devaluation
2. Impulsiveness in at least two areas that are potentially self-damaging, such as spending, sex, substance use, shoplifting, reckless driving, binge eating (not including suicidal or self-mutilating behavior covered in No. 5, below)
3. Affective instability: distinct shifts from baseline mood to depression, irritability, or anxiety, usually lasting a few hours and only rarely more than a few days
4. Inappropriate, intense anger or lack of control of anger, for example, frequent displays of temper, constant anger, recurrent physical fights
5. Recurrent suicidal threats, gestures, or behavior, or self-mutilating behavior
6. Marked and persistent identity disturbance manifested by uncertainty about at least two of the following: self-image, sexual orientation, long-term goals or career choice, type of friends desired, preferred values
7. Chronic feelings of emptiness or boredom
8. Frantic efforts to avoid real or imagined abandonment (not including suicidal or self-mutilating behavior covered in No. 5, above)

From American Psychiatric Association (1987) Diagnostic and statistical manual of mental disorders III-R, Washington, DC, The Association.

Professionals who care for these adolescents respond with countertransference and succumb to disagreements with coworkers, a sense of failure, and frustration and anger with the adolescent.

To avoid these reactions, interventions for the adolescent with borderline personality disorder include appointing a primary nurse or therapist and requiring the adolescent, family, and treatment team members to refer to the primary person for all requests and treatment planning (Gossett and others, 1983). Treatment team members support one another and check discrepancies in the plan. The adolescent requires structure for each day, with specific, scheduled times when contact with the inpatient primary nurse, therapist, and/or parent or school nurse or counselor occurs. A contract to avoid self-injurious acts, with concrete plans for alternative behaviors, including self-soothing techniques, is important in helping the adolescent manage destructive impulses. Medication may be used, usually to treat the depression that accompanies this disorder.

Antianxiety agents may be administered during periods of extreme destructiveness, especially if disorientation occurs. Careful long-term coordination of the adolescent often results in significant improvement (Masterson, 1985; Durkin, 1975).

EATING DISORDERS

Eating disorders are characterized by gross disturbances in eating behavior. They include anorexia nervosa, bulimia nervosa, pica, and rumination disorder at infancy (APA, 1987) (see box below). The most common eating disorders of adolescence are anorexia and bulimia.

The most visible and immediately noticeable symptom of anorexia nervosa is an excessive loss of weight (see box on p. 105). The onset of this disorder is seen most frequently in females between 12 and 18 years of age. The incidence of anorexia may be as high as 1 in 20 teenage girls, with mortality of 10% to 21% (Halmi, 1974; Kalucy and others, 1977). Anorexia is a disturbance of body image—a consistent fear of being or becoming overweight. Because body image and body concept are changing during adolescence, anorexia may be due to the conflict of an emerging body concept complicated by enormous social pressure to maintain an acceptable image. Diagnostic criteria for anorexia nervosa include a refusal to maintain body weight at a minimal normal weight for age and height; intense fear of gaining weight or

---

Medical and Nursing Diagnoses Related to Eating Disorders

Medical diagnoses (DSM-III-R)

307.10   Anorexia nervosa
307.51   Bulimia nervosa

Nursing diagnoses (PMH)

7.4.2   Altered eating processes
       7.7.2.2   Anorexia
7.7.9.9   Nutrition processes not otherwise specified

Eating Disorders

Anorexia nervosa

A. Refusal to maintain body weight over a minimal normal weight for age and height, for example, weight loss leading to maintenance of body weight 15% below that expected or failure to reach expected weight

Bulimia nervosa

A. Recurrent episodes of binge eating (rapid consumption of a large amount of food)
B. A feeling of lack of control over eating behavior during the eating binges
C. Regular engagement in self-induced vomiting, use of laxatives or diuretics, strict dieting or fasting, or vigorous exercise to prevent weight gain
D. A minimum average of two binge-eating episodes per week for at least 3 months
E. Persistent overconcern with body shape and weight

From American Psychiatric Association (1987) Diagnostic and statistical manual of mental disorders DSM-III-R, Washington, DC, The Association.

---

becoming fat even though underweight; disturbance in perception of body weight, size, or shape; and in females, absence of at least three consecutive menstrual cycles (American Psychiatric Association, 1987). Severe anorexia nervosa should be considered a life-threatening disorder because of critical body tissue waste and dehydration.

Bulimia nervosa is characterized by self-induced vomiting or excessive use of laxatives alternating with periods of binge eating. Because of this behavior, bulimia also is known as the "binge and purge" syndrome. The incidence of this disorder is about 5% in young women (Hart and Ollendick, 1985). Bulimia may be related to anorexia nervosa. When it is not associated with anorexia, the behavior is less life-threatening; however, the weight fluctuations still must be regarded as serious. Common physical problems include dental erosion (because of vomiting), electrolyte imbalance, dehydration, cardiac arrythmias, and occasionally, sudden death. DSM-III-R criteria for diagnosis include recurring episodes of binge eating, a lack of control over binge behavior, regular self-induced vomiting, two binge episodes per week for at least 3 months, and persistent overconcern with body shape and image.

Behaviors associated with eating disorders frequently continue undiscovered for long periods of time. Denial of these disorders is common. Even on an inpatient unit the behaviors associated with these disorders may be hidden or disguised. Adolescents frequently hide their malnourished bodies by wearing oversized or layered clothing. Close observation should be given to the type and amount of food ordered and consumed. Persons with anorexia are particularly aware of the caloric value of food. Adolescents with anorexia and bulimia may be very clever in disguising their vomiting behavior, particularly if they feel they are being observed. Anorexic adolescents frequently resort to excessive exercise to lose weight.

In anorexia and bulimia, control may be a common issue. The family that tends to be controlling can become dominated by the conflict with the anorexic teenager

(Miller, 1980). Control of body image and even denial of body maturation by controlling the menses can occur. By vomiting and purging, the person with bulimia can regulate weight and reverse the perceived lack of control over binging.

Interventions. These long-term problems can be successfully treated. Behavioral techniques, psychological counseling, family therapy, and medication to relieve underlying symptoms are commonly used. This adolescent requires patience and close observation during treatment.

ADOLESCENT CHEMICAL DEPENDENCY

Chemical dependency (alcohol and other psychoactive drug dependencies) (see box on p. 107) is a disorder characterized by a compulsion to use a chemical or chemicals in spite of serious physical and social consequences of the use. The disorder is progressive and can lead to serious health problems and death. A chemically dependent person experiences an increasing tolerance for the drug(s), blackouts, and withdrawal symptoms if the drug is unavailable. A psychosocial and spiritual deterioration occurs as the disease progresses. The psychological defense mechanisms of denial, projection, and rationalization make the disease difficult to identify and treat. Adult chemical dependency develops over a number of years, but in adolescents the course is very rapid, probably because of physical immaturity.

About 73% of high school students drink. Approximately 30% of adolescents drink to drunkeness more than four times per year (Rachal and others, 1975, 1980, 1982; Zucker, 1986); 22% of adolescents drink to drunkenness once per week or more; 7% once per month; 7.8% two to four times per month (Zucker, 1986). A survey of south suburban high schools in the Dayton, Ohio, area showed that almost 70% of secondary students drank once per week.

Adolescent chemical dependency is caused by genetic and psychosocial factors. Current research into the biological basis of alcoholism demonstrates several trait markers that indicate a predisposition to alcoholism. A study of sons of alcohol abusers showed decreased intensity of reaction to alcohol; two types of brain wave changes; and the presence of biochemical markers: an enzyme and several blood antigens (Schukit, 1987). In children of alcohol abusers the disease is three times more likely to develop than it is in the children of nonalcoholic parents.

The overwhelming socially significant factor in teenage drinking is peer pressure and the expectation among parents that teenage drinking is developmentally normal. Studies have shown that there are a number of predictors of problem drinking (see box on p. 108).

The psychosocial characteristics of adolescents who have been in a chemical dependency treatment program (National Institute on Alcohol Abuse and Alcoholism, 1986) include the following:

1. Family relationships characterized by stress, physical and psychological abuse, or indifference
2. Social alienation, isolation from peers, and lack of adequate stable relationships
3. Deficiencies in the social competencies necessary for building and maintaining peer relationships and for dealing effectively with emotions
4. Uncertainty of values, goals, and priorities; difficulty in making sound decisions

---

Medical and Nursing Diagnoses Related to Adolescent Chemical Dependency

Medical diagnoses (DSM-III-R)

Alcohol
303.90   Dependence
305.00   Abuse
Amphetamine or similarly acting sympathomimetic agent
304.40   Dependence
305.70   Abuse
Cannabis
304.30   Dependence
305.20   Abuse
Cocaine
304.20   Dependence
305.60   Abuse
Hallucinogen
304.50   Dependence
305.30   Abuse
Inhalant
304.60   Dependence
305.90   Abuse
Nicotine
305.10   Dependence
Opioid
304.00   Dependence
305.50   Abuse
Phencyclidine (PCP) or similarly acting arylcyclohexylamine
304.50   Dependence
305.90   Abuse
Sedative, hypnotic, or anxiolytic
304.10   Dependence
305.40   Abuse
304.90   Polysubstance dependence
304.90   Psychoactive substance dependence not otherwise specified
305.90   Psychoactive substance abuse not otherwise specified

Nursing diagnoses (PMH)

5.3.2   Altered conduct/impulse processes
     5.3.2.9   Substance abuse
5.5.3   Ineffective individual coping
     5.5.3.2   Ineffective denial

---

5. Low self-esteem and self-awareness and an unstable identity
6. Lack of self-control
7. Undue peer influence

In addition to these problems, affected adolescents experience a dependence and craving for alcohol and other drugs and the physical side effects of the drugs. To

---

Characteristics That Predict Problem Drinking Among Youth

Influenced greatly by friends
Parents who drink
Greater approval, more models, and increased pressure to drink by peers and parents
Parents who are not involved
Accessibility to alcohol
Lacking parental affection
Feelings of being isolated
Unstable relationships
Inadequate social skills
Transient and undefined values
Difficulty making decisions
Exaggerated desire for independence
Lacking self-control
Tolerant of deviance
Attaching little importance to religion
Focus on positive aspects of drinking
Low value on academic achievement
High value on self-determination and autonomy from parents
Positive family history of alcoholism

Modified from National Institute on Alcohol Abuse and Alcoholism (1986). In Felstad C, editor, Youth alcohol and abuse, Phoenix, Oryx Press.

---

obtain larger amounts of the illegal substances to satisfy their increasing tolerances, teenagers often resort to criminal behaviors, beginning with stealing money and objects from home.

Because the adolescent hides and denies the use, the family has difficulty determining what the problem is and often seeks inappropriate treatment. In addition, the chemically dependent adolescent often has other diagnoses, especially depression and attention deficit disorder. Families often struggle with this problem for 2 to 2½ years before seeking help.

Interventions. Interventions for chemically dependent adolescents include education regarding the illness, help in recognizing the symptoms in their own life, and making plans for lifelong abstinence from chemicals through the 12-step program of Alcoholics Anonymous/Narcotics Anonymous. The family must undergo the same educational process. Unfortunately many chemically dependent adolescents live in families with parents or siblings who are active users. Conditions that coexist with the dependency must be treated concurrently. All the aforementioned treatment therapies must be adapted to the developmental level of the adolescent.

CODEPENDENCE

Codependence is a term created by alcoholism counselors that was developed by clinicians working with the adult children of alcoholics to describe a set of behaviors that develop in those who live with addicted persons. Codependence is present in young children, as well as in adult children of addicts and has been found to continue in the child or adult child when the parent addict is cured. Codependent behaviors are comparable to older diagnoses and behaviors described by the psychiatric and mental health disciplines. Depression, borderline posttraumatic stress syndrome (Cermak, 1986), and some personality disorders exhibit characteristics of codependence. Codependence includes the following patterns: intense, clinging relationships that have an addictive quality; shaping thoughts, behaviors, and feelings on the basis of perceived expectations of others; excessive caretaking; stress-related physical illnesses; self-centeredness ("I cause and can fix everything"); serious problems with attempts to control people and situations; lack of self-awareness; dishonest (white lies) communication; fears; being judgmental; and problems with intimacy (Shaef, 1986; Cermak, 1986). Adolescents who have grown up in alcoholic families also have been abused psychologically and often physically.

Interventions. Interventions for codependence are directed toward encouraging the adolescent or parent to accept appropriate roles relative to another person's dysfunction, focusing on the individual's issues as opposed to others', education about chemical dependency, counseling related to guilt feelings and resentment toward others, and referral to support groups for codependent persons, such as Al-Anon or Alateen.

Posttraumatic Stress Disorder

The diagnosis of posttraumatic stress disorder (PTSD) first appeared in the 1980 edition of DSM-III. It was developed in response to the need for an official DSM diagnosis that described the clinical symptoms of Vietnam veterans who had been traumatized during their military service. Posttraumatic stress is defined as a group of maladaptive responses to an overwhelming event lasting at least 6 months; it may continue for up to 25-30 years after the trauma (American Psychiatric Association, 1987).

Until recently, limited information was available on traumatic stress in children and adolescents. The current proliferation of literature on this disorder in children and adolescents marks the growing recognition that a discrete event can have a severe and lasting effect on the developing child. The widely publicized primary intervention programs for children who have survived disasters, such as the program provided after the kidnaping at Buffalo Creek and the loss of teacher Christa McAuliffe on the space shuttle (Lyons, 1987) emphasize that PTSD has become a diagnostic entity in this age-group.

Current statistics verify the occurrence of an astonishing incidence of trauma, including physical and sexual abuse, during the childhood and adolescence of both psychiatric patients and the general population and that traumatic experiences during childhood and adolescence constitute a major public health problem (Chu and Dill, 1990).

The damaging effects of trauma through abuse on the growth and development of youth has been well documented and strongly associated with many later adult psychiatric difficulties, including depression, anxiety, affective, eating, and personality disorders, identity disturbances, social isolation, self-destructive, codependence behaviors, and substance abuse (Chu and Dill, 1990). The prevalence of traumatic events has prompted prudent clinicians to include a history of traumatic events in their diagnostic interviews with all children and adolescents, regardless of the "chief complaint" and presenting problems.

DEFINITIONS AND CONCEPTS

Assessment of symptoms of PTSD is based on an interaction model in which both an extreme situation and a symptom-laden response to the situation are necessary for a person to be considered "traumatized" (see boxes). Four main categories comprise the diagnostic criteria for PTSD: (1) exposure to or direct involvement in a traumatic event, (2) persistent reexperiencing of a traumatic event in a variety of ways, (3) persistent attempts to avoid stimuli associated with the trauma, and (4) persistent symptoms of increased physiological arousal (hyperarousal) that were not present before the trauma (American Psychiatric Association, 1987). The two major symptoms that distinguish PTSD from other DSM disorders are (1) exposure to an event that could be traumatic and (2) intrusive reexperiencing of the trauma. Other DSM-III-R criteria include numbing of responsiveness to or reduced involvement with the external world and at least two of the following symptoms: hyperalertness/startle, sleep disturbance, survivor guilt, impaired memory and concentration, behavioral avoidance of trauma-related cues, and intensification of a traumatic event. The DSM-III-R (1987) added a new symptom, "sense of shortened future," based on work with children involved in the Chowchilla bus kidnaping (Terr, 1983).

Reexperiencing is the hallmark and core symptom of PTSD. Repeated and intrusive reexperiencing of the traumatic event occurs through nightmares and through recurrent and unbidden waking recall and flashback experiences, during which the person actually acts or feels as if the event is recurring. The reexperiencing usually recreates the traumatic event with little symbolic transformation; it contrasts starkly with nightmares and other altered states of consciousness in which there are symbolic distortions such as snakes and monsters. The realism of intrusive reexperiencing accounts for the internal, self-perpetuating imagery that cast the traumatic event in an ever-present context that can be continually disturbing and self-reinforcing.

Events that children and adolescents witness as bystanders, which threaten their personal safety, also can result in PTSD. The traumatic situation can be a near-miss experience, one in which the youth identifies with persons who did suffer loss or injury, such as witnessing, indirectly experiencing, or having intimate knowledge of parental, sibling, or peer abuse or suicide. A classic example of a near-miss case described in the literature (Terr, 1983) reports the treatment of a boy who had gotten off a school bus just before the others on the bus were kidnaped; 4 years after the event the boy continued to present posttraumatic stress symptoms.

PTSD also develops as a result of traumatic events caused by actions of the persons themselves. These acts are in conflict with their value system, such as soldiers committing combat atrocities or accidentally harming civilians. One case study, which describes the treatment of a 13-year-old boy who accidentally shot and killed another child with a gun when he was 6 years old (Hoffman and Kuperman, 1990), illustrates that traumatic events occurring during early childhood often resurge in adolescence.

Posttraumatic Stress Disorder

A. The person has experienced an event that is outside the range of usual human experience and that would be markedly distressing to almost anyone, e.g., serious threat to one's life or physical integrity; serious threat or harm to one's children, spouse, or other close relatives and friends; sudden destruction of one's home or community; or seeing another person who has recently been, or is being, seriously injured or killed as the result of an accident or physical violence.

B. The traumatic event is persistently reexperienced in at least one of the following ways:
   (1) recurrent and intrusive distressing recollections of the event (in young children, repetitive play in which themes or aspects of the trauma are expressed)
   (2) recurrent distressing dreams of the event
   (3) sudden acting or feeling as if the traumatic event were recurring (includes a sense of reliving the experience, illusions, hallucination, and dissociative [flashback] episodes, even those that occur upon awakening or when intoxicated)
   (4) intense psychological distress at exposure to events that symbolize or resemble an aspect of the traumatic event, including anniversaries of the trauma

C. Persistent avoidance of stimuli associated with the trauma or numbing of general responsiveness (not present before the trauma), as indicated by at least three of the following:
   (1) efforts to avoid thoughts or feelings associated with the trauma
   (2) efforts to avoid activities or situations that arouse recollections of the trauma
   (3) inability to recall an important aspect of the trauma (psychogenic amnesia)
   (4) markedly diminished interest in significant activities (in young children, loss of recently acquired developmental skills such as toilet training or language skills)
   (5) feeling of detachment or estrangement from others
   (6) restricted range of affect, e.g., unable to have loving feelings
   (7) sense of a foreshortened future, e.g., does not expect to have a career, marriage, or children, or a long life

D. Persistent symptoms of increased arousal (not present before the trauma), as indicated by at least two of the following:
   (1) difficulty falling or staying asleep
   (2) irritability or outbursts of anger
   (3) difficulty concentrating
   (4) hypervigilance
   (5) exaggerated startle response
   (6) physiologic reactivity upon exposure to events that symbolize or resemble an aspect of the traumatic event (e.g., a woman who was raped in an elevator breaks out in a sweat when entering any elevator)

E. Duration of the disturbance (symptoms in B, C, and D) of at least one month. Specify delayed onset if the onset of symptoms was at least six months after the trauma.

From American Psychiatric Association (1987) Diagnostic and statistical manual of mental disorders III-R, Washington, DC, The Association.

Medical and Nursing Diagnoses for Posttraumatic Stress Disorder

Medical diagnoses (DSM-III-R)

309.89   Posttraumatic Stress Disorder

Nursing diagnoses (PMH)

5.1.2.   Altered abuse response
5.1.2.1.   Post trauma response
5.1.2.2   Rape trauma response
1.4.2.4   Nightmares/terrors
2.5.2.1   Amnesia
2.6.2.11   Thought insertion (?)
2.6.99   Thought processes NOS: flashbacks
4.1.2.1   Anger
4.1.2.2   Anxiety
4.1.2.5   Fear
4.1.2.7   Guilt
4.1.2.9   Shame
5.5.3.1   Defensive coping: dissociation

Contagion or secondary traumatizing frequently occurs in young persons, and it is often necessary, in the diagnostic process, to explore who actually had the experience. Case studies of contagion reported in the literature emphasize that the young clients did not claim to be victims; however, their behavioral symptoms supported the diagnoses of PTSD. A case study that provides an excellent example of contagion (Rosenheck and Nathan, 1985) describes the treatment of a boy whose father suffered PTSD as a result of Vietnam combat. The boy, who witnessed his father's flashbacks and nightmares, exhibited symptoms of PTSD, such as a preoccupation with war games and death fantasies. For diagnostic clarity and case finding, clinicians need be alert to the possibility of contagion. When contagion occurs in young clients, their peers, siblings, and other associates, such as classmates, need evaluation. Assailants frequently abuse more than one child, and the child's social network may be at risk (Lyons, 1987).

Gender differences in the prevalence of PTSD indicate that boys show stronger responses to potential traumatic events. Boys have higher anxiety scores in predisaster and postdisaster studies and also exhibit more codependency symptoms of trauma as a result of witnessing parents being beaten by partners than do girls (Chu and Dill, 1990).

DEVELOPMENTAL AGE AND STAGE DISTINCTIONS

A major problem in developing knowledge of child and adolescent PTSD is the lack of agreement among clinicians and researchers as to what constitutes a traumatic event and at what age and stage of childhood and adolescence it occurs. The DSM-III (American Psychiatric Association, 1980) stated that to qualify as a traumatic event, the identified stressor must be "outside the range of such common experiences as simple bereavement and chronic illness." Although experts in the area of child and adolescent PTSD have further defined that the traumatic experience generally is surprising, unanticipated, and piercingly intense and that it must be real, not imagined (Terr, 1981, 1985), the term "traumatized" is used to describe any pathological response to an extreme event. This vague definition is due, in part, to the fact that PTSD has been available as a diagnostic category only since 1980 and that the criteria delineated for adults apply to children and adolescents (Fairbank and Nickelson, 1987).

A second obstacle to understanding traumatic disorders in children and adolescents is that most professional health care workers and adults in general have been extremely slow in accepting the idea that traumatic events are even experienced by children and adolescents. Researchers became aware of this professional denial during the development of life stress scales for children and adolescents in the 1960s. Parents, teachers, and mental health professionals were asked to identify, rank, and assign weights of importance of life stressors they perceived children and adolescents to experience. Remarkable discrepancies were found between the traumatic events identified as stressful by adults and by children. These differences have been found repeatedly (Lyons, 1987), which suggests that adults are unaware of, deny, or ignore the presence and impact of traumatic experiences in childhood and adolescence (Offer and others, 1981).

Many adults believe that children and adolescents do not experience events as traumatic because understanding trauma-inducing situations requires high levels of cognitive mediation and processing skills that young children lack. However, even though young children have not developed the capacity to assimilate, accommodate, and interpret concretely, there is evidence that even newborn infants experience and respond to trauma. Because emotions are present at birth when emotional responses occur before language development, infants and small children experience trauma in intensified distortions since their cognitive processes are immature and often inaccurate (Piaget, 1972).

The person's developmental stage at the time of trauma is critical information for assessment because it identifies important links between the level of social development and the symptoms of PTSD. However, no human is immune to the effects of traumatic events, and some posttraumatic stress symptoms have been found to be independent of age. For example, all clinical studies indicate that after a traumatic event, adjustments and changes in the person's trust and autonomy occur regardless of age. In infants and small children, because trust and autonomy are in the process of being developed, these qualities are less consolidated developmentally. Considerable research data suggest that dissociative experiences characteristically seen in adult PTSD are linked to early childhood traumas. Clearly, such trauma is worse if it results from actions of family members. Abuse by a family member compromises the young person's most intimate social environment, resulting in difficulties in the establishment of basic trust. Trauma at this time has profound outcomes for the child's developing personality (Swartz, 1985).

Adult denial of childhood trauma has been attributed to the unconscious guilt many adults experience for not shielding or buffering youngsters from the traumatic experiences. A clinical study of staff nurses working in an inpatient child and adolescent psychiatric unit when John Kennedy was assassinated (Harrison and others, 1967) illustrates a lack of staff awareness of the patients' response to this event. When interviewed, nursing staff members reported that the patients were unaffected by the assassination; direct observations of the patients' behaviors, however, revealed remarkable behavioral changes in response to the event, including increased behavioral disruptions, changes in sleep patterns, increased incidents of nightmares, night terrors, hyperviligance, hyperactivity, and an increase in somatic complaints. Staff denial of these changes was attributed to the nurses' preoccupation with their own shock and grief responses and their unconscious conflicts over their inability to protect or buffer the patients from knowledge of and effects of this traumatic event.

It is not unusual for children in the latency stage and for adolescents to discuss a previous traumatic childhood experience that their parents deny or of which they were unaware before the family interview during the assessment session. In some cases this lack of information occurs because small children seldom discuss traumatic experiences and the parents may, indeed, be unaware or deny events, which often occurs in cases of child molestation. Parents also may negate the importance of the event, reacting defensively to the introduction of new information about their child of which they had no former knowledge. Many parents carry the out-dated notion that children do not remember, cannot feel, and/or their emotions are transient and their memories inaccurate (Kemp and Kemp, 1984).

When adolescents and older children report a traumatic experience during an assessment interview that their parents deny, the nurse needs to defer exploration of the event until the individual interview with the child. At that time, the adolescent's report of the traumatic event and changes in their behaviors can be reviewed. For example, during the family assessment session, an adolescent vividly described an attack by a vicious dog that occurred while he was walking to school with a friend when he was in the first grade. He attributed his earlier problems, his school phobia, enuresis, nightmares, sleep walking, and eating and learning problems to this traumatic experience. His parents denied the event and attributed his "story" to his "wild imagination." The mother reported that during his first year of school, he had a fight with an older "bully" on the way home from school; she described his crying, cuts, and bruises, and his disheveled, torn clothes. She rejected the dog attack incident and claimed it was a story the boy fabricated at the time to avoid punishment for fighting. She did, however, acknowledge that the symptoms the boy reported concerning his early childhood years were true. The nurse was able to draw on her knowledge of the developmental changes in the signs and symptoms during earlier childhood years and confirmed the boy's story by reviewing the pediatrician's record.

A third reason for the lack of recognition of PTSD in children and adolescents is that this age-group does not respond to trauma or reexperience trauma in the same manner as do adults, although the same criteria are used. Adults with PTSD reexperience the distressing aspects of traumatic life events in a number of ways (Wilson, 1985):

1. Intrusive or unbidden imagery present during the day or night
2. Affective (emotional) flooding either with or without trauma-associated intrusive imagery

3. Flashback or dissociative episodes in which the trauma is directly, partially or symbolically relived or reenacted in behavior
4. Hallucinations that contain trauma-related cognitive material or affect
5. Anniversary reactions, which can be conscious or unconscious
6. Intensification of various syndrome symptoms by exposure to events that in some way resemble the traumatic event
7. Unconscious behavioral reenactments that have a parallel psychological structure to the behavior during the trauma

The intrusion of imagery has been attributed to external cues related to the traumatic event in the environment. Although they are consciously unaware of these trigger factors, victims respond automatically to these trigger factors. Denial is used as a defensive measure against painful feelings caused by perceptions of reality. By the use of denial or refusal to accept the reality of certain experiences, the person isolates the traumatic experience or experiences and thus is protected from reexperiencing the feelings, reactions, anxieties, and memories of the trauma.

As a defense mechanism, denial rarely is absolute in its effectiveness to negate external traumatic events and to ward off psychological responses in small children, whose defensive apparatus is immature. Traumatic incidents often are vividly recreated in children's dramatic play, "as if" the themes emerged from the experience of others. Children vividly recall traumatic experiences through symbolism in dreams, which fail to disguise the trauma. Frequently phobias develop in small children concerning environmental cues or stimuli perceived during trauma, of which the child may have been unaware at the time (Krener, 1985). For example, a child physically abused may not recognize the abuser when he or she sees them, just as adults often fail to recognize and remember the names of other adults who have embarrassed them or caused them trauma.

The flashbacks characteristically seen in adults usually do not occur in younger adolescents; however, cognitive perceptual distortions regarding the event, such as the sequencing of events, and the belief that unheeded omens warned of the coming traumatic event are common in children (magical thinking).

Many children and adolescents report dreams in which they experience their own death, a phenomenon seldom seen in adult PTSD. It is common for traumatized children and adolescents to have a limited view of themselves in the future, and often they are unable to make plans for their lives. Although there are inconsistent reports as to the effects of posttraumatic stress on academic performance, deterioration in job performance commonly is seen in adult clients.

Small children exhibit sleep disorders, irritability, diarrhea, and separation anxiety. Elementary school–aged children show more adult behaviors associated with PTSD. Somatization occurs less frequently as children grow older, and these symptoms seldom are seen in the school-aged child.

Denial mechanisms provide older adolescents and adults powerful defenses against the reexperiencing of trauma, and adolescents often use reaction formation or partial denial of the anxiety aroused by the traumatic experience (Saigh, 1987). Adolescents traumatized by sexual or physical abuse, for example, exhibit tendencies to recreate the traumatic experience, manifesting seductive mannerisms when they are with adults whose behaviors are similar to the behaviors their abusers exhibited toward them; some are frankly promiscuous.

The dissociative symptoms that characterize PTSD provide defenses used to escape the overwhelming pain of the traumatic experience (Chu and Dill, 1990). Painful psychological and physical experiences are made less intense through dissociation and alterations in perceptions. These unconscious dissociative defenses include the mechanisms of depersonalization and derealization, which make it possible for the person who experienced the traumatic event to forget it (psychogenic amnesia) or to completely disown the experience, as if it were someone else's experience. Defensive dissociation is also characteristic of multiple personality disorders, which have been strongly related to early childhood physical, sexual, and emotional abuse.

Dissociative symptoms of PTSD can be misinterpreted as psychotic behaviors. The auditory hallucinations of adolescents with multiple personality disorders, for example, may be due to the fact that split-off personalities are attempting to speak to other personalities. Some experts link the posttraumatic stress symptoms of dissociation with dissociative multiple personalities disorders (Potham, 1989; Lowenstein and others, 1988).

According to Freudian theory, when dissociation is used, the repressed and dissociated experiences do not remain dormant but are reexperienced in dreams, nightmares, flashbacks, and the flooding of feelings and sensations related to the initial experience. The traumatic effects of childhood sexual abuse are seen in self-destructive behaviors these victims of abuse act out as coping mechanisms against the sequel of psychic pain and unconscious self-blame the sexual trauma causes (Shapiro, 1987). Acting out in the context of trauma is defined as a direct expression of an unconscious wish or impulse to avoid being conscious of the affect that accompanies the trauma. Thus it provides a pathological outlet for avoidance of underlying affects and tensions resulting from trauma (Vaillant, 1978).

Often sexual experiences, such as incest, are not acknowledged or viewed as traumatic by parents or caretakers until adolescent acting out behavior leads to therapeutic intervention. Young children often are able to successfully deny or encapsulate their traumatic pain, or they act out in hyperactivity, conduct, and learning disorders; these problems often are ignored or viewed as part of growing up that the child will grow out of. Thus PTSD seldom is identified during early childhood, but as the child becomes an adolescent, the earlier defense mechanisms are retained, which results in unsuccessful negotiation of puberty and subsequent adolescent psychosocial roles and behavioral expectations. Usually, during adolescence—often years after the traumatic childhood experience occurred—the victim enters treatment, usually for apparently unrelated reasons. At that time the story of the trauma, such as sexual abuse, and reactions to it unfold. Only after the history is disclosed in the context of treatment can clinicians relate the presenting symptoms and psychopathology to the traumatic sexual-abuse experience (Orzek, 1985).

In contrast to the younger child, more defense mechanisms to deny trauma are available to the adolescent's psychic structure. For example, splitting is a defense mechanism used by adolescents and adults. Although available from infancy, it seldom is demonstrated by younger children. Splitting is a predominant mechanism during adolescence, best known for its role in borderline personality disorder (Kernberg, 1985). Splitting, which is particularly detrimental to adolescent psychosocial development, contributes to the development of a true-self/false-self dichotomy. In posttraumatic disorders, splitting provides the adolescent a means of creating a separation, distance, or dissociation from unwanted memories, affects, or anxieties. It serves the victim in warding off an inner sense of "badness" and a profound sense of shame. Thus negative self-experience is "split off," which results in a self-representation filled with the bravado of narcissism and apparent complete self-control (false self) that the adolescent presents publicly. Splitting allows psychological distancing from trauma; it often functions so efficiently that in many sexually traumatized adolescents it results in promiscuity, prostitution, and other forms of sexual acting out (Shapiro and Dominiak, 1990). The powerful, unconscious splitting mechanism also explains why many traumatized adolescents are described as extremely compliant (false self) while internally feeling helpless rage (true self).

Adolescents with PTSD and borderline personality disorders are noted for their impaired identity formation. According to Erikson's theory (1963), the defense mechanism of splitting, which may be in place earlier to protect the younger child from feeling trauma, causes disruptions in mastery of the adolescent's developmental tasks of establishing identity.

Another crucial adolescent task is the development of intimacy. The traumatic ending of an adolescent's first intimacy experience is another example of an experience parents often ignore, negate, or view as inconsequential "puppy love" (Jacobsen and others, 1986). Conflicts that center on early romantic experiences have been identified as one of the major reasons for adolescent suicide. This illustration of the adolescent's tendency to act out in response to traumatic events should be an ever-present concern of supportive adults (Shapiro, 1987).

Trauma during the critical adolescent developmental stage results in remarkable changes in behavior, for example, becoming overly compliant and withdrawn or aggressive, abusing substances, and acting out sexually (Newman, 1981). Guilt is more pronounced among adolescents, who tend to be highly secretive about the trauma and their symptoms. Adolescents often attribute posttraumatic stress flashbacks to their self-medication with street drugs to alleviate psychic pain. Drug-related flashbacks can be terrifying and can also cause posttraumatic stress responses. Careful history taking is critical to identify the cause of the flashbacks; substance abuse and PTSD often coexist (Friedman, 1985; Rey and others, 1990).

In contrast to adults with PTSD, children and adolescents seldom show psychogenic amnesia, nor do they have the same degree of numbing. Denial and splitting, which support defensive displacement behaviors, are more common in youths. Displacement allows the individual to be temporarily distracted by focusing attention on some seemingly distant matter of importance unrelated to core conflicts. Distortions help create false perceptions of self and others, and interpersonal events and interactions are experienced in ways that serve the individual's defensive needs. Reality is distorted, which is seen in adolescent idealization of peers or parents, or in the devaluations of others and exaggerated self-blaming and self-depreciation.

In addition to understanding psychosocial developmental differences in the symptoms that character PTSD in adolescents, the distinctions between PTSD and similar adolescent psychiatric mental disorders are important, including distinctions from adjustment disorders, major depression, closed head injuries, and spinal cord lesions (Lyons, 1985).

Nurses need to be alert to behaviors that indicate traumatic stress symptoms that may not have been present on the adolescent's admission. Nurses who work in general hospital settings with adolescents with closed head injuries, with injuries resulting from physical and sexual abuse, or with serious life-threatening diseases such as cancer (Koocher, 1985; Nir, 1985) need be attentive to the possibility that these conditions may reactivate dormant traumatic experiences.

The negative aftermath of traumatic experiences correlates directly with the establishment of maladaptive defense mechanisms discussed in this section. As higher levels of defenses become more pronounced as the child grows older, it is important that nurses assess the psychological defenses on which adolescents rely. Because parents and mental health clinicians have special difficulties in observing and interpreting the dissociative symptoms that characterize PTSD, these symptoms often are overlooked. It is recommended that simple evaluation questions about depersonalization, derealization, psychogenic amnesia (lost time), flashbacks, and switches in ego states be included in all adolescent assessment protocols. Multimethod evaluations should include both the parent's version and the youth's report of event, as well as the parent's and adolescent's recall of the youngster's behaviors before and after the experience. At this time there are no standardized interview schedules or psychometric tests that specifically assess PTSD. In light of the high incidence of child physical and sexual abuse, some experts suggest the use of various gauges of stress and life change, as well as the Dissociate Experience Scale (Ross and others, 1988), in assessment for additional confirmation of PTSD diagnosis. Fortunately, psychological defenses, either primitive or neurotic, once diagnosed, are extremely responsive to treatment.

INTERVENTIONS

Interventions include behavioral deconditioning, hypnosis, play and games therapies, psychodynamic psychotherapy, group therapy, family therapy, parental counseling, and pharmacological techniques.

The client's acknowledgment of the traumatic experience is emphasized as the most important goal in almost all treatment techniques. Some clinicians claim that for improvement to occur, the traumatic events must be reexperienced and abreacted, whereas others believe that acknowledgment of the trauma often is sufficient. In most instances the client's recognition of the traumatic experience profoundly shifts the attitudes of both the adolescent and the professionals providing the care.

For effective treatment of PTSD, there is a need to establish the cognitive and affective connections so that the original trauma is worked through. For traumas in which abuse has occurred, residual guilt and shame need to be resolved. When controlled reexposure to traumatic cues is the treatment of choice, the individual therapists, nursing staff members, and parents and teachers must be prepared for the considerable turmoil adolescents undergo as they work through the traumatic memories. During the initial phase of working through, increases or intensifying of symptoms often occurs, a response that should be expected; in inpatient settings, the nursing staff needs to be alerted to this possibility. This intensification does not indicate a negative response to the treatment but a sign that an increased range of traumatic cues are being reexperienced. Some experts hold that reexposure to all facets of the traumatic memory is required for extinction of the traumatic response (Wilson, 1985; Rosenbeck, 1985; Saigh, 1987). However, when the psychogenic pain, which has been encapsulated and held in check by defense mechanisms, is released, it may cause the person to retreat to an acute regressive state. Regression can occur during psychotherapy, and these treatment interventions should be undertaken only by skilled, experienced therapists.

The best predictor for positive outcomes for traumatized adolescents is the ability of significant adults, including parents, teachers, and nurses, to assist them in dealing with the traumatic event. Teaching parents and teachers to address traumatic events honestly and openly with the young person is an important treatment goal that can be achieved by role modeling in family meetings and through direct instruction.

Self-blame is a coping strategy many trauma victims use to minimize their sense of helplessness and to restore feelings of control. Because guilt often is a major symptom of PTSD in adolescents, an effective strategy is to shift the adolescent's self-blaming global comments, such as "I'm a terrible person," to comments such as "I should not have hitched a ride and gotten in a car with a stranger." It also is therapeutic to emphasize that the youngster may not have had sufficient life experiences at the time of the traumatic incident to know how to handle it (Shapiro and Dominiak, 1990).

Teaching ways to deal with possible future stressors and to understand that different choices can be made if the traumatic event were to recur has been found therapeutically valuable. The adolescent's sense of self-efficacy can be promoted by providing knowledge of and fostering active coping strategies to help deal with intrusive reexperiencing. These include teaching adolescents to anticipate anniversary reactions and increases in symptoms in response to other reminders of traumatic events. Relaxation training also is an effective treatment and provides them a sense of self-control (Figley, 1985).

Groups of youngsters who experience traumatic events appear to be able to provide one another peer support. However, there is little information in the literature on the use of group therapy in adolescent PTSD intervention.

In contrast, there are many articles and texts available on interventions with traumatized families. On the basis of the premise that traumatic events involve the family, not just the young person, Figley (1989) has developed a conceptual framework for interventions that has an important preventive component. Detailed descriptions of cases, assessment tools, and an intervention framework for a "healing theory" include many of the usual family therapeutic techniques, such as reframing, improving communication skills, sharing perceptions and feelings, and empowering the family to develop a "health theory." Families likely to have difficulties dealing with trauma can be assessed in advance. These families are characterized by denial or misperceptions of stressors who use blame-oriented problem solving, low family cohesion, and have rigid family roles.

Family Disorders

In the recent past there was a common belief among family therapists that families caused the problems of the adolescent. Today, because of societal conditions, it is very easy to blame the family or society for the teenager's problems. Recent research, however, points to the existence of genetic predisposition toward certain disorders, as well as the occurrence of neurochemical and other biological changes in an individual with a psychiatric illness or diagnosis. The important thing to keep in mind when studying a family is how this family functions in the nine categories proposed by Beavers and others (noted in Chapter 3) and how the functioning differs from that of less troubled families. Systems theory, communication theory, and biological theories are relevant to the study and treatment of the family.

Family health may be viewed on a continuum from optimal to troubled (Table 5-3). In this chapter the midrange and troubled family is discussed. (Optimal and adequate families are discussed in Chapter 3.)

MIDRANGE FAMILIES

Midrange families include persons with mental health problems. The "identified patient" in the family is likely to be neurotic or behaviorally disordered, depending on the family style. Family members also may have physical illnesses. Although family members are reasonably effective, they are restricted. An *open system orientation* is absent in these families; family members need others only under certain conditions. The family tends to believe that there are causes for events, but members are not sure what they are. They continuously strive to find answers and to do well.

Boundaries remain fairly clear in these families, although when under pressure, the family will solidify its boundaries and turn inward (that is, keep the trouble inside), or the family may lose its boundaries and the problems may spill into the environment. Interaction among family members (intrasystem interaction) is restricted.

Links to society are present, but they are disrupted when the family is under unusual pressure. Families that tend to externalize trouble (that is, push it into the environment) usually become involved with law-enforcement agencies.

Midrange families also have difficulty with *contextual clarity.* Oedipal issues are not resolved because expressions of sexuality are stereotyped and stifled. The parental coalition is present but weak, and other coalitions develop that undermine the effectiveness of the parents. *Communication* in these families generally is clear but expressed with fear, guilt, or anger.

Power is the central problem in midrange families. The family confuses love and power. Love is a feeling that moves one person to care about the life and growth of another. Midrange families often believe that caring is *controlling* the life of another, and by means of overt or covert coercion, they apply a system of "oughts" and "shoulds." The "shoulds" are often sex-stereotyped. The parents believe in doing the "right" thing and are constantly struggling for control of the children through discipline, money, and other means. Children become powerful by manipulating the parents, not by learning to assume power and responsibility. Family roles are defined by sex or by other beliefs about the family member, such as "She's so good and never causes any trouble," or "He's the athletic one." The family behaves as if someone is judging their actions, thoughts, and feelings in terms of their goodness or badness.

Encouragement of autonomy is not found in midrange families; children are expected to adhere to the family's norms. The constant power struggles and repression of feelings and ideas within the family sap family members' creativity.

Table 5-3   Family Mental Health Continuum

Family	Characteristics of children
Troubled	Process schizophrenia
	Severe behavior disorder
	Borderline personality disorder
Midrange	Neuroses
	Behavior disorders
Adequate	No obvious pathology
Optimal	Unusual individual competence

Children tend to stay in the parental home well into adulthood or to leave home very early, in pursuit of a kind of pseudoautonomy.

The *affective issues* that characterize midrange families are depression, anxiety, and anger. The resultant conflicts may be overtly expressed in angry exchanges or repressed through submission to the oughts and shoulds. As a result, members display little empathy, have conflicts over rules and norms, feel considerable frustration, and express caring that is controlling rather than growth-producing. *Self-esteem* of the family members is low, and the identified patient has very low self-esteem.

Although the work of the family is accomplished, *negotiation and task performance* occur through coercion because the parental team cannot agree on responsibilities. Midrange families do not hold family meetings.

Transcendent values of hope and altruism are lacking in midrange families. Family members eventually accept change and loss but with a great deal of pain, anger, and frustration. They look toward the future as if to say, "What difficulty will present itself?" Martyrdom is not an unusual role for members of these families.

Health problems in midrange families include excessive use of alcohol, prescription tranquilizers, and other drugs for relief of the pain of daily living. The stressful existence of midrange families produces some psychophysiological illnesses such as headaches, ulcers, and obesity. Because the family is concerned with doing the "right" things, they meet their basic health needs. The family attempts recreation and exercise, but the conflict that surfaces during the planning of events reduces their pleasure. In some families the presence of a great deal of anger leads to dangerous activities, such as hitting, driving at excessive speeds, and running away. The midrange family is too preoccupied with daily events to explore health promotion and wellness activities.

TROUBLED FAMILIES*

Families that function on the more entropic end of the family health continuum tend to include members who exhibit antisocial or borderline personality disorders,

---

*Parts of this section are modified from Johnson BS, editor (1988) Psychiatric mental health: adaption and growth, Philadelphia, JB Lippincott Co.

psychotic disorders, and chemical dependencies. Troubled families display qualities that are the opposite of the optimal family's characteristics. The family tends to be highly rigid or disordered rather than open and flexible.

The *boundary* issues in troubled families are problematic. The family system boundary is rigid, with minimal social links that are tentative and mistrustful, and that generate limited outside input. Troubled families also may have diffuse boundaries, which means that family business tends to spill over into the environment. Interpersonal boundaries in these families also are diffuse, resulting in family members' global response to input. Distancing between people is prevalent.

Contextual clarity is blurred in troubled families. Because of a weak parental coalition, cross-generational clinging occurs and Oedipal issues remain unresolved. The parents deal with their personal pain by reaching across generational boundaries for comfort and control of the situation. Often this cross-generational clinging takes the form of a triangle, for example, the mother and son may form a coalition against the father. Often covert or overt incestuous behavior occurs. The child who is "triangled" usually is the symptom-bearer in the family. This child (or young adult) responds to these pressures with mental disorder, physical illness, or delinquent behavior (Johnson, 1988).

Communication in troubled families is not clear, congruent, specific, direct, or honest. Because persons in troubled families have low self-esteem, they fear rejection from others and are embarrassed about it. To cover up their fear of rejection, members of troubled families tend to use the four following patterns of communication described by Satir (1988):

1. Placating or doing anything to prevent others from getting angry
2. Blaming or attempting to look strong and reject others first
3. Computing or treating others as insignificant by using big words
4. Distracting or eliminating the possibility of rejection by changing the subject or talking in a "crazy way"

Another characteristic of communication in troubled families is incongruence between verbal and nonverbal communication, or the lack of congruence between the content of what is said and the feeling beneath it, for example, smiling when talking in an angry tone of voice. Double-bind communication occurs when an incongruent message is sent that includes a direction to do one thing, with a nonverbal message to do the opposite, and with the understanding that the receiver of the message is not permitted to comment on the messages. For example, a father says to his child, "Come here and let me hug you. You know Daddy loves you" (in an angry tone of voice). The child answers, "You sound mad." The father responds, "I don't know what you're talking about." The child is then faced with the dilemma of choosing how to respond. A child faced with continuous double-bind communication is unable to determine the true meaning of verbalizations and to identify and name normal feelings. As the ability to test reality becomes impaired, the child may invent a personal language and peculiar explanations for events. In some troubled families, anger is communicated through hitting and other forms of assault.

Another communication difficulty found in troubled families is *disqualifying*. Disqualifying occurs when an individual fails to attend to another's message by being silent, by ignoring the other, or by changing the subject. Evasiveness in communication also is common in these families.

Power, which is diffuse in the troubled family, does not flow from the parents. *Autonomy* is discouraged; in fact, the troubled family does not tolerate differentness. Paradoxically, the family tends to view one of its members as "different" and therefore the cause of its trouble; this process is called *scapegoating*.

The *affective tone* in troubled families with diffuse boundaries tends to be exaggerated. The members react inappropriately to threats or to one member's difficulties. In families with rigid boundaries the affective tone is restricted, depressed, despairing, and lacking in empathy; great distance exists between the members. Undue attention, which can be confusing, smothering, or rejecting, is paid to one member. *Self-esteem* in troubled families is low, and hate, inability to respond empathically, loneliness, and hopelessness predominate. Negotiation is not accomplished, and performance of tasks varies widely. Conflict may be a constant, overt, and unresolved presence in families with diffuse boundaries; in families with rigid boundaries it may be denied, not commented on, and left unresolved. *Transcendent values* are absent. The inability of troubled families to tolerate loss or differences leads to a cynical, hopeless outlook rather than to an altruistic, hopeful one. The stresses of unhappy family life often produce serious physical illness, usually in one member.

CHEMICAL DEPENDENCY AND THE FAMILY

The high incidence of alcoholism and other chemical addictions and their effects on families require a separate discussion. For example, there is a separate body of literature that addresses alcohol abuse in families. This focus is a result of the development of treatment for chemical dependency that is outside the traditional psychiatric or mental health treatment approaches and literature dealing with them. The failure of traditional psychiatric therapy to help alcohol abusers and their families led to this separation. Although the breach is narrowing, addiction treatment is based primarily on clinical experience and the principles of Alcoholics Anonymous (AA), with a clinical jargon of its own. It is very important that nurses thoroughly understand the AA and Al-Anon programs and the disease model of alcohol abuse if they expect to gain the trust of and intervene in families with this very difficult problem. Wegscheider (1981) explains the dysfunction by describing the roles family members take in an alcoholic family system (Table 5-4).

The Troubled Community

A troubled community, compared with a "good" community, has problems in one or more functional areas or in the areas responsible for the quality of life described in Chapter 3. A peculiar phenomenon in suburban community life is that the problems of adolescents tend to be simply ignored. A community may be concerned about academic and athletic excellence at the local high school, but citizens will not even mention at a city council meeting or school board meeting concerns about teenage drinking, drug use, pregnancy, crime, or discipline problems in school. Most school systems provide services for troubled youths, but the initiative comes from the school staff, not the community. Community concerns are related to the provision of goods and services, zoning regulations, services and recreation for adults and young

Table 5-4   Roles and Dynamics of an Alcoholic Family

Role	Motivating feeling	Identifying symptoms	Payoff		Possible price
			For individual	For family	
Dependent	Shame	Chemical use	Relief of pain	None	Addiction
Enabler	Anger	Powerlessness	Importance; self-righteous-ness	Responsibility	Illness; martyr-dom
Hero	Inadequacy; guilt	Overachievement	Attention (positive)	Self-worth	Compulsive drive
Scapegoat	Hurt	Delinquency	Attention (negative)	Focus away from depen-dent	Self-destruction; addiction
Lost child	Loneliness	Solitariness; shy-ness	Escape	Relief	Social isolation
Mascot	Fear	Clowning; hyper-activity	Attention (amused)	Fun	Immaturity; emotional illness

From Wegshieder S (1981) Another chance: help and hope for the alcoholic family, Palo Alto, Calif, Science & Behavior Books.

children, and services for senior citizens. Two main factors contribute to this problem: one is parent apathy and the other is governmental self-protection. If the schools and community appear to be "excellent" on the surface, then citizens will vote for the taxes, bond issues, and officials associated with the excellence.

Urban communities are rife with serious, overwhelming problems of safety, crime (especially related to drug problems), and urban flight. Pollution of all kinds is a serious issue for cities.

Rural communities may have problems obtaining goods and services because of distances in the horizontal and vertical patterns and because of inadequate tax bases.

Interventions in the community by adolescent psychiatric nurses and school nurses on behalf of adolescents are described in Chapters 8 and 9.

REFERENCES AND SUGGESTED READINGS

Abt AL and Weissman LE, editors (1987) Acting out: theoretical and clinical aspects, ed 2, Northvale, NJ, Jason Aronson, Inc.

Adams PL and Fras I (1988) Beginning child psychiatry, New York, Brunner/Mazel, Inc.

American Nurses' Association (1974) Standards of psychiatric mental health nursing practice, Kansas City, Mo, The Association.

American Psychiatric Association (1980) Diagnostic and statistical manual of mental disorders, Washington, DC, The Association.

American Psychiatric Association (1987) Desk reference to the diagnostic criteria from diagnostic and statistical manual of mental disorders, ed 3, Washington, DC, The Association.

American Psychiatric Association (1987) Diagnostic and statistical manual of mental disorders, ed 3 , revised, Washington, DC, The Association.

Anderson J, Williams S, McGee R, and Silva PA (1987) DSM-III disorders in preadolescent children: prevalence in a large sample from the general population, Archives of General Psychiatry 44:69-76.

Andreasen NC, Rice J, Endicott J, and others (1987) Familial rates of affective disorder, Archives of General Psychiatry 44:461-469.

Andrews H and Roy C (1985) Essentials of the Roy adaptation model, Englewood Cliffs, NJ, Prentice-Hall, Inc.

Babigan HM (1985) Schizophrenia: epidemiology. In Kaplan HI and Sadock BJ, editors, Comprehensive textbook of psychiatry, ed 4, Baltimore, Williams & Wilkins.

Barkley RA (1987) Defiant children: a clinician's manual for parent training, New York, The Guilford Press.

Barkley RA (1988) Attention deficit disorder with hyperactivity. In Mash EJ and Terdal LG, Behavioral assessment of childhood disorders, ed 2, New York, The Guilford Press.

Baxter LR, Phelps ME, Mazziota JC, and others (1987) Local cerebral glucose metabolic rates in obsessive-compulsive disorder: a comparison with rates in unipolar depression and in normal controls, Archives of General Psychiatry 44:211-218.

Berkowitz MS, editor (1985) Peer conflict and psychological growth, San Francisco, Josey-Bass Inc, Publishers.

Bernstein G (1990) Anxiety disorders. In Garfinkel BB, Carlson GA, and Weller EB, editors, Psychiatric disorders in children and adolescents, Philadelphia, WB Saunders Co.

Bernstein GA and Garfinkel BD (1986) School phobia: overlap of affective and anxiety disorders, Journal of the American Academy of Child and Adolescent Psychiatry 25:235-241.

Bernstein GA and Garfinkel BD (1988) Pedigrees, functioning and psychopathology in families of school phobic children, American Journal of Psychiatry 145:70-74.

Bernstein GA, Garfinkel BD, and Hoberman H (1989) Self-reported anxiety in adolescents, American Journal of Psychiatry 146:384-386.

Blatt SJ (1987) The Wechsler scales and acting out. In Abt LE and Weissman SL, editors, Acting out, ed 2, Northvale, NJ, Jason Aronson, Inc.

Blos P (1962) On adolescence: a psychoanalytic interpretation, New York, The Free Press of Glencoe.

Bowlby J (1973) Attachment and loss, vol 2, Separation, New York, Basic Books.

Brent DA, Kerr MM, Goldstein C, Bozegar J, Wartella M and Allan MJ (1989) An outbreak of suicide and suicidal behavior in a high school, Journal of the American Academy of Child and Adolescent Psychiatry 28:918-924.

Brent DA and Kolko DJ (1990) Suicide and suicidal behavior in children and adolescents. In Garfinkel BD, Carlson GA, and Weller EB, editors, Psychiatric disorders in children and adolescents, Philadelphia, WB Saunders Co.

Brody C and Forehand R (1986) Maternal perceptions of child maladjustment as a function of the combined influence of child behavior and maternal depression, Journal of the Consulting and Clinical Psychology 54:237-242.

Brown F (1987) The Bender gestalt and acting out. In Abt LE and Weissman SL, editors, Acting out, ed 2, Northvale, NJ, Jason Aronson, Inc.

Brunstetter RW and Silver LB (1985) Attention deficit disorder. In Kaplan H and Sadlock BJ: Comprehensive textbook of psychiatry IV, Baltimore, Williams & Wilkins.

Bunney WE, Pert A, Rosenblatt J, Pert CB, and Gallaper S (1979) Mode of action of lithium: some biological considerations, Archives of General Psychiatry 36:898-901.

Calabrese RL (1987) Adolescence: a growth period conducive to alienation, Adolescence 22:929-938.

Cancro R (1985) History and overview of schizophrenia. In Kaplan HI and Sadock BJ, editors, Comprehensive textbook of psychiatry, ed 4, Baltimore, Williams & Wilkins.

Cantwell DP and Baker L (1989) Stability and natural history of DSM-III childhood diagnoses, Journal of the American Academy of Child and Adolescent Psychiatry 28:691-697.

Cantwell DP and Carlson GA, editors (1983) Affective disorders in childhood and adolescence: an update, New York, Spectrum Publications.

Carlson GA and Cantwell DP (1980) Unmasking masked depression in children and adolescents, American Journal of Psychiatry 137:445-449.

Cermak TL (1986) Diagnosing and treating codependence, Minneapolis, The Johnson Institute.

Chess S and Thomas A (1986) Temperament in clinical practice, New York, The Guilford Press.

Chethink M (1986) Levels of borderline functioning in children: etiological and treatment considerations, American Journal of Orthopsychiatry 56:109-119.

Chu JA and Dill DL (1990) Dissociative symptoms in relation to childhood physical and sexual abuse, American Journal of Psychiatry 147:887-892.

Cohen P, Valez N, Kohn JM, Schwav-Stone M, and Johnson J (1987) Child psychiatric diagnosis by computer algorithm: theoretical issues and empirical tests, Journal of the American Academy of Child and Adolescent Psychiatry 26:631.

Crowe RR, Noyes R, Pauls DL, and Slyman D (1983) A family study of panic disorder, Archives of General Psychiatry 40:1065-1069.

Cytryn L and McKnew DH (1974) Factors influencing the changing clinical expression of the depression process in children, American Journal of Psychiatry 131:879-880.

Durkin RP and Durkin AB (1975) Evaluating residential treatment programs for disturbed children. In Guttentag M and Struening EL, editors, Handbook of evaluation research, vol 2, Beverly Hills, Calif, Sage Publications.

Edelbrook E (1985) Conduct problems in childhood and adolescence: developmental patterns and progressions, Unpublished manuscript.

Erikson EH (1963) Childhood and society, New York, WW Norton Co.

Eth S and Pynoos RS, editors (1985) Posttraumatic stress disorder in children, Washington, DC, American Psychiatric Press.

Fairbank JA and Nicholson RA (1987) Theoretical and empirical issues in the treatment of posttraumatic stress disorder in Vietnam veterans, Journal of Clinical Psychiatry 43:44.

Farrington DP (1986) Stepping stones to adult criminal careers. In Olweus D, Block J, and Yarrow MR, editors, Development of antisocial and prosocial behavior, New York, Academic Press.

Figley CR (1989) Helping traumatized families, San Francisco, Jossey-Bass Inc, Publishers.

Figley CR, editor (1985) Trauma and its wake, New York, Bruner/Mazel, Inc.

Flament MF, Rapoport JL, and Berg CJ (1985) Clomipramine treatment of childhood obsessive-compulsive disorder, Archives of General Psychiatry 42:977-983.

Flament MF, Rapoport JL, and Murphy DL (1987) Biochemical changes during clomipramine treatment of childhood obsessive-compulsive disorder, Archives of General Psychiatry 44:219-225.

Freud A (1965) Normality and pathology in childhood, New York, International Universities Press, Inc.

Freud A (1969) Adolescence as developmental disturbance. In Kaplan G and Lebovici S, editors, Adolescence: psychological perspectives, New York, Basic Books.

Freud S (1953) Remembering, repeating and working through. The standard edition of the complete psychological works of Sigmund Freud, vol 132, London, Hogarth Press (originally published in 1914).

Friedman MJ (1985) Toward rational pharmacotherapy for posttraumatic stress disorder: an interim report, American Journal of Psychiatry 145:281.

Galanter M (1990) Cults and zealous self-help movements: a psychiatric perspective, American Journal of Psychiatry 147:543.

Galanter M editor (1989) Cults and new religious movements: a report of the American Psychiatric Association, Washington, DC, American Psychiatric Association.

Gershon ES, Hamovit J, and Juroff JJ (1982) Family study of psychoaffective, bipolar I, bipolar II, unipolar and normal control probands, Archives of General Psychiatry 39:1157-1167. Reprinted in Stiffman AR and Feldman RA (1988) Advances in adolescent mental health, vol 3, Greenwich, Conn, JAI Press, Inc.

Glaser K (1987) Suicide in children and adolescents. In Abt LE and Weissman SL, editors, Acting out, ed 2, Northvale, NJ, Jason Aronson Inc.

Goldstein MJ, Baker BL, and Jamison KR (1980) Abnormal psychology: experiences, origins and interventions, Boston, Little, Brown & Co.

Gomes-Schwartz B, Horowitz JM, and Sauzier M (1985) Severity of emotional distress among sexually abused preschool, school-age and adolescent children, Hospital and Community Psychiatry 36:503.

Gossett J, Lewis J, and Barnhart D (1983) To find a way out: the outcome of hospital treatment of disturbed adolescents, New York, Brunner/Mazel, Inc.

Harnett NE (1989) Conduct disorder in childhood and adolescence: an update, Journal of Child and Adolescent Psychiatric and Mental Health Nursing 2:74-77.

Harrison SI, Davenport CW, and McDermott JF (1967) Children's reactions to bereavement: adult confusions and misperceptions, Archives of General Psychiatry 17:593-597.

Hart K and Ollendick T (1985) Prevalence of bulimia in working and university women, American Journal of Psychiatry 142:857-854.

Hendren RL, Sholevar GP, Weinberger DR, and Wiener JM (1990) Grand rounds: schizophrenia in a fourteen-year-old boy, Journal of the American Academy of Child and Adolescent Psychiatry 29:141-148.

Hoffman S and Kuperman N (1990) Indirect treatment of traumatic psychological experience: the use of TAT cards, American Journal of Psychotherapy vol XLIV, no 1, Jan., 107-115.

Izard CE and Schwartz GM (1986) Patterns of emotion in depression. In Rutter M, Izard CE, and Read PB, editors, Depression in young people: developmental and clinical perspectives, New York, The Guilford Press.

Jacobson MS, Rubenstein EM, and Bohannon WE (1986) Follow-up of adolescent trauma victims: a new model of care, Pediatrics 77: 113-116.

Jensen JB (1990) Obsessive-compulsive disorder in children and adolescents. In Garfinkel BD, Carlson GA, and Weller EB, Psychiatric disorders in children and adolescents, Philadelphia, WB Saunders Co.

Johnson BS, editor (1988) Psychiatric mental health nursing: adaptation and growth, Philadelphia, JB Lippincott Co.

Josselyn I (1987) Acting out in adolescence. In Abt LE and Weissman SL, editors, Acting out, ed 2, Northvale, NJ, Jason Aronson, Inc.

Kallman F and Roth B (1956) Genetic aspects of preadolescent schizophrenia, American Journal of Psychiatry 112:599-606.

Kay RL and Kay J (1986) Adolescent conduct disorders. In Frances AJ and Hales RE, editors, Annual review, vol 5, Washington DC, American Psychiatric Association.

Karson CN, Kleinman JE, and Wyatt RJ (1986) Biochemical concepts of schizophrenia. In Millon J and Klerman G, editors: Contemporary directions in psychopathology, New York, Guilford Press.

Kazdin AE (1985) Treatment of antisocial behavior in children and adolescents, Homewood, Ill, Dorsey Press.

Kazdin AE, Esveldt Dawson K, Sherick RB, and Colbus D (1985) Assessment of overt behavior and childhood depression among psychiatrically disturbed children, Journal of Consulting and Clinic Psychology 53:201.

Kemp R and Kemp H (1984) The common secret, New York, WH Freeman & Co Publishers.

Kernberg OF (1985) Neurosis, psychosis, and the borderline states. In Kaplan HI and Sadock BJ, editors, Comprehensive textbook of psychiatry, Baltimore, Williams & Wilkins.

Khouri PJ and Akiskal HS (1986) The bipolar spectrum reconsidered. In Miller T and Klerman GL, editors, Contemporary directions in psychopathology, New York, The Guilford Press.

Kimmel DC and Weiner IB (1985) Adolescence: a developmental transition. Hillsdale, NJ, Lawrence Erlbaum Associates, Inc.

Klerman GL (1978) Long-term treatment of affective disorders. In Lipton MA, DiMascio A, and Killan KF Psychopharmacology: a generation of progress, New York, Raven Press.

Klerman GL (1986) Historical perspectives on contemporary schools of psychopathology. In Millon T and Klerman GL, editors, Contemporary directions in psychopathology, New York, The Guilford Press.

Klorman R (1986) Attention deficit disorder in adolescence, Advances in Adolescent Mental Health, vol 1, part A, Greenwich, Conn, JAI Press, Inc.

Koocher GP (1985) Psychosocial care of the child cured of cancer, Pediatric Nursing 11:91.

Kovacs M, Feinberg TL, Crousse-Novack MA, and others (1984) Depressive disorders in childhood, Archives of General Psychiatry 41:229-237, 643-649. Reprinted in Stiffman AR and Feldman RA (1988) Advances in adolescent mental health, vol 3, Greenwich, Conn, JAI Press, Inc.

Krener P (1985) After incest: secondary prevention? Journal of the American Academy of Child and Adolescent Psychiatry 24:231-234.

Kutscher SP, Marton P, and Korenblum M (1990) Adolescent bipolar illness and personality disorder, Journal of the American Academy of Child and Adolescent Psychiatry 29:355-358.

Leckman JF, Dolnansky ES, Hardin MT, and others (1990) Perinatal factors in the expression of Tourette's syndrome: an exploratory study, Journal of the American Academy of Child and Adolescent Psychiatry 29:220-226.

Leckman JF, Weissman MM, Merikangas KR, Pauls DL, and Prusoff BA (1983) Panic disorder and major depression, Archives of General Psychiatry 40:1055-1062.

Levi J (1987) Acting out indicators on the Rorschach. In Abt LE and Weissman SL, editors, Acting out, ed 2, Northvale, NJ, Jason Aronson, Inc.

Levy R (1982) The new language of psychiatry, Boston, Little, Brown & Co.

Lewis D, Lewis M, Unger L, and Goldman C (1985) Conduct disorder and its synonyms. Diagnosis of dubious validity and usefulness. In Annual progress in child psychiatry and child development, New York, New York University Progress.

Lieberman J (1984) Evidence for a biological hypothesis of obsessive-compulsive disorder, Neuropsychobiology 11:14-21.

Loeber R (1988) Natural histories of conduct problems, delinquency and associated substance use. In Lahey BB and Lazdin AD, editors, Advances in clinical child psychology, vol 11, New York, Plenum Press.

Loeber R and Schmaling KB (1985) Empirical evidence for overt and covert patterns of antisocial conduct problems: a meta-analysis, Journal of Abnormal Child Psychology 13:337.

Loewenstein R, Hornstein N, and Faber B (1988) Open trial of clonazepam in the treatment of posttraumatic symptoms in multiple personality disorder Dissociation 1(3):3-12.

Lyons JA (1987) Post-traumatic stress disorder in children and adolescents: a review of the literature, In Chess S, Thomas A, and Hertzig ME, Annual progress in child psychiatry and adult development, New York, Bruner/Mazel, Inc.

Mahler M (1968) On the concepts of symbiosis and separation individuation, vol 1, New York, International Universities Press Inc.

Masterson JF (1985) Treatment of the borderline adolescent: a developmental approach, New York, Brunner/Mazel Inc.

McClennan JM, Rubert MP, Reichler RJ, and Sylvester CE (1990) Attention deficit disorder in children at risk for anxiety and depression, Journal of the American Academy of Child and Adolescent Psychiatry 4:534.

McEnany GW (1990) Psychobiological indices of bipolar mood disorder: future trends in nursing care, Archives of Psychiatric Nursing 4:29.

McGee B, Feehan M, Williams S, Partridge F, Silva PA, and Kelly J (1990) DSM-III disorders in a large sample of adolescents, Journal of the American Academy of Child and Adolescent Psychiatry 4:611.

McMahon RJ and Forehand R (1988) Conduct disorders. In Mesh J and Terdal LG, editors, Behavioral assessment of childhood disorders, ed 2, New York, The Guilford Press.

Miller D (1974) Adolescent psychology, psychopathology, psychotherapy, New York, Jason Aronson, Inc.

Miller D (1980) Family maladaptation reflected in drug abuse and delinquency. In Sugar M, Responding to adolescent needs, Jamaica, NY, Spectrum Publications.

Miller D (1983) The age between: adolescents and therapy, New York, Jason Aronson, Inc.

Miller D (1986) Attack on the self: adolescent behavioral disturbances and their treatment, Northvale, NJ, Jason Aronson, Inc.

National Institute on Alcohol Abuse and Alcoholism (1986). In Felsted C, editor: Youth, alcohol and abuse, Phoenix, Oryx Press.

Newman J (1981) Children of disaster: observations following the Chowchilla school-bus kidnaping, American Journal of Psychiatry 138:14.

Nichtern S (1982) The sociocultural and psychodynamic aspects of the acting out and violent adolescent, Adolescent Psychiatry 10:140-146.

Nir Y (1985) Post-traumatic stress disorder in children with cancer. In Eth S and Pynoos RS, editors, Post-traumatic stress disorder in children, Washington, DC, American Psychiatric Press.

Offer D and Offer J (1975) Three developmental routes through male adolescence, Adolescent Psychiatry 4:121-125.

Offer D, Ostrov E, and Howard K (1981) The mental health professional's concept of the normal adolescent, Archives of General Psychiatry 38:149-153.

O'Toole AW and Loomis ME (1989) Revision of the phenomena of concern for psychiatric mental health nursing, Archives of Psychiatric Nursing 3:288-299.

Orvashel H (1990) Early onset psychiatric disorder in high risk children and increased familial morbidity of depression and anxiety in their second degree relatives, Journal of the American Academy of Child and Adolescent Psychiatry 29:184.

Orvashel H, Thompson WD, Belanger A, Prusoff BA, and Kidd KK (1982) Comparison of family history method to direct interview factors affecting the diagnosis of depression, Journal of Affective Disorders 4:49.

Orzek AM (1985) The child's cognitive processing of sexual abuse, Journal of Child and Adolescent Psychotherapy 2:110-217.

Papanek E (1987) Management of acting out adolescents. In Abt LE and Weissman SL, editors, Acting out, ed 2, Northvale, NJ, Jason Aronson, Inc.

Patterson GB and Stouthamer-Loeber M (1984) The correlation of family management practices and delinquency, Child Development 55:1299.

Patterson GR (1976) The aggressive child: victim and architect of a coercive system. In Mash EJ, Hamerlynck LA, and Handy LC, editors, Behavior modification and families, New York, Brunner/Mazel, Inc.

Patterson GR (1982) Coercive family process, Eugene, Ore, Castalina.

Pauls DL, Towbin KE, Leckman JF, and others (1986) Gilles de la Tourette's syndrome: an obsessive compulsive disorder—evidence supporting a genetic relationship, Archives of General Psychiatry 43:1180-1182.

Peck ML, Farberow ML, and Litman RE, editors, (1985) Youth suicide, New York, Springer Publishing Co, Inc.

Piaget J (1972) Intellectual evolution from adolescence to adulthood, Human Development 15:1.

Poal P and Weisz JR (1990) Therapists' own childhood problems as predictors of their effectiveness in child psychotherapy, Journal of Clinical Child Psychology 18:202-208.

Puig-Antich J (1985) Affective disorders. In Kaplan HI and Sadock BJ, editors, Comprehensive textbook of psychiatry IV, Baltimore, Williams & Wilkins.

Putnam FW (1989) Diagnosis and treatment of multiple personality disorder, New York, The Guilford Press.

Quay HC (1986) A critical analysis of DSM-III as a taxonomy of psychopathology in childhood and adolescence. In Millon T and Klerman GL, editors, Contemporary directions in psychopathology, New York, The Guilford Press.

Rachal JV, Maisto SA, Coness LL, and Hubbard RL (1982) Alcohol use among youth. In U. SD. National Institute on Alcohol Abuse and Alcoholism. Alcohol and Health Monograph No 1, Alcohol consumption and related problems (Department of Health and Human Services Pub No ADM 82-1190), Washington, DC, US Government Printing Office.

Rapoport JC (1986) Childhood obsessive compulsive disorder, Journal of Child Psychology and Psychiatry 27:289-295.

Rashkis HA and Wallace AFC (1959) The reciprocal effect: how patient disturbance affects and is affected by staff attitudes, Archives of General Psychiatry 1:489-498.

Rasmussen SA (1986) Childhood obsessive-compulsive disorder, American Journal of Psychiatry 138:1545-1554.

Reid JB, Hinojosa-Rivera G, and Lorber R (1981) A social learning approach to the outpatient treatment of children who steal, Eugene, Oregon Learning Center, unpublished manuscript.

Reid WH and Wise MG (1989) DSM-III-R training guide, New York, Brunner/Mazel, Inc.

Rey JM and Plapp JM (1990) Quality of perceived parenting in oppositional and conduct disordered adolescents, Journal of the American Academy of Child and Adolescent Psychiatry 3:382-385.

Rey JM, Plapp JM, and Stewart GW (1990) Reliability of psychiatric diagnosis in referred adolescents, Journal of Child Psychology and Psychiatry and Allied Disciplines 30:879-888.

Robbins DR and Alessi NE (1985) Depressive symptoms and suicidal behavior in adolescents, American Journal of Psychiatry 142:588-592.

Robertiello RC (1987) "Acting out" and "working through." In Abt LE and Weissman SL, editors, Acting out, ed 2, Northvale, NJ, Jason Aronson, Inc.

Rodriguez CM and Routh DK (1989) Depression, anxiety and attributional style in learning disabled and non-learning disabled children, Journal of Clinical Child Psychology 18:299-304.

Rome HP and Barry MJ (1987) Problems of therapeutic management of acting out with hospitalized patients. In Abt LE and Weissman SL, editors, Acting out, ed 2, Northvale, NJ, Jason Aronson, Inc.

Rosen JN (1987) The concept of "acting-in." In Abt LE and Weissman SL, editors, Acting out, ed 2, Northvale, NJ, Jason Aronson, Inc.

Rosenberg ML, Smith JC, Davidson LE, and Conn JM (1987) The emergence of youth suicide: an epidemiologic analysis and public health perspective, Annual Review of Public Health 8:417.

Rosenheck R and Nathan P (1985) Secondary traumatization in children of Vietnam veterans, Hospital and Community Psychiatry 36:538-539.

Ross CA, Norton GR, and Anderson G (1988) The dissociative experiences scale: a replication study, Dissociation 1:21-32.

Ross DM and Ross SA (1982) Hyperactivity: research, theory and action, ed 2, New York, John Wiley and Sons, Inc.

Rutter M, Graham IP, Chadwick F, and Yule W (1976) Adolescent turmoil: fact or fiction, Journal of Child Psychology and Psychiatry and Allied Disciplines 17:35.

Safer JD and Allen RP (1976) Hyperactive children: diagnosis and management, Baltimore, University Park Press.

Saigh P (1987) In vitro flooding of an adolescent posttraumatic stress disorder, Journal of Clinical Child Psychology 16:147-150.

Satir V (1988) The new peoplemaking, Mountain View, Calif, Science & Behavior Books.

Satterfield JH, Satterfield B, and Cantwell D (1981) Three-year multimodality treatment study of hyperactive boys, Journal of Pediatrics 98:650-658.

Schaif AW (1986) Codependence: misunderstood – mistreated, San Francisco, Harper & Row, Publishers, Inc.

Schildkraut JJ, Green AI, and Mooney JJ (1985) Affective disorders: biochemical aspects. In Kaplan HI and Sadock BJ, editors, Comprehensive textbook of psychiatry, IV, Baltimore, Williams & Wilkins.

Schukit M (1987) Biological vulnerability to alcoholism, Journal of Consulting and Clinical Psychology 55:301-309.

Sgroi SM (1982) Handbook of clinical intervention in child abuse, Lexington, Mass, Lexington Books.

Shafii M, Carrigan S, Whittinghill JR, and Derrick A (1985) Psychological autopsy of completed suicide in children and adolescents, American Journal of Psychiatry 142:1061-1064.

Shapiro S (1987) Self-mutilation and self-blame in incest victims, American Journal of Psychotherapy 41:46-55.

Shapiro S and Dominiak G (1990) Common psychological defenses seen in the treatment of sexually abused adolescents, American Journal of Psychotherapy 44:68-74.

Silver LB and Brunstetter RW (1986) Attention deficit disorder in adolescents, Hospital and Community Psychiatry 36:608-613.

Spirito A, Stark L, Fristad M, Hart K, and Owens-Stively J (1987) Adolescent suicide attempters on a pediatric unit, Journal of Pediatric Psychology 12:171-178.

Spitzer R and Cantwell D (1980) The DSM-III classification of psychiatric disorders of infancy, childhood and adolescence, Journal of the American Academy of Child and Adolescent Psychiatry 19:356-370.

Stanton AH and Schwartz MS (1949) The management of a type of institutional participation in mental illness, Psychiatry 12:13-26.

Stuart GW and Sundeen SJ (1983) Principles and practice of psychiatric nursing, ed 2, St Louis, Mosby-Year Book, Inc.

Stuart GW and Sundeen SJ (1991) Principles and practice of psychiatric nursing, ed 4, St Louis, The CV Mosby Co.

Sullivan HS (1953) Interpersonal theory of psychiatry, New York, WW Norton & Co Inc.

Terr LC (1981) Psychic trauma in children: observations following the Chowchilla school bus kidnapping, American Journal of Psychiatry 138:14-19.

Terr LC (1983) Chowchilla revisited: the effects of psychic trauma four years after a school bus kidnapping, American Journal of Psychiatry 140:1543-1550.

Terr LC (1985) Children traumatized in small groups. In Eth S and Pynoos RS, editors, Posttraumatic stress disorders in children, Washington DC, American Psychiatric Press.

Thomas A and Chess S (1981) The role of temperament in the contribution of individuals to their development. In Lerner RM and Busch-Rossnagel NA, editors: Individuals as producers of their development, New York, Academic Press.

Wegscheider S (1981) Another chance, help and hope for the alcoholic family, Palo Alto, Calif, Science & Behavior Books.

Weissman MM, Gammon GD, Merikangas KR, John K, Warner V, Pausoff BA, and Sholomakas D (1987) Children of depressed parents, Archives of General Psychiatry 44:847-853.

Wicks-Nelson R and Israel AC (1984) Behavior disorders of childhood, Englewood Cliffs, NJ, Prentice-Hall, Inc.

Wilson JP, Smith WK and Johnson SK (1985) A comparative of PTSD among various survivor groups. In Figley CR, editor: Trauma and its wake, New York, Bruner/Mazel, Inc.

Zametkin AJ and Rapoport JL (1987) Neurobiology of attention-deficit disorder with hyperactivity: where have we come in 50 years? Journal of the American Academy of Child and Adolescent Psychiatry 26:676-687.

Zubin J (1985) Psychobiological markers for schizophrenia: state of the art and future perspectives, Psychopharmacology Bulletin 21:490-496.

Zucker Rand Hartford T (1986) National study of the demography of adolescent drinking practices in 1980. In Felstead C, editor: Youth and alcohol abuse: readings and resources, Phoenix, Oryx Press.

Chapter 6

Assessment of the Adolescent

Patricia Clunn

Adequate assessment is the cornerstone of intervention for adolescents seen in all psychiatric mental health care settings. It requires knowledge of personality theory, psychopathology, family dynamics, communication skills, and adolescent development. The comprehensive evaluation of adolescents, in contrast to that of adult clients, includes assessment of their families or the significant adults upon whom the adolescent is economically and psychologically dependent. Teachers, peers, and community and environmental factors have an impact on adolescents' psychological well-being and are essential considerations in a thorough assessment.

In most situations, a multiple assessment approach is used with adolescents that draws on the special skills of clinicians from a variety of disciplines; physicians, neurologists, psychologists, nurses, teachers, and social workers are major contributors to an interdisciplinary team assessment. A comprehensive assessment usually includes family and individual interviews, observations, and physical, neuropsychological, and mental status examinations. The social world of the adolescent is more complex and extensive than that of the younger child, but early and mid-aged adolescents continue to depend on their families emotionally, economically, and socially. Thus, assessment of the structure and functioning of the adolescent's family is essential. Teachers and peers also can provide important information in understanding the adolescent's problem. Given the importance of environment, assessment of the school and community is critical. Knowledge of the community's assets, resources, and limitations is critical in understanding many of the behavioral problems and characteristics of these young people.

The tools and techniques used in assessing adolescents, families, and environments are undergoing constant change and refinement because of the rapid advances in scientific knowledge. The expansion of knowledge in the field of adolescent mental health has occurred rapidly in the past few decades, and clinicians now need to conduct initial assessment interviews to gather a phenomenal amount of data in a brief amount of time to determine an effective treatment plan.

The outcome of the initial assessment interview depends on how the clinician collects the critical data. The interview is the foundation of all mental health interventions, and reliable diagnosis, effective treatment planning, and family support and compliance with the therapeutic interventions all hinge on the clinician's ability to engage the adolescent and family creatively. The clinician must gain the adolescent's cooperation in a therapeutic alliance (Shea, 1988) — one of the most challenging and inventive tasks of mental health professionals.

Nurses participate in two kinds of adolescent interviews: DSM-III-R (1987) diagnostic structured interviews and nursing assessment interviews. When a DSM-III-R diagnosis is the goal of the assessment, the same components, tools, and procedures (such as the mental status examination) are assessed similarly by all members of the core mental health professions. In contrast, nursing diagnostic assessment interviews are conducted by and for the nursing staff to establish nursing diagnoses and to provide the basis for nursing care management.

The validity of the baseline data depends on the clinician's ability to establish the therapeutic alliance, to direct and focus the communication, and to use empathic interviewing skills. Clinicians need be aware of their role in the assessment interview, and nurses who wish to develop their diagnostic interviewing skills further will find it helpful to videotape their interviews and obtain a critique from a more seasoned nurse or clinical specialist. There are also a number of guidelines clinicians can use for evaluation of their assessment interview skills, such as the protocol by Sattler (1988) and the checklist included at the end of this chapter.

Variations in Assessment Situations

Assessment of adolescents is conducted for a variety of reasons: clinical problems, psychoeducational purposes, eligibility for special programs, and evaluation of progress and change. The clinical assessment interviews have significant consequences for adolescents and their families and are planned for a definite purpose. They require the clinician to be responsible for the interaction — to take the initiative, to face unpleasant facts or feelings, and to document the context and history of the adolescent's difficulties. They require the adolescent's and family's sustained attention. In many cases the reports are given the adolescents and families and treatment goals are mutually agreed upon.

In accord with Public Law 94-142, the Education for All Handicapped Children Act (1975, 1984), many nurses participate as members of the psychoeducational assessment team — as independent agents in outpatient and community settings or as team members in inpatient settings — for psychoeducative assessments and team development of young adolescents individualized educational programs (IEPs).

Although procedures for conducting diagnostic interviews with emotionally disturbed adolescents vary according to the purpose of the assessment, most mental health agencies are usually careful in their management of referrals and contacts by adolescents and their families before the initial assessment interview. It is estimated that more than 50% of adolescents and their families who are referred for psychological assessment and treatment do not follow through on it (Call, 1985). Professionals are concerned that many troubled adolescents identified to be in need of psychiatric services do not receive initial care because of the family's or adolescent's resistance to seeking psychiatric treatment. Thus, problems are ignored until they become full-blown crises.

A vast amount of literature suggests how to handle the initial contacts so that the adolescent and family follow through. In some settings, for example, telephone calls from parents or adolescents seeking help are referred directly to the professional staff. The opportunity to speak directly to a clinician during the first contact has proved to be highly beneficial because the initial contact is made at a time of crisis for the caller; reassurance (as well as considerable clarifying information) can be provided. The problem can be evaluated, the time and procedure of the assessment interview can be briefly conveyed, and costs and financial arrangements can be discussed. Most important, clinicians can advise parents how to prepare the adolescent in advance for the initial interview. Many authorities recommend that the parental explanations be rehearsed with parents before the diagnostic assessment interview, recognizing that adolescents often are unwilling to participate in evaluations, and by the time parents seek professional help, many other resources and efforts have been exhausted (Call, 1985; Dodds, 1985).

During the initial telephone contact, parents also can be requested to bring medical records and other pertinent information with them. Because of denial or the duress of the interview situation, frequently families cannot recall some important baseline data during the initial encounter. When the situation is not a crisis and the assessment is scheduled at a later time, some agencies mail forms to the families to complete at home prior to the scheduled interview. Information that is available in advance, such as the adolescent's health and developmental profile, provides the clinicians some prior information enhancing rapport with the family and usually alleviates some of the family's misgivings and apprehensions about the assessment procedure and the kinds of information needed. This in addition to various reports from school, courts, and other professionals needs to be incorporated with the information gained from interviewing after parental permission has been given.

Diagnostic tools and techniques have become highly complex. Many large health facilities serve as diagnostic centers and provide comprehensive diagnostic evaluations and then return their results to the clinicians who referred their clients for diagnosis. These large facilities generally have the equipment and staff for more sophisticated neuropsychological assessment techniques, such as neuroimaging and biological brain studies. These agencies follow prescribed procedures for highly sophisticated interdisciplinary evaluation of adolescents and their families. Some take 2 or 3 days for all members of the interdisciplinary team to complete their evaluations while others require the adolescent and family to reside several days in the facility's family apartment for comprehensive study. Nurses working in these settings have a major role in the interdisciplinary assessment procedures and, in addition to their psychological assessment responsibilities, expand their roles to include nursing clinical techniques that support biophysical brain and enzyme studies.

Assessment Interviewing Techniques with Adolescents

The clinical assessment interview and the psychotherapeutic interview have differences and similarities in many critical areas. The ability to distinguish between them and to develop clinical skills in both nursing functions is essential for effective psychiatric nursing with adolescents.

The major distinctions between diagnostic and psychotherapeutic techniques are in the goals, direction, structure, and contact time. The objectives of an assessment interview are (1) to obtain the information needed to arrive at a diagnosis, the need for referral, and the kind of treatment or remediation needed, (2) to cover specific content areas, such as the developmental history and mental status, and (3) to limit contact time, usually to 1 or 2 hours. The objectives of the psychotherapeutic interview are (1) to foster change, focusing on therapeutic goals and affective change and (2) to maintain contact with the client for the time needed to accomplish that change. The similarities are (1) to establish rapport and facilitate communication, (2) to communicate respect, genuineness, and empathy, (3) to listen for feelings and information, (4) to provide an environment in which the adolescent can reveal concerns, preoccupations, and feelings, and (5) to assess verbal and nonverbal communications. The techniques are not mutually exclusive. Often during a psychotherapeutic interview, continuing assessment techniques are needed, and the adolescent may be so disturbed during the assessment interview that psycho-therapeutic interventions are required to encourage the patient to talk and to concentrate (Sattler, 1988).

When to see the adolescent individually during the initial assessment has been widely discussed in the literature, given the importance of adolescent developmental considerations and the family's distress. Some experts (Barker, 1990; Esman, 1988) suggest that if more than one assessment session is to be held, it is best to schedule the first interview directly with the adolescent rather than the parents, inasmuch as adolescents are usually unwilling participants under pressure. When parents are interviewed first or participate in the initial arrangements, adolescents surmise that unfavorable things have been said about them, and this increases their negativism and unwillingness to cooperate. This obstacle can be minimized if contact with the parents occurs after the adolescent has been interviewed.

Others advocate that the best time for the initial contact with the adolescent is with the family. These experts claim that the family intake interview opens up a great deal of material quickly and is valuable in learning about family feelings and dynamics. This intake interview provides the nurse an excellent opportunity to establish an immediate rapport with the adolescent, especially those who are in the late latency stage. If the family session is followed by the individual evaluation session with the adolescent, when the nurse is alone with the adolescent for the first time, a good method of forming an alliance with the adolescent is to comment on the vibrations picked up in the family session (Dodds, 1985).

Generally it is productive to have a brief family session initially so that the adolescents can hear what the parents are saying and can offer alternative points of view and their versions of the situations presented by parents. In crisis situations—for example, when the adolescent is out of control or unaware of what is going on—the initial interview is brief and extensive evaluation is deferred until the crisis has been stabilized.

Perhaps the best situation is one in which the approach is open and the decision about how to proceed with the initial assessment of the adolescent and family can be based on the clinician's observations of their waiting room behaviors and their initial responses after the formalities of introductions have been completed. Adolescents tend to be self-conscious, and the goal of the initial contact is to enlist their cooperation without coercion. The clinician considers the adolescent's developmental level and presenting behaviors when initiating and conducting the interview and adjusts the procedures accordingly. The adolescents can be asked if they prefer to talk separately first or to wait until the family interview has been completed. In this approach the clinician conveys that the adolescent's point of view is valued (Call, 1985).

Regardless of the decision for an initial individual or family session, communication with the adolescent, especially the younger adolescent, should be framed within the adolescent's developmental stage and presenting behaviors. It is important that the adolescent is clear about the reason for the interview, and this reason needs to be addressed initially in family or individual interviews. The nurse needs to address the adolescent first and to ask who it is they believe requested the assessment, the reasons they believe the person had for the request, and if they agree with that opinion. It is important for the nurse to convey respect for adolescents' confidentiality and privacy. They might not want to talk about some areas with the nurse when the family is present or want other materials or evaluations included in their records (such as the school counselor). The topics to be covered in the initial interview, besides the reason for referral, include interests, peers, school, family, fears and worries, self-image, mood, feelings, thoughts, fantasies, aspirations, relationships, sexual activities, and drug and alcohol abuse.

There are many interviewing strategies: using descriptive comments, using reflection, praising frequently, using open-ended questions, formulating questions in the subjunctive mood; exercising tact; using props that help young adolescents to communicate verbally; and using special techniques that facilitate the expression of culturally unacceptable or sensitive responses (such as using general references like "most young people do such-and-such"). It is important to clarify episodes of reported misbehavior by having the adolescent recount them, to handle uncommunicative adolescents by clarifying the interview procedures, and to treat resistance and anxiety by giving support. The clinician needs to use understandable language and avoid psychiatric jargon — use the adolescent's cultural or "hip" language cautiously or judiciously (Shea, 1988).

Clinicians need to participate actively, keep control of the encounter, and focus on the task at hand, regulating their own verbal and nonverbal behaviors to facilitate the data-gathering process (Sattler, 1988; Shea, 1988). The clinician usually determines what kind of information is needed to make an appropriate disposition and needs to be flexible in collecting a valid data base.

The individual interview with the adolescent may be combined with the mental status examination. The interview becomes a relationship that undergoes changes as the evaluation progresses and information unfolds to delineate problem areas. An effective way to begin the individual interview with an adolescent is to clarify again that the next hour or so will be spent in determining what the problems are and that the clinician will ask a number of questions and will need to record the responses for the assessment report.

If the adolescent has had previous contacts with mental health care workers, those interactions need be explored early in the interview, and details of previous episodes of psychopathology should be noted. If this is the first encounter the differences between conversations and interviewing, professional and social, and relationships and responsibilities need to be established. During the interview, the nurse assumes responsibility for controlling, setting limits, focusing, and directing and maintaining the communications. Even if the nurse does not agree, the adolescent's point of view should be respected. The nurse controls the activity and goals of the interview, asking questions and continuing to explore topics until satisfied that misinterpretations and misunderstandings, as well as the adolescent's point of view, are fully understood. The nurse has the right to probe, but the adolescent has a right to privacy and may not respond.

Many adolescents come to the interview with a long history of talking with adults and professionals about conflict and problems — discussions that have been frustrating and unproductive. They may express a disinterest in going over the same old story with the nurse. These past experiences may lead them to expect contradictions, fault-finding, blaming, and efforts to control their behavior. Their resistance is usually high, and this resistance needs be resolved before the evaluation process begins, if it is to be a constructive process. The management of angry, unwilling adolescents, such as those who refuse to talk or who walk out of the interview room, is similar to the management of adolescents who leave or refuse to attend one-to-one therapeutic sessions. It is best not to stop them or try to make them return to the interview room. In these situations, clinicians need to explain to the family in the waiting area or to members of the floor staff (if in an inpatient setting) that the interview ended before it was completed and that the adolescent being interviewed did not want to discuss the information needed at this particular time. It is best to suggest calmly that the meeting be rescheduled to another time and avoid power struggles.

Developmental Considerations

Adolescents whose cognitive processes have matured within normal ranges of expectations are capable of thinking abstractly. These cognitive processes enable them to have more ideas and complex explanations for their problems. However, adolescents often are more resistant and unmotivated during an assessment than are children in the prelatency stage. Many teenagers referred for evaluation have been severely criticized by the adults in their lives, and their ability to think abstractly and argue hypothetically and deductively makes them powerfully resistant when they feel distrustful or defensive (Goldman and others, 1983). Intellectual abilities, maturing drives for self-esteem, autonomy, and the following features of adolescent development need to be considered in the assessment interview include (Barker, 1990):

1. Identity formation, which includes feelings of self-worth, competence, social skills, and prospects for the adult work world. Adolescents usually are considering various vocational choices, difficult decisions requiring the adolescents to plan ahead, as well as self-evaluate.

2. Dependence-independence conflicts with the family results as teenagers gradually learn to live their own lives and make more and more decisions about their activities. This transition is uneven and difficult, and usually peer group affiliations,

pressures, and values are substituted for former family power and influence.

3. Physical and sexual development, the development of sexual identity, and the adoption of adult sexual roles are major tasks of adolescence. Physical development, an aspect of identity formation, is based on biological maturation, and is extremely uneven and causes many conflicts and problems among adolescents of the same chronological age. Sexual and intimate feelings develop and become the basis for intense sexual relationships.

4. The influence of peer groups increases in importance as the family's influence decreases, and there are often conflicting value systems. Peer influences may be beneficial if the teenager is accepted by a good group or detrimental to self-esteem if the teenager falls in with a bad crowd (Bierman and Schwartz, 1986).

5. The demands of contemporary society and adolescent developmental tasks are often in conflict. For example, the extended period of formal education now required for many adult roles requires adolescents to be financially dependent on their parents into their twenties, which may cause dependency conflicts.

6. Adjustments in the family system are necessary as children reach adolescence. These changes challenge the family system, structure, and functioning. Child-management techniques that worked before puberty are no longer effective, and many family systems cannot adjust to the adolescent developmental changes.

Components of Assessment

Diagnostic assessment interviews usually involve the following 10 general content areas (Shea, 1988):

1. The diagnostic areas of the DSM-III-R criteria
2. History of present illness
3. Formal mental status examination
4. Social history, including family, community, stressors, and substance abuse
5. Family history
6. Determination of suicidal/homicidal potential
7. Past psychiatric history, previous mental health problems, and treatment, such as medications therapy, hospitalization, and counseling
8. Developmental and psychogenetic history from birth onward, including birth trauma, developmental milestones, toilet training, academic progress and difficulties, and early object relationships
9. Medical history
10. The interviewer's perspective

HISTORY OF PRESENT ILLNESS

The history of present illness (HPI) includes the presenting problem or chief complaint and the events leading to the current problem. The HPI includes the chronological development and characteristics of the symptoms, the reason for referral, and the names of the referring persons.

Pertinent historical aspects of the adolescent's behavior up to the time of the interview usually are compiled from reports from the family, teachers, previous clinicians, and the sources the family may bring to the initial interview. Most

DSM-III-R diagnostic criteria emphasize the duration and frequency of the problem, and the onset of the first signs of behavior change and when the first full symptom presented are essential. These two points in time help clarify the interaction between events and psychopathology (Skodol, 1989).

Most experts claim that the presenting complaints are of greater importance for adolescents and children than they are in adult psychiatry. It is suggested by Adams and Fras (1988) that the clinician ask the following questions of the family in the first stage of contact:

1. What concerns you about your adolescent?
2. When did these problems start?
3. Are they getting worse?
4. Have the problems been noticed in school as well as at home?
5. What makes the behaviors better? worse?
6. How have these problems affected the adolescent's life with you, siblings, peers, teachers?
7. Has the adolescent's school performance suffered?

MEDICAL HISTORY

The medical history may be acquired through the parents from the child's pediatrician; if that is not available, a complete review of the systems (including a neurological examination) is essential. Past and present illness, medications, and known food and medication allergies should be recorded. The DSM-III-R has an axis for noting physical disorders relevant to understanding and managing the patients (Axis I).

As the advances in psychobiological understandings (discussed in Chapter 5) are integrated into practice, assessment and tests of areas such as circadian patterns, disorders of appetite and weight, and psychoendocrinological disorders have been included in the medical evaluation. Nurses need to add these to the nursing assessment protocols, as well as to explore new interventions that support these advances (McEnany, 1990).

FAMILY HISTORY AND THE FAMILY INTERVIEW

Information needed for the family history includes medical illnesses in blood relatives and the incidence of schizophrenia, affective disorders, suicide, drug abuse, alcoholism, seizure disorders, dyslexia, and attention deficit disorders—mental disorders currently viewed as having strong genetic imbalances in brain structure, functioning, or biochemistry. These data are collected from the parents, often in advance of the interview, through checklists with yes or no questions.

Many clinicians prefer to use genograms for the initial organization of both physical and psychological family data and for the ongoing monitoring of the adolescent and family. Inasmuch as family therapists and general family practice clinicians frequently use genograms both for family therapy and for medical management and preventive medicine, the nurse needs to ascertain if the family already has an established genogram and should request a copy to add to the family records.

Genograms are based on system theories that view the family as persons who function as an interrelated group, with the adolescent, parents, and their problems existing within the same biological and social context. They are schematic representations of information on the family structure, life cycle fit, pattern repetition across generations, life events, family functioning, relational patterns and triangles, and family balances and imbalances (Woolf, 1983). By viewing themselves and their children within a broad intergenerational context, parents often feel less guilty and will more readily discuss their relationships.

Developing a genogram, which facilitates the therapeutic relationship with parents and helps alleviate their initial anxiety, usually requires several sessions. In many cases, adolescents are interested in learning the health history and intergenerational data—roots about which they had been unaware. Clinicians who use genograms will find the text by McGoldrick and Gerson (1985) useful, inasmuch as it includes guidelines for developing genograms with reconstituted and single-parent families. The computer-generated genogram of Gerson (1984) is another useful tool and has special appeal to adolescents interested in expanding their own computer skills and participating in the genogram development.

Process observations to be made during the family interview include family behaviors, such as spontaneous seating, verbal and nonverbal communication, the dominant communicator, and the time communication occurs. Exploration and clarification of recurring communication themes help to put the parents at ease.

Parents often come to the assessment interview experiencing frustration, helplessness, embarrassment, fear, and guilt because of what they perceive to be their failure to produce a capable teenager. They may appear defensive and angry—behavior that often disguises a great deal of pain. Parents and other closely involved family members may themselves be experiencing emotional disorders or chemical dependence.

In an inpatient admission assessment, the family structure and communication patterns are usually seriously disrupted, and feelings are intense. Because the situation is a crisis, the family will respond to crisis intervention techniques, as well as to a warm, caring, empathic approach by the nurse. The initial interview sets the tone for the family's comfort with the staff and program and significantly affects the family's compliance and treatment and contributes to the social and school functioning needed for the DSM-III-R diagnosis. The presence of the adolescent's psychosocial stressors relating to the problem are indicated on Axis IV of the DSM-III-R and the level of adaptive functioning on Axis V and the work toward Axis VI (Morrison and others, 1985).

The interview begins with the nurse making introductions, shaking hands with each family member, and arranging for comfortable seating. An uninterrupted hour or so is required for the process. If the meeting is an assessment, the nurse may begin with comments such as the following:

We are meeting today to determine what kind of assistance will best meet your family's needs. I will meet with the whole family, then with the adolescent and parents separately. We'll then get back together and decide on a plan. Let's begin with the thought that no one is to blame for the problems but everyone in the family can participate in the solutions. We can start by talking about what's been happening that caused you to make this appointment today. Who would like to start?

If the interview is an admission assessment, the nurse might say:

Welcome to the adolescent program. We know you are going through a very difficult time and are probably feeling pretty upset right now. After we go through the admission process together, I hope you will feel reassured that your problems are being addressed. What we will do for the next hour or so is explain the program to you and complete a nursing assessment and health history. We will spend most of the time together, but some time will be with just Mom and Dad and some time just with you. Let's start with what happened to cause the referral.

The family interview flows from the problem areas the family members identify. If the family states that the adolescent has problems at school, then the assessment proceeds to the family's and adolescent's relationships with school and other community groups, as well as to their relationships with each other. The family interview includes the assessment of the family system dynamics and the parents' view of the adolescent's difficulties (Table 6-1).

MENTAL STATUS EXAMINATION

The focus of the mental status examination (MSE) is on information gathered directly from the adolescent and collected in an individual interview alone with the adolescent. The general MSE format used in psychiatric evaluations is similar for adults and adolescents in that it is an objective description of the presenting behaviors and functioning at the time of the encounter. It does not include diagnostic assessment opinions or possible explanations about the adolescent's problem. The interviewer should take into account that the adolescent's reasoning ability, maturation level, and developmental attainment vary according to the early, middle, and late adolescent stages. Conducting a fruitful MSE requires a sound knowledge of adolescent development (Barker, 1990), and all observations should be presented within a developmental framework using age-appropriate norms.

The MSE routinely covers 10 areas: appearance, behavior, mood, affect, thought process, thought content, orientation, memory, judgment, and insight (Skodol, 1989). The purpose of the MSE is to organize observations so that the results of the interaction are presented in a clear, succinct, and systematic format that can be understood by other participants in the diagnostic work-up and treatment team. Comparing the MSE to the physical examination, Shea (1988) noted that only the current blood pressure — not past blood pressure readings — is to be noted. Nurses and other mental health clinicians often waste excessive amounts of time repeating themselves in writing these documents, and repetitions obscure the purpose of the current status.

The initial assessment establishes baseline data, providing a benchmark against which later diagnostic possibilities can be evaluated (see boxes on pp. 146-148). A brief unstructured MSE for older adolescents is presented in the box on p. 149. Many agencies prefer to use the structured Mini-Mental State Examination, which is a 30-item standard format with scoring and interpretive guidelines (Forslen and others, 1975).

SOCIAL HISTORY

The social history includes interpersonal and environmental information, such as assessment of the adolescent's friends, school, teachers, schoolmates and other

Table 6-1 Family Assessment Guidelines

Assessment categories	Sample questions
Open-system orientation	
Multiple causation of events	What do you believe are the reasons for the difficulty?
Need for each other and other people	What do you think the solution is?
Boundaries	
Touching	(Notice who touches whom, who talks to whom, presence of eye contact.)
Interaction between family members	(Notice whether the touching is parental, kind, loving, seductive, rough, violent.)
Allocation of space in household	Where does everyone sleep?
	Do you all have time alone?
Links to society	How do you get along with the adolescent's teacher? Scout leader? Other significant people in the adolescent's life?
	How do you like the adolescent's friends? Are you in touch with their parents?
Contextual clarity	
Clear generational lines	Who's in charge in this family?
Strong parental coalition	Who gets along best with whom?
	Who does what around the house?
	(Notice whether parents agree on what is happening)
Oedipal issues resolved	(Notice whether there is unusual closeness between child and opposite-sex parent.)
Communication	
Clear, direct, honest, specific	(Is communication clear, honest, specific? Do members make "I" statements or blaming "you" statements?)
Congruent	(Can the interviewer get an answer to a question? Can family members get an answer?)
	Can the interviewer follow the family conversation?)
	(Are verbal and nonverbal communications congruent?)
	How much is your television turned on?
Power	
Flows from parental coalition	(Do the parents set the tone for the interview; set limits on children's behaviors? Are the limits reasonable, not just talk or punitive?)(Does one person control the group by talking or distracting?)
Delegated to children appropriate to age	
Clear role definition	
Not sex-defined	(Does everyone talk or at least seem involved?)
Rules	Tell me your rules. What happens if they are broken?
	What are everyone's jobs at home?

Modified from Hogarth C (1987) Families and family therapy. In Johnson BS, editor, Psychiatric mental health nursing, Philadelphia, JB Lippincott Co. *Continued.*

Table 6-1   Family Assessment Guidelines—cont'd

Assessment categories	Sample questions
Encouragement of autonomy	
Differentness accepted	If you, the mother, like to stay home and read and you, the father, like to go to parties, how do you deal with these different desires?(Are members stereotyped as "the angel," "the wild one," "just like his Uncle Joe," and so on?)
	What kinds of things are you, the adolescent, interested in?
	How are you different from your siblings?
Affective issues	
Warmth and caring	(Can the interviewer feel warmth and caring, or does the
Empathy	interviewer feel uncomfortable, fearful?)
Feelings attended to	(What do you think the adolescent is feeling? What are
Amount of conflict	you feeling as you listen to the adolescent?)
	(Notice whether family members feel ashamed or embarrassed.)
Resolution of conflict	(Are conflicts resolved?)
Self-esteem of members high	What do you do when you get angry?
Negotiation and task performance	
Amount of conflict	Do you argue about household chores?
Led by parents	(Can the family solve a problem with parents having final say in the issue?)
Input from all members	Do you have meetings?
Transcendent values	
Expect loss	(Do family members believe that problems can be solved?)
Recover from and prepare for loss	
Hopeful	What do you think and feel about the adolescent going to camp? Getting married? (and so on)
	What do you (parents) do for fun?
	(Do family members accept that life is complicated, difficult, joyous, and routine?)
Altruistic	What kinds of community activities are you involved in?
	(Do family members laugh at themselves, have a sense of humor?)
Health measures	
Healthy diet	When and where do you eat meals? Do you eat one meal
Freedom from drugs and chemicals	each day together? What kinds of things do you eat?
	How often do you have a drink? Does anyone take medications?

Continued.

Table 6-1   Family Assessment Guidelines—cont'd

Assessment categories	Sample questions
Regular exercise and recreation	Tell me how you have fun.
Concern for the environment	Do you participate in sports or other
Abstinence from dangerous	exercise?
activities	What do you do to relax?
Family history of health	What illnesses have family members had?
	Grandparents, aunts, uncles?
	Any suicide, mental illness, drug or
	alcohol addictions?

friends, living conditions, neighborhood, and community. Current and past stressors, including abuse or the use of drugs, are components of this section.

The social history is gathered from the adolescent, family, and teachers. Social assessment takes into account the adolescent's social skills and social support system, including the number and quality of peer and adult supports (other than parents), relationships, and social, work, and school activities.

An evaluation of how the adolescent relates to peers of both sexes is very important, as is the style of relating to adults, such as teachers, parents, friends, and employers. School attendance and academic achievement are the major work of adolescents, and it is important to determine how the adolescent fills school as well as nonschool time. Interviews with teachers and peers may be indicated in addition to the self-reports of the adolescent and family.

Activities such as sports, music, community groups, scouts, and 4-H clubs should be listed. If the adolescent works, the type of work performed, the hours, and the pay are recorded. The adolescent's career goals should be noted, as well as how the adolescent views and is preparing for adult work and future social roles.

The adolescent's spiritual area also is explored, including the belief in and relationship with God or a supreme being or force, church affiliation and participation, and sense of hope and transcendence. Esthetic sensibilities are best noted and reported in this section.

Personality traits and signs of personality disorders often are revealed in the adolescent's social history; however, personality functioning and personality disorders to be rated on the DSM-III Axis I are seldom confirmed in the initial interviews. Antisocial and asocial behaviors, such as conduct problems, running away, run-ins with the law, gang membership, school truancy, vandalism, and frequent fighting, indicate interpersonal/social difficulties, limited impulse control, and problems in managing anger and rage should be noted. The adolescent's potential for suicide or violence toward others needs be evaluated within this social context and additional assessments such as suicide or violence potential should be made.

Personality is shaped by the interaction of physiological, psychological, and environmental/interpersonal factors. Thus, the adolescent's temperament and disposition often can be traced as it is socially and environmentally reinforced in the developmental and social histories. For example, adolescents who live in dysfunc-

Text continued on p. 148.

Areas Covered in the Mental Status Examination (MSE) of the Adolescent

Appearance and behavior

Accurate descriptions of the adolescent's outward behavior and presentation usually begin with a general description of the adolescent's clothes and self-care. Interpretations about clothing and presentation however, need be avoided, inasmuch as "stylish," "preppie," "conservative," or "punk" are subjective interpretations that lack consensus among professionals (Wallace, 1983). General appearance notations include height, weight, cleanliness, facial appearance, posture, and gait. Special characteristics, such as scars, tattoos, and the appearance of being older or younger than the chronological age, are important observations. The appropriateness of behavior for the adolescent's age and educational level is recorded.

Specific details — not generalities — about behaviors to be noted during the interview include eye contact, bizarre gestures, repetitive movements, abnormal posture, inappropriate facial expression, abnormally slow or excessive movements, and special or unusual mannerisms, such as tracking of eyes or shaking head as if shutting out unwanted voices. The last may represent responses to hallucinations.

Motor behavior observations usually are described as edgy, impatient, defiant, restless, worried, aggressive, inattentive, agitated, subdued, shaking, tremulous, rigid, pacing, or withdrawn.

The way the adolescent relates to the nurse during the interview can be described as cooperative, submissive, attentive, friendly, manipulative, approval-seeking, excessively conforming, hostile, wary, suspicious, superficial, negative, challenging, ashamed, embarrassed, or guilty.

Speech and communications

This section focuses on aspects of the adolescent's speech: rate, volume, tone of voice, and speech flow (rapid, controlled, hesitant, slow, pressured). One also looks for over- or under-productivity, paucity of ideas, clang associations, responses that are tangential, preserverative, irrelevant, neologistical, and misleading such as answering "no" to all questions.

Specific descriptions of thought process relate to the way the adolescent's words are organized and the form and organization of thought content as presented in speech are noted. Terms describing these observations include pressured speech, tangential thoughts, loosening of associations, flight of ideas, thought blocking, and illogical thoughts. The relationship and congruence between verbal and nonverbal communication, tone and content, and how interested the adolescent appears to be in communicating are also noted. Speech impediments, such as lisping or stuttering, are also described.

Modified from Sattler JM (1988) Assessment of children, ed 3, San Diego, Jerome M Sattler, Publisher.

Continued.

Areas Covered in the Mental Status Examination (MSE) of the Adolescent — cont'd

Content of thought

In this section, ruminations, delusions, obsessions, and suicidal or homicidal ideation are evaluated. Ruminations suggest anxiety and depressive states and are demonstrated by preoccupations with worries and feelings of guilt. Usually the adolescent views these thinking processes as normal, and they are caught up in and talk at length about their problems. Obsessions — the going over and over of a problem to seek an answer — are usually recognized by the teen as unusual and painful and he or she may describe efforts to try and stop them. Common themes are thoughts of violence, homosexual fears, issues of right and wrong, compulsions, recurrent ideation, fantasies, images, and impulses. The presence of suicidal or homicidal wishes or plans and the degree of intent to follow up on them should be precisely and specifically described. Delusions (strong beliefs different from others in the person's culture) also need be noted. Hallucinations or delusions may be present, but the client denies their existence at this time.

The content the client spontaneously introduces and discusses and recurring themes should be specifically described.

Sensory and motor functioning

Observations and cues about how intact the adolescent's senses are — such as hearing, sight, touch, and smell — are assessed at this time. Adequacy of gross and fine motor coordination and signs of motor difficulties, such as exaggerated movements and repetitive movements (tics, twitches, tremors, bizarre posturing, grimaces, rituals), are noted.

Cognitive functioning

Cognitive functioning can be informally assessed during the interview by observing the way the adolescent responds to questions about orientation to time, place and person, concentration, and long- and short-term memory. Formal cognitive examinations include a battery of tests with age-appropriate norms. During the interview, the nurse needs to observe and note general cognitive functioning, such as the ability to concentrate, alertness, memory for recent and remote events vocabulary, general fund of information, and age-appropriate cognitive competence relating to educational background (such as the ability to read, write and spell).

Continued.

Areas Covered in the Mental Status Examination (MSE) of the Adolescent — cont'd

Emotional functioning

Whereas mood is a subjective symptom to be recorded as reported by the adolescent, affect is a physical indicator of the immediate feelings of the client as demonstrated in facial expressions and nonverbal behaviors during the interview. This should be described by the nurse. Affect is often transient; it may be demonstrated even as the adolescent denies it (for example, while yelling aggressively). It is important that the behaviors be specifically described: for example, "denies feeling angry while frowning and banging on the table with clenched fists." Notations to be made include sad, elated, indifferent, angry , irritable, changeable, anxious, tense, suspicious, perplexed, mood swings during interview, and affect appropriate (or inappropriate) for the content of communication.

Insight and judgment

In this section the adolescent's insight and basic level of functioning and motivation are recorded. The adolescent's insight or beliefs about why he or she came to the interview and the mental health care agency and perception of the problem and the concerns of others and reasons for referral are noted. Adolescents' ideas about what caused the problem, what they can do, and how it can be alleviated are recorded. Evidence of good judgment in carrying out everyday activities of living is assessed and how the adolescent solves his or her problems in everyday living are described in terms such as impulsively, independently, responsibly, or through trial and error. The extent to which the adolescent makes use of advice and assistance from others and desires help is explored and noted.

tional, abusive, violent families or in communities where the crime rates are high frequently reflect the behaviors of their environment. Violence and acting out beget violence and acting out.

Assessment of the community is an essential component of the social assessment. Providing adequate care for adolescents and their families requires a working knowledge of the communities in which adolescents live. A continuum of care is not possible without an intimate knowledge of the community. If the adolescent is receiving services in the hospital, knowledge of follow-up services is necessary for successful completion of treatment. For the nurse who works with adolescents in school and in outpatient settings, knowledge of services, problems, and supports in the community is helpful for linking adolescents and their families to services or for modifying the therapeutic approaches. Nurses who are interested in prevention and crisis intervention must understand all aspects of the community, including the power structure, to effect change. (The boxes on pp. 150-151 present a community assessment guide that is based on the discussion in Chapter 3.)

DSM-III-R AND NURSING DIAGNOSES

Diagnostic interviews for DSM-III-R and nursing diagnoses require the interviewing skills noted earlier. The last part of the diagnostic assessment interview is the

---

Brief MSE for Adolescents*

1. What is today's date?
2. What day is it?
3. What month is it?
4. What year is it?
5. Where are you?
6. What is the name of this city?
7. What is the name of this hospital (or clinic or office)?
8. What is your name?
9. What do you do?
10. How old are you?
11. Who is the president of the United States?
12. Who was the president before him?
13. What are two major news events in the last month?
14. How did you get to this hospital (or clinic or office)?
15. What is your father's name?
16. What is your mother's name?
17. When is your birthday?
18. Where were you born?
19. [If appropriate] When did you finish elementary school?
20. [If appropriate] When did you finish high school?
21. Say these numbers after me: 6-9-5, 4-3-8-1, 2-9-8-5-7.
22. Say these numbers backwards: 8-3-7, 9-4-6-1, 7-3-2-5-8.
23. Say these words after me: pencil, chair, stone, plate.
24. What does this saying mean: "A stitch in time saves nine"?
25. What does this saying mean: "Too many cooks spoil the broth"?
26. Read these words: pat, father, setting, intervention.
27. Write these words: pat, father, setting, intervention.
28. Spell these words: spoon, cover, attitude, procedure.

From Sattler JM (1988) Assessment of children, ed 3, San Diego, Jerome M Sattler, Publisher.

*Note: Questions *1-4*, *5-7*, and *8-10* test general orientation to time, place, and person, respectively; *11-16* test recent memory; *17-20* test remote memory; *21-23* test immediate memory; *24-25* test insight and judgment; and *26-28* test oral reading, writing, and spelling skills.

---

interviewer's diagnostic perspective and identification of the major DSM-III-R syndromes that correspond to the adolescent's problems based on the materials gained from the diagnostic interview. In some cases, the data gathered is not sufficient for a definite diagnosis, and the tentative formulation usually suggests which kinds of additional tests and evaluations are needed to round out the picture, such as those described in the following clinical disorder section.

There are many excellent, comprehensive nursing assessment tools for the establishment of the related nursing diagnoses. Many excellent, comprehensive nursing assessment formats for adolescent clients have been developed and incorporate most of the DSM-III-R areas. For example, Sedgewick's holistic assessment tool for adolescents (Sedgwick, 1988), which is presented in the box on pp. 152–155 incorporates DSM-III and nursing diagnoses areas. In contrast to the clinical assessment data required for the DSM-III-R diagnoses, this tool is useful to nurses who are the primary care clinician in outpatient settings and is of special value in inpatient settings.

Text continued on p. 155.

Community Assessment Guide

Public safety

Police budget
Number of officers per population and geographical area
Type I crime rate: number of cases of murder, forcible rape, robbery, and aggravated
    assault reported per 100,000 per age-group
Type II crime rate: number of cases of burglary, larceny ($50 and over), and auto theft
    reported per 100,000 population per age-group
Police and justice services for minors

Strong economy

Retail sales: $ per 1000 population
Percentage of heads of households within census tract claiming no occupation
Unemployment rate: percentage of total work force
Number of assistance payment welfare cases
Number of income tax returns claiming adjusted gross income: under $3000, $3000 to
    $5000, $5000 to $10,000, $10,000 to $15,000, $15,000 or more
Vacancy rate: percentage of housing units in an area that are vacant or abandoned
Median assessed value of single-family units
Percentage total of subsidized starts placed in each census tract

Health care

Suicide rate: number of suicides per 100,000 population per age-group
Communicable disease index: number of cases of venereal disease, tuberculosis, and
    hepatitis reported per 1000 population
Infant mortality rate: number of deaths of children younger than 1 year old per 1000
    births
Teen pregnancy rate
Alcohol-related deaths and accidents
Mortality rates for accidents and diseases

Education

Number of high school seniors taking college board examinations (SAT/ACT)
Average per-pupil expenditures
Pupil/teacher ratio

Population

Size
Heterogeneity
Categorical equality

Modified from Lyndon B. Johnson School of Public Affairs (1987) Community analysis research
project, University of Texas at Austin. In Lyon, L, editor, The community in urban society, Chicago,
The Dorsey Press.

Continued.

Community Assessment Guide — cont'd

Social interaction

Heterogeneity
Individual liberty
Local identification
Attendance at community celebrations
Percentage voting in local elections compared with state and federal elections
Communal fraternity

Representative responsive government

Community government is proactive in dealing with social and economic problems for
    all citizens
Content of council meetings
Task forces
Response and voting records of council members

Land use

Acres of park and recreation space available per 1000 population

Transportation and distribution of goods and services

Percentage of public street miles served by public transportation
Number of traffic accidents per 100,000 population
Number of complaints submitted to city sewer, water, and garbage collection agencies
per 1000 population
General obligation bond rating
Location of services relative to consumers' work and residence
Types of services and goods available

Power structure

Business leaders
Government
Association leaders

Holistic Assessment Tool for Adolescents

Physical

Genetic history
Who in your family has had any of the following mental or emotional illnesses?
>   Depression
>   Suicide
>   Drug addiction, alcoholism
>   Schizophrenia

Health history
What illnesses, injuries, hospitalizations, or surgeries have you had?
Obtain developmental landmarks from parents.

Activities of daily living
Describe your typical day, beginning with when you get up in the morning and moving
    through the day until you go to bed at night.

Diet and elimination
What changes in your appetite and weight have occurred and over what period of time?
What problems are you having with elimination?

Exercise and activity
What kinds of activities do you participate in? How often? For how long? Any change?
What kind of exercise do you participate in? How often? For how long? Any change?

Sleep and rest
How many hours of sleep do you get? Is it adequate?
What difficulties do you have going to sleep, staying asleep, or waking up?

Tobacco, drugs, alcohol
How much do you smoke?
What drugs or medications do you take?
How much alcohol do you drink? What kinds of alcohol?
In what ways do drugs or alcohol interfere with your daily activities?

Leisure activities
What do you do for fun and recreation?

General appearance
Note any unusual physical characteristics, the style of dress, grooming, gait, posture, and
    general behavior

Body image
Describe yourself physically. What do you think about your body?
How do you feel about your body?
Do you see yourself as normal?
What would you change about your body if you could?

Sexuality
What are your worries or concerns about your sexual self?
What problems are you having with menstruation, birth control, erections, intercourse,
    or masturbation?
What is your sexual preference?

Modified from Sedgewick R (1988) The adolescent. In Beck CK, Rawlins RP and Williams SR
Mental health—psychiatric nursing, ed 2, St Louis, The CV Mosby Co.

Continued.

Holistic Assessment Tool for Adolescents — cont'd

Emotional dimension

Affect
What is the adolescent's affect?
How appropriate is the adolescent's affect to the situation?
Mood
What is your predominant mood?
Does the adolescent have mood swings?
How well do you control your emotions?
How well does the adolescent express feelings?
What are your fears and anxieties?
Are you depressed, suicidal, angry?
Do you feel hopeless?
What are your coping skills?

Intellectual dimension

Sensation and perception
Do you see, hear, feel, smell, or taste things that others do not?
Do you believe that your actions are outside your control?
How realistically does the adolescent perceive events and situations?

Memory

Immediate
Ask adolescent to repeat a question you asked.
Recent
Ask for events leading up to the adolescent's seeking help.
Remote
Ask for descriptions of events in the adolescent's early childhood.

Cognition

Is the adolescent oriented to time, place, person?
What is the adolescent's knowledge of current events?
How well is the adolescent functioning academically?

Judgment

How does the adolescent make decisions?

Insight

Does the adolescent recognize that he or she is ill and needs help?
How much does the adolescent blame others for his or her difficulties?
How much awareness does the adolescent have of the impact of his behavior on others?

Abstract thinking

What is the adolescent's style of thinking, concrete or abstract?

Attention

What is the adolescent's ability to listen and concentrate?

Continued.

Holistic Assessment Tool for Adolescents — cont'd

Communication

What is the rate of speech?
What is the tone of speech?
Does the adolescent have any speech impediments?
Is the adolescent verbally active?
Does the adolescent respond freely to questions?
Are responses relevant?
How well are thoughts organized?
Is there evidence of blocking, circumstantiality, tangentiality, flight of ideas, loose associations, neologisms?

Flexibility — rigidity

How open to new ideas and alternatives is the adolescent?
Is the adolescent upset when routine is disrupted?

Social

Self-concept

Describe yourself, including your strengths and limitations. What kind of person would you like to be?

Interpersonal relations

Who is your best friend?
How do you get along with your parents, your brothers and sisters, your peers, people at school, at work, and in the community?
How much time do you spend with your family?
Who is supportive for you?
How do you get along with authority figures?

Cultural factors

What traditions do you and your family observe?
What conflicts arise from these traditions?

Environmental factors

What situations or events are stressful for you?
What risk-taking events do you participate in?

Level of socialization

How conforming or nonconforming is the adolescent?
What evidence is there of legal difficulties?
How well does the adolescent accept responsibility?

Trust-mistrust

How suspicious is the adolescent?
How naive is the adolescent?

Dependence-independence

What evidence is there of dependence-independence conflicts?
In what areas does the adolescent demonstrate autonomy?
In what areas does the adolescent demonstrate dependence?

Continued.

Holistic Assessment Tool for Adolescents — cont'd

Spiritual

Philosophy of life
What is your purpose in life?
What is important about life to you?
Who is your hero?
Sense of transcendence
Are you an optimist or a pessimist?
Do you think life can be better?
What can you do to make it better?
Concept of deity
What is your view of God or a higher power?
How similar is it to your parents' or family's views?
How comforting is your relationship with God or a higher power?
Spiritual fulfillment
What is beautiful to you?
What are your creative abilities?
What do you believe about life and death?
Are you preoccupied with religion?
What conflicts arise from your religious beliefs?
How much do you question or reject your parents' beliefs?
How do you implement your own belief system?

The boxes on pp. 156-162 are an example of a format for comprehensive nursing admission assessment. It compiles pertinent information in a consistent and comprehensive format and has been found to be a useful tool in adolescent inpatient settings.

Other Special Evaluation Procedures

NEUROPSYCHOLOGICAL EVALUATIONS

The recent development of computed tomography (CT) has remarkably altered traditional assessment procedures. New techniques have been especially important in the diagnosis of the disorders historically known as the major psychoses, schizophrenia and depressive disorders. These objective diagnostic techniques provide observable evidence that verifies many theoretical explanations set forth prior to brain study for these major mental disorders (Behar and others, 1984; Gilberg and Svendsen, 1983).

Advances in tomographical techniques have contributed information that has led to important changes in the diagnosis and treatment of many adolescent disorders. The results of laboratory studies of brain function and structure have affected diagnostic decision making and theoretical explanations. According to Behar and others (1984), research findings based on studies in endoscopic retrograde pancreatography (ERP) have challenged traditional underarousal and maturational lag theories of hyperactivity. In addition, organic brain changes have been found in

Text continued on p. 163.

Nursing Admission Assessment

General history

Section A: Must be completed by RN, LPN, or MHT

From: Home ____   Mode: Ambulatory _____

AM   Other ____   Wheelchair _____

Date: ____   Time: ____ PM   Nursing Home: ____   Stretcher _____

Religious preference: _____

Referral source: _____

Patient's rights: Voluntary _____   Involuntary _____   Basic: minor/legal __

Patient's rights explained: _____

Legal guardian's name: _____

Parent/guardian rights explained: _____

Male/female:

Vital signs   Temperature: ____ Pulse: ____ Respiration: ____ BP: Right arm _____

Left arm _____

Height: _____ Weight: _____ Hair color: _____ Eye color: _____

Allergies   NKA: _____   Drugs: _____

Food: _____   Other: _____

Smoking Habits: _____

Informed of Smoking Policy: Yes _____ No_____

Valuables checked: Yes _____ No _____ Envelope No. _____

Car on premises: Yes _____ No _____ If yes, give reason: _____

Patient's belongings searched: Yes _____ No _____ If yes, give reason:

Aids for daily living: N/A, hearing, glasses, contact lenses, dentures, dental appliances

Describe _____

Ambulation needs: N/A, walker, crutches, wheelchair, cane, other _____

_____

Describe: _____

Patient's ID band on: Yes ____ No ____ Admission forms signed: Yes ____ No _____

Oriented to unit Yes: _____ No _____   Signature/title: _____

Section B: Must be completed by RN

Patient's/parents reason for hospitalization: _____

From Dettmer Hospital, Troy, Ohio.

Continued.

Nursing Admission Assessment — cont'd

Patient stressors: Parental illness, divorce, separation, death of significant other,
   moving, change of school, loss of peers

Support system: mother, father, siblings, teachers, friends, pastor, physician,
   other _____

Patient's strengths: Patient's weaknesses:

Patient's goals during hospitalization:

History of previous psychiatric treatment:

History of medical/physical problems:

Current medical/physical problems:

Current Drug Therapy: Does patient have medication
Yes ____ No ____   here? Yes _____ No _____
Medication: _____
Dose: _____
Frequency: _____
Last taken: _____

Section C: Nutrition and sleep

Appetite   Weight gain: Yes ____ No ____
change: Yes ____ No ____   Weight loss: Yes ____ No ____
Eating problems: _____
Diet restrictions: _____
Caffeinated beverage: _____
Food allergies: _____
Overall physical appearance: Well nourished ____ Obese ____ Poorly nourished ____
                             Frail __ Run down __ Other _____
Regular hours of sleep: Yes _____ No_____
Difficulty falling asleep: Yes ____ No____ Restlessness:Yes ____ No ____
Early AM awakening: Yes ____ No ____ Nightmares: Yes ____ No ____

Continued.

Nursing Admission Assessment — cont'd

Section D: Developmental and school history

Immunizations up-to-date? Yes _____ No _____ Other _____

Family physician _____

History of alcohol and/or drug abuse:

Developmental and school history

Problems during pregnancy and birth? _____

Birth weight _____   What number is the child in the family? _____

Approximate age at which child accomplished activity during toddler stage; yes/no in other stages:

<u>Toddler stage</u> (12 mo-3 yr)	<u>Juvenile 6-9 yr)/ preadolescent (9-12 yr) stages</u>	<u>Adolescent stage</u>
____ Feeds self	____ Peer importance vs. family importance	____ Shows concern for appearance
____ Walks alone	____ Friends are of same peer group	____ Normal rebellion vs. acting out
____ Says first word (15 mo)	____ Hormonal and physical characteristics	____ Member of peer group
____ Dresses himself	____ Competitive in all activities	____ Selection of future occupation/college
____ Becomes toilet trained trained (1-3 yr)		

Current school address: _____

Current grade level: ____	LD classes: Yes ____ When ____ No ____	SBH classes: Yes ____ When ____ No ____

Schoolwork is: _____ Below average   ____ Average   ____ Above average

Extracurricular activities: _____

What psychological or achievement tests have been administered? _____

School contact person _____

Overactivity: fidgeting, inability to sit still, slowed movement or speech, teachers complaining of distracting behavior in class

Age of onset: ____

Treatment for attention deficit disorder _____

Circle those that apply: stealing, lying, destructiveness of property, temper tantrums, cruelty to people, cruelty to animals, self-mutilation, extreme sibling rivalry, overly sensitive, overly dependent, shyness, anxiety, tension, social withdrawal, truancy, depression, sadness, mood swings, defies authority, fire setting, sexual acting out, runaway history

Explanations: _____
_____

Nursing Admission Assessment—cont'd

Section E: Review of systems: (enter "C" for current problem, "P" for past problem)

General
____ Fever/chills
____ Weakness
____ Fatigue
____ Diabetes
____ Anemia

Respiratory
____ Smoker
____ Dyspnea
____ Cough
____ Wheezing
____ Pain
____ Asthma
____ TB/emphy-
sema

Head
____ Headaches
____ Dizziness/
infection
____ Ear pain/
infection
____ Tinnitus
____ Diplopia
____ Double vision
____ Head injuries
when ____
____ Nose bleeds

Neurological
____ Seizures/
convulsions
First-
____ last ____
how fre-
quent _____
____ Temper out-
burst
____ Facial tics
____ Blackouts
when ____how
often ____
____ Unconscious-
ness
how
long _____
____ EEG
when _____
where _____
____ CT scan
when _____
where _____

Gastrointestinal
____ Nausea/
vomiting
____ Constipation
____ Diarrhea
____ Melena
____ Indigestion

Cardiovascular
____ Chest pain
____ Palpitations
____ Orthopnea
____ Heart murmur
____ BP high/low
____ EKG
when _____
where_____

Genitourinary
____ Pain/burning
____ Urgency/
hesitancy
____ Discharge
____ Discoloration
____ Enuresis
____ Encopresis

Skin
____ Rashes/hives/
lesions
____ Burns
____ Abrasions
____ Bruising
____ Lacerations
when _____
where _____

Musculoskeletal
____ Scoliosis
____ Skull fracture
____ Sports injury
____ Childhood ar-
thritis
____ Muscle pain/
weakness

Gynecological
____ Breast lumps
____ Amenorrhea
____ Dysmenorrhea
____ Pregnancy
____ Abortions
____ Last menstrual
period
____ Birth control

Section F: Mental status

Level of consciousness: Responds to: ____ Verbal stimuli/alert
                                             ____ Touch
                                             ____ Pain
                                             ____ Nonresponsive

Appearance and behavior: _____

Posture: normal rigid limp bizarre ill at ease other

Gait: normal brisk shuffling swaggering slow other _____

Continued.

Nursing Admission Assessment — cont'd

Section F: Mental Status — cont'd

Movements:
____ Coordinated
____ Agitated
____ Clumsy
____ Hyperactive
____ Jerky
____ Graceful
____ Immobile
____ Posturing
____ Quick
____ Retarded
____ Restless
____ Rituals
____ Tremors
____ Smooth
____ Fidgeting
____ Picking
____ Purposeless
____ Hand-wringing
____ Uncoordinated
____ Effeminate
____ Other

Grooming:
____ Neat
____ Well-groomed
____ Poor
____ Meticulous
____ Other

Facial Expression:
____ Appropriate
____ Dazed
____ Perplexed
____ Staring
____ Grimacing
____ Lip smacking
____ Masked
____ Other

Dress
____ Appropriate
____ Neat
____ Unkempt
____ Soiled
____ Torn
____ Bizarre
____ Other

Eye contact:
____ Direct
____ Glaring
____ No contact
____ Fixed
____ Indirect
____ Darting
____ Other

Continued.

Nursing Admission Assessment — cont'd

Section F: Mental Status — cont'd

Speech (circle those that apply)

Pace: normal pressured retarded blocking mute stuttering other ___
Volume: normal very loud very soft monotonous whisper yelling other ___
Form: logical coherent illogical rambling circumstantial other ___
Clarity: clear slurred garbled other ___
Content: normal flight of ideas loose associations echolalia obscene
          word salad neologisms rhyming other ___

Attitude and sensorium

Patient's statement of mood: _____
Examiner's evaluation — Affect:

___ angry	___ depressed	___ hopeless	___ inappropriate
___ anxious	___ euphoric	___ helpless	___ sad
___ appropriate	___ fearful	___ hostile	___ suspicious
___ blunted	___ flat	___ irritable	___ indifferent
___ calm	___ guarded	___ labile	___ other
___ cheerful	___ happy	___ manic	

Attention: (circle those that apply): normal span, alert, hyperalert, easily distracted,
fluctuating, short span, other _____
Orientation: Person Yes ___ No ___;   Place Yes ___ No ___;
          Time Yes ___ No ___
Memory — intact for: Remote events Yes ___ No ___
          Immediate recall Yes ___ No ___
          Recent events Yes ___ No ___
Judgment (overall): Good ___   Fair ___ Poor _____
Insight: Complete denial ___   Intellectual awareness ___
          Minimal awareness ___ Intellectual and emotional awareness ___
Intelligence: Below average ___   Average ___ Above average ___

Signs and symptoms

Hallucinations: Yes ___ No ___ Type: auditory, visual, tactile, olfactory,
                                        gustatory
                                        Specify: _____
Delusions: Yes ___ No ___ Specify: _____
Illusions: Yes ___ No ___ Specify: _____
Homocidal ideation: Yes ___ No ___ Specify: _____
Grandiose ideation: Yes ___ No ___ Specify: _____
Paranoid ideation: Yes ___ No ___ Specify: _____
Phobias: Yes ___ No ___ Specify: _____
Suicidal ideation: Yes ___ No ___ Specify: _____
Obsessions/compulsions: Yes ___ No ___ Specify: _____
Ideas of reference: Yes ___ No ___ Specify: _____
Somatic complaints: Yes ___ No ___ Specify: _____
Abstract thinking: Yes ___ No ___ Specify: _____

Continued.

Nursing Admission Assessment — cont'd

Section F: Mental status — cont'd

Impulse control:
Current control ____ Good   ____ Fair   ____Poor   ____Uncertain
History of violence

History of abuse:

Past history of suicide attempts:

Present suicidal ideation:

Availability of method: _____   Lethality of method: _____

Section G: Nursing problems identified

Identified problems — prioritized
(nursing diagnosis)

1. _____
   _____
2. _____
   _____
3. _____
   _____
4. _____
   _____
5. _____
   _____

Patient/family teaching needs (general,
academic, health teaching)

1. _____
   _____
2. _____
   _____
3. _____
   _____
4. _____
   _____
5. _____
   _____

Discharge planning needs: _____
_____
_____
_____

Signature/title _____

adolescents with obsessive-compulsive disorders, resulting in more accurate diagnostic and treatment decisions. Abnormalities in brain structure and function have also been identified that support the diagnosis of dyslexia and learning disabilities in adolescents. Furthermore, differences in brain structure and function have been shown to occur in many disorders, such as autism, adolescent alcoholism, Tourette's syndrome, depression, and schizophrenia (Callaway and others, 1983).

At this time two main areas of brain imaging techniques are widely used. The first area focuses on brain anatomy and uses CT and magnetic resonance imaging (MRI). The second area deals with various brain functions: blood flow; metabolism; receptor status, for which positron emission tomography (PET) and single photon emission computed tomography (SPECT) are used, and electrophysiology, for which computerized electroencephalography (CEEG) is used. Each contemporary brain imaging technique examines the brain in a distinctive way (see box on p. 164).

PSYCHOLOGICAL EVALUATIONS

Psychological evaluations are indicated in complex psychological situations, for example, if psychosis, suicide, or loss of control is suspected (Adams and Fras, 1988). Most psychological tests are "norm-referenced," that is, psychologists have identified norms of response for various ages and diagnostic groups. Although there are a limited number of tests developed specifically for the adolescent age-group, adaptations of adult tests are available that have proved somewhat clinically useful. Most psychological tests require that a clinical psychologist administer and interpret results. Nurse clinicians, however, need to be familiar with tests generally used with adolescents, the behaviors they measure, and the normal expectations and their implications for diagnoses and management.

One of the most widely used psychological tests of intelligence or cognition used with children aged 6 to 15 years is the Wechsler Intelligence Scale for Children, Revised (WISC-R). The test consists of verbal and performance scales and detects the presence of learning disabilities and some behavior disorders. Interpretation of the tests results, however, requires a skilled psychologist, inasmuch as initial scores can obscure more serious problems. For example, youngsters with perceptual or perceptual-motor dysfunctions and with developmental language or reading disorders usually show combinations of deficiencies on one or both of the subscales. Of interest is the classic WISC-R finding: a performance IQ of 15 points above (conduct disorder) or below (attention deficit disorder with hyperactivity) the youngster's verbal IQ (Adams and Fras, 1988).

Personality tests provide structured data on a person's conflicting motives, impulses, and inner conflicts, as well as the psychological defenses that have been developed against them. Most personality or projective tests provide the adolescent an ambiguous stimulus, such as a picture or an incomplete sentence, and request that the person respond to the stimulus. It is expected that examinees will "project" their personality in response. These tests are used to provide hints on the young person's psychological needs, impulses, affects, reality testing, self-image, self-esteem, relationship to parents, defense mechanisms, and coping devices. The following are the most frequently used projective tests:

1. Thematic Apperception Test (TAT) consists of a series of unstructured picture

---

Neuroimaging Techniques

Computed tomography (CT scan)

Brain structure is examined by the differential absorption of x-rays in the gray matter, white matter, and cerebrospinal fluid. Cross-sectional images are produced from various angles. Used to detect lesions and calcified tissue. Limited studies suggest neuropathological differences in some disorders.

Positron emission tomography (PET scan)

With the use of various biochemical tracers with radioactive isotope labels of carbon, oxygen, and fluorine, cross-sectional images of the brain show regional brain metabolism or hypermetabolic areas around seizure foci. Not used in children and adolescents as yet.

Magnetic resonance imaging (MRI scan)

Detailed anatomical images of brain structures are obtained without ionizing radiation. This method provides more detailed information than does the CT scan. Although limited studies have been conducted with the use of this scan in children and adolescents, young children diagnosed with infantile autism have been reported to have larger fourth ventricular area than do their normal counterparts. No definite findings at this time.

Single photon emission tomography (SPECT)

Blood flow studies that use isotopes thought to contribute to premature aging of brain and to cardinal features of antidiuretic hormone deficiency. No definite findings as yet.

Electrophysiology computerized electrocephalography (CEEG)

Compared to other forms of functional neuroimgaing (PET or SPECT), easier to perform, noninvasive does not involve radiation. Nonspecificity, artifacts, and other confounding variables limit usefulness and applications.

Modified from Kuperman S, Gaffney GR, Hamdan-Allen G, Preston DF, and Venkatesh L (1990) Neuroimaging in child and adolescent psychiatry, American Academy of Child and Adolescent Psychiatry 29(2):159-172.

---

cards showing the people in various ambiguous situations so that the pictures can be interpreted in a variety of ways. The Symonds Picture Story Test (SCT), specifically designed for adolescents, is based on the same unstructured stimulus principles as those of the TAT.

2. The Rorschach test, the least structured and most ambiguous of all projective tests, is famous for its inkblots that stimulate interpretations that provide information about interpersonal relationships, reality testing, imagination, and how the person manages affect.

3. Incomplete sentence tests, which require the person to complete the sentences and provide cues to immediate stresses, coping mechanisms, and defenses.

Personality inventories consist of questions the examinee answers as true or false. They measure personality traits that can be compared with normative samples. Since the Minnesota Multiphasic Personality Inventory (MMPI), widely used with adults, is not suitable for youngsters, the Personality Inventory for Children (PIC), was developed from the MMPI. The PCI can be interpreted on the basis of adolescent scales. These and other psychological tests frequently used with adolescents are noted in Table 6-2.

A number of diagnostic instruments have been developed during the past decade that assist in the formulation of psychiatric diagnoses for adolescents. These interviews cover a range of psychiatric disturbances. Some of the instruments in use that have psychometric support are the Diagnostic Interview for Children and Adolescents (Wellner and others, 1987), the Diagnostic Interview Schedule for Children (Costello and others, 1985), and the Children's Version of the Schedule for Affective Disorders and Schizophrenia (Puig-Antich, 1983).

Many experts attribute the "underdiagnosis" of many adolescent disorders, such as depression and suicide potential, to the limited number of psychological diagnostic measurements that have been specifically developed for use with the adolescent age-group. Because of the lack of developmentally relevant age-specific psychological tests, it has been customary to use adult psychological measures. Thus the recently developed Millon Adolescent Personality Inventory (MAPI) has been well-received and is being widely used by clinical psychologists. Its availability is expected to improve the ability to identify the adolescent personality that is prone to depression, suicide, and other psychopathological disorders. Several published research projects based on the MAPI suggest two depressive dimensions: the withdrawn, socially disengaged adolescent who is easily recognized and the adolescent whose depression is overshadowed by acting out tendencies and is thus more difficult to recognize (Ehrenberg and others, 1990) and missed in earlier MAPI adaptations.

Tests that measure social adjustment and adaptive behaviors also have been limited in number. The Vineland Social Maturity Scale has been widely used, and the Vineland social quotient (SQ) score can be used on the DSM-III-R adaptive functioning Axis V. The recently developed Children's Global Assessment Scale (CGAS) also provides an adaptive rating for Axis V.

Behavior-rating scales, in contrast to psychological tests, are not the exclusive domain of psychologists. They are used by members of the interdisciplinary team. These scales focus on observable actions, rather than inferred psychopathological factors and are frequently used with parents, teachers, and self-administered adolescents. A wide variety of rating scales are available, and most have been developed for a specific behavioral diagnostic category. The best known behavioral scales used in educational settings have been developed by Connors (1985) for specific disorders, such as hyperactivity, and for specific populations, such as the Connors' Parent Symptom Questionnaire and the Connors' Teacher Rating Scale (1985). Three frequently used behavioral rating scales in inpatient settings are the Brief Psychiatric Rating Scale, the Massachusetts Adolescent Level of Functioning Scale, and the Beck Depression Scale for Children (Beck, 1974; Carlson, 1980; Kovacs, 1985).

Text continued p. 168.

Table 6-2   Commonly Used Psychological Tests

Name	General classification	Description	Special features
Bender (Visual-Motor Gestalt Test)	Graphomotor technique; may be used as projective technique	Geometric designs that the patient is asked to draw or copy, with design in view	Useful for detecting psychomotor difficulties usually correlated with brain damage
California Personality Inventory	Objective personality test	Seventeen scales developed presumably from normal populations for use in guidance	Less emphasis on mental illness than MMPI scales; measures dominance, responsibility, socialization
Cattell 16 Personality Factor Questionnaire (16 PF)	Objective personality test	Questionnaire covering 16 personality factors derived from factor-analysis	Bipolar variables allow for interpretation of scores varying either above or below the norm, such as reserved vs. outgoing; trusting v. suspicious, timid vs. venturesome
Draw-a-Person Test	Graphomotor projective technique	Patient draws a person and then one of the sex opposite to their first drawing	Projects body image, how the body is conceived and perceived; useful for detecting brain damage; modifications include: draw an animal; draw a house, a tree and a person (H-T-P); draw your family; draw the most unpleasant memory you can think of
Millon Adolescent Personality Inventory (MAPI)			In process of testing. Newly developed
Minnesota Multiphasic Personality Inventory (MMPI) (forms: individual, group, and shortened R)	Objective personality test	Questionnaire yielding scores for 9 clinical scales in addition to other scales	Includes scales related to test-taking attitudes; empirically constructed on basis of clinical criteria; computer interpretation services available
Rorschach technique	Projective technique	Ten inkblots used as basis for eliciting associations	Especially revealing of personality structure; most widely used projective technique

Modified from Freedman AM, Kaplan HI and Sadock BJ editors, (1981) Comprehensive textbook of psychiatry, ed 3, Baltimore, The Williams & Wilkins Co.   *Continued.*

Table 6-2   Commonly Used Psychological Tests—cont'd

Name	General classification	Description	Special features
Rosenzweig Picture Frustration Test	Projective technique	Carton situations, dialogue to be completed by subject	Designed specifically to assess patterns of reaction to typical stress situations; child, adolescent, and adult forms
Sentence completion test (SCT)	Varies from direct response questionnaire to projective technique	Incomplete sentence stems that vary as to their ambiguity	Highly flexible; may be used to tap specific conflict areas; reveals generally more conscious, overt attitudes and feelings
Symonds Picture Story Test	Projective technique	Pictures of adolescents	Designed specifically for adolescents
Thematic Apperception Test (TAT)	Projective technique	Ambiguous pictures used as stimuli for making up a story	Especially useful for revealing personality dynamics; some pictures are designed specifically for women, men, adolescent girls, and adolescent boys
Wechsler Adult Intelligence Scale (WAIS)	Intelligence test	Eleven subtests: vocabulary, comprehension, information, similarities, digit span, arithmetic, picture arrangement, picture completion, object assembly, block design, and digit symbol	Most commonly used intelligence scale that yields a measure of intelligence expressed as IQ scores; differences in subtests can also be used clinically
Wechsler Intelligence Scale for Children (WISC)	Intelligence test	Similar to the WAIS	Standardized for children ages 5 to 15
Wechsler Preschool and Primary Scale of Intelligence (WPPSI)	Intelligence test	Similar to the WAIS and WISC	Standardized for children ages 4 to 6½
Word-association technique	Projective technique	Stimulus words to which patient responds with first association that comes to mind	Flexible; may be used to tap associations to different conflict areas; generally not as revealing as SCT responses

Behavioral rating scales are used for assessment and also for measuring changes in behavior as treatment progresses. The scales provide important documentation of changes in behavior as a result of interventions—documentation that is important in that it increases knowledge of effective nursing interventions, provides data for quality assurance programs, and justifies quality treatment to third-party payers.

Assessment of Specific Clinical Disorders

ACTING OUT

Although acting out is not a diagnostic label in itself, it is a behavioral component of the many adolescent mental disorders and is discussed in Chapter 5. Assessment of the adolescent's potential for acting out is essential to determine when acting out behavior is inappropriate and requires intervention. Clinicians need to assess the actions or symptoms in the context of the relationship the behaviors pose to normal development. The social consequences of acting out are the most important assessment considerations. Violations of social rules via acting out are major concerns, and prudent nurses are especially alert to the adolescent's increased potential to act out in the days immediately after admission.

In addition to clinical observations of verbal and nonverbal behaviors, several psychological tests are used routinely in comprehensive diagnostic work-ups. When administered to adolescents before hospitalization, these tests contribute to the assessment of the adolescent's potential for acting out.

The Wechsler scales (Blatt, 1986) provide many indications of potential for acting out. They also summarize the acting out profiles presented earlier (Blatt, 1987):

1. Imbalance between performance scale and verbal scale, with the performance scale IQ exceeding the verbal scale
2. Behavior and responses during tests that are impulsive and unreflective
3. Action-oriented verbalization rather than conceptual and abstract definitions
4. Impaired judgment, defiance of social conventionality, or lack of anticipation and planning as reflected in low scores in the category of Comprehension or Picture Arrangement
5. Qualitative aspects of response to items in Comprehension or in story response to Picture Arrangement sequences that indicate impaired judgment or a defiance of social conventionality
6. Impulsiveness indicated by heightened anxiety and a diminished tolerance for anxiety
7. Negativism

Other psychological tests provide and confirm assessment concern about acting out. Four patterns found in Rorschach test responses relate acting out to personality structure and emphasize alterations in areas of inner controls, resourcefulness, depression, behavior patterns, obsessive-compulsive behavior, and overattention to unimportant details (Levi, 1987). When projective drawing assessments are used with young adolescents, such as the Draw-a-Person (DAP) test, some cues to potential acting out are also found, as in drawings of aggressive characters in the composition, in forceful strokes, and in use of color (Wadeson, Durkin, and Perach, 1989).

BEHAVIOR AND CONDUCT DISORDERS

Defiant, conduct, and attention deficit with hyperactivity disorders are categorized under disruptive behavior disorders in the DSM-III-R and, as noted earlier, are the most prevalent acting out behavior disorders of adolescence.

Longitudinal, comparative behavioral studies of nonreferred (normal) and referred conduct of youngsters and their parents were conducted at the Oregon Social Learning Center (Patterson and others, 1982, 1983). These findings provide a developmental framework for assessing some of the social differences among and between these adolescents and their parents, findings useful for clinicians during the screening process and in planning interventions. In these studies a variety of psychological tests and data collection methods were used, such as parent, peer, and teacher interviews; parent and child self-reports; sociometric studies; and observations of behaviors in classrooms, at home, and in formal and informal community settings and activities.

These researchers found two additional constructs, which they added to the usual model of parenting behaviors: inept parental discipline and inept parental monitoring (Patterson, 1982). Inept discipline is failure of parents to back up threats, persistence of nagging in response to both trivial and significant deviant behaviors, and use of extreme forms of physical punishment. Inept monitoring refers to the parents' failure to be aware of or to believe reports of their youngsters' conduct disorder.

The following statements summarize some of the findings of the Patterson report (1982) and of other psychological studies that identify parental behaviors of youngsters with conduct disorders (aged 6 to 16 years) that appear to contribute to and reinforce the noncompliant behaviors and that differ from the behaviors of parents of adolescents who do not have conduct disorders. An assessment of the family characteristics of adolescents with conduct disorders usually reveals parents who exhibit the following patterns:

1. They are more commanding and critical of their children.
2. They use poor disciplinary measures and inadequately monitor their adolescent and school-aged children's activities, as shown by court records and self-reports of delinquency behaviors.
3. They monitor younger children with less concern and attention than they monitor adolescent children, indicating a developmental change in the significance most families attribute to this important developmental period.
4. They manage the children in their family differently. These fathers take a secondary role less frequently than do fathers of nonreferred children and adolescents.
5. They experience more depression, anxiety, and personal, interparental, and marital conflict, and extrafamily distress than do parents of children and adolescents without behaviors, that reflect conduct disorders.
6. Marital distress is directly related to the parents' biased perceptions of the child or adolescent's noncompliance. This rejecting or scapegoating of youngsters when there is marital discord is more frequently directed at boys than at girls.

7. They have higher frequencies of stressful events in their lives.
8. They are more isolated, distant, critical, and dissatisfied with friends, neighbors, and the community than are nonreferred children. Family interactions with relatives and helping agencies are more negatively perceived, and there is a low level of positively perceived support from friends. Findings reflect the "insularity construct" (Dumas and Wahler, 1984) that identifies those parental attitudes found in persons who are unable to sustain the positive effects of treatment. Parents with aversive relationships outside the home have aversive interactions with their children.
9. Their personal distress, depression, and anxieties are associated with misperceptions of the child's behavior. Maternal depression is a significant factor in misperceptions and the mislabeling of the child's problems in the referral process.
10. They experience depression that influences parenting behaviors. The youngster's behavior is perceived as deviant by depressed parents, and depression changes parenting behaviors. As the number of parental commands directed at the child increases, the level of noncompliant responses by the child increases (Furey and Forehand, 1986).

The following statements reflect some of the clinical distinctions that distinguish children and adolescents with referred and non-referred conduct disorders:

1. Family interactions. Youngsters with behavior disorders were found to exhibit more adverse behaviors in family interactions.
2. Peer interactions. Children with conduct disorders exhibit more adverse behaviors with their peers. Parents reported them to be less socially competent than other children and more likely to be rejected by their peers.
3. Cognitive distortions. Children with conduct disorders were found to misread or misperceive hostile intentions in others. Aggressive children and adolescents distort social cues in interactions and perceive others to have hostile intentions toward them. This attribution bias also is held by other family members.
4. Social problem-solving skills. Aggressive youths are more deficient in social problem-solving skills; they evaluate aggressive interpersonal styles as more desirable than nonaggressive. Aggressive youths were found to be less empathic than were nonaggressive youths.
5. Depression. A close association among conduct disorders, depression, and attention deficit hyperactivity disorder was noted. The relationship of depression and conduct disorders has been found to be much higher in males.
6. Academic achievement. Children with conduct disorders have poorer academic achievement than do their counterparts, starting in elementary grades. It was found that low academic performance and being held back, beginning at the third grade, occurred three times as often in adolescents with behavior disorders in junior high school than it did in matched control groups. In addition, reading disabilities were highly associated with conduct disorders.

The assessment of adolescents with oppositional, defiant, and conduct disorder, and attention deficit hyperactivity disorder includes many similar techniques. Problem behaviors occur most often in the adolescent's social interactions with familiar adults and peers. Because clinicians initially lack this familiarity, many of the disruptive behaviors reported by others may be missed during first encounters and initial screening. Thus several assessment interviews need to be conducted. Further, to complete this assessment, the clinician needs to use the various psychological and behavioral scales developed for teachers and parents.

ATTENTION DEFICIT HYPERACTIVITY DISORDER

During the last decades, valuable research has provided remarkable expansions in the assessment tools for attention deficit hyperactivity disorder (ADHD). In addition to these scientific advances in assessment, reliable, valid tools and techniques now measure treatment intervention outcomes, marking the many positive advances in care.

Theoretical explanations and DSM-III-R diagnostic criteria have a number of significant implications for the clinical assessment of young adolescents with ADHD. On first encounter, the clinician needs to be sensitive to the distress and guilt most parents are experiencing and should avoid blaming and focus on seeking solutions. Lack of empathy can push the parents into defensive behavior. All too often these parents have been exposed to the myth that "there are no problem children, only problem parents." This prevalent attitude reinforces guilt feelings and causes parents to believe that they are responsible for their child's ADHD. At one time or another most clinicians encounter parents whose expectations of adolescent behavior are overly demanding or who are naive about normal adolescent development.

In most cases the mother, who has known the youngster longer than anyone else and is the one who has the most contact with the child, is the most reliable source of the adolescent's and family's history. However, it is often difficult to obtain a factual history rather than a report of what mother thinks or a defensive response to criticism by others. Areas such as the adolescent's degree of distractibility, attention deficit, overall life-style, and characteristic ways of reacting are important information to gather.

1. Explore the parent's report of the adolescent's attention span in detail. This is a central symptom and may include behavior descriptions such as "fidgeting, can't sit still, can't stay with things." This behavior reflects the youngster's inability to screen out incidental stimuli, both external (for example, sights and sounds) and internal (for example, impulses and stimulus hunger). Evidence of stimulus barrier deficits are revealed when clients are easily distracted by irrelevant stimuli, when their focus is constantly shifting, and when their attention span improves in one-to-one contact in a quiet environment such as the clinical interview.

2. Hyperactivity is erratic and random, and the parents' report of a high activity level is not diagnostic of ADHD, although the most prominent feature is gross motor overactivity. The youngster appears "driven," "like a tornado," moving actively from one thing to another. This "perpetual motion" is without apparent purpose to the observing, reporting parent. However, for the adolescent these manifestations may be self-stimulating actions to further motor activity.

3. Impulsive behavior is a major concern. Parents may report the youngster's violence toward siblings, peers, and animals. Actions occur on the spur of the

moment, as do picking fights and tormenting and beating others up. Killing of animals is the most ominous sign of defect in impulse control.

During the interview the attention span of these adolescents deteriorates after 15 minutes of watching and looking. They display many nonverbal extraneous movements that reflect restlessness, such as shifting their legs, twisting their hair, and drumming their fingers. These activities usually are signs of the need for sensory input and a search for distractions. They also can indicate that the adolescent is distraught, unhappy, anxious, or depressed. Their verbal communication reveals a use of language that is superficial and concrete. Some experts claim that these adolescents experience less than average psychic pain and react differently from their peers to social rejection and negative parental and adult disappointments. It is clear, however, that the considerable negative reactions they experience in their environment cause the development of low self-esteem. Thus low self-esteem is one of the major areas clinicians focus on during one-to-one psychotherapy with ADHD adolescents.

Nurse clinicians who work with hyperactive youngsters need to become familiar with the many behavior checklists and rating scales that are essential tools for the evaluation and management of ADHD. Table 6-3 presents evaluation instruments useful in the assessment of adolescent difficulties with compliance.

Research indicates that disagreements between the parents of hyperactive youngsters are more frequent than they are between the parents of normal youngsters or those with different psychopathological conditions. The stress that the hyperactive child places on the family system often is the reason why marriages break down. Therefore, from the first encounter, the clinician needs to assist parents with the adolescent and with other weakened family interactions, and family therapy may be necessary.

The following areas, which describe the adolescent's behavior during activities of daily living, also require immediate attention: mealtimes, while parents are on the telephone, when watching television, while visitors are at the home, while visiting other homes, in public places such as supermarkets, while the mother is occupied with chores or activities, when the father is at home, when asked to do a chore, at bedtime, and during other daily life situations such as in the car and in church. For each of these situations, the parents should be asked the following "probe" questions (Barkley, 1981):

1. Is this a problem area?
2. What does the adolescent do in this situation that bothers you?
3. What is your response?
4. What will the adolescent do next?
5. If the problem continues, what will you do next?
6. What usually is the outcome of this interaction?
7. How often do these problems occur in this situation?
8. How do you feel about these problems?
9. On a scale of 0 to 10 (0 = no problem; 10 = severe), how severe is this problem for you?

Behavior modification interventions based on operant conditioning that rewards the delay of gratification and self-control are among the most widely and successfully used interventions. Thus the collection of the aforementioned data during the initial

Table 6-3   Evaluation Instruments for Assessment of Adolescent Difficulties with Compliance

Rating scale	Author(s), date	Brief description
Child Behavior Checklist	Achenback and Edelbrock, 1979, 1981, 1986, 1987	Scale that identifies 20 social competency and 118 behavior problem–items. Normative data and profiles for adolescents aged 12-16 years for both sexes. Attention to developmental changes. Factor scales for schizoid, depressed, uncommunicative, somatic complaints, obsessive, social withdrawal, hyperactive, aggressive and delinquent behaviors. Parent respondent (1979). Youth respondent (1981). Teacher respondent (1986).
Conners' Parent Rating	Conners, 1985; revised	48-item rating scale with five factors: conduct, learning, psychosomatic, impulsive, hyperactive, anxiety. Used most to evaluate hyperactive youngsters and treatment responses. Briefer than CBCL, sensitive to medication and parent training interventions. Used for baseline pretreatment measures.
Home and School Questionnaire	Barkley, 1987	Evaluates areas in which children have problems, in contrast to the type of problem, as in the scales above. Has 16 situations and discriminates ADHD behavior from that of normal children; sensitive to drug and parent training intervention changes.
Self-Report Rating Scales for Children	Achenback and Edelbrock, 1981, 1986	Similar to CBCL; for children aged 11-18 years; first-person wording. Reliability and validity norms not established as yet; however, very useful for clinician's comparisons of perception differences among child, parents, and teachers.
Behavior Problems Checklist	Quay and Peterson, 1987	Consists of 89 items completed by parents and teachers; measures conduct and personality problems, such as inadequate, immature and socially delinquent. Composed of six factors: conduct disorder and socialized aggression; attention problems, anxiety, withdrawal, psychotic behavior, and motor excess. Used for screening, evaluating dimensions of deviant behavior and treatment outcomes.

Continued.

Table 6-3   Evaluation Instruments for Assessment of Adolescent Difficulties with Compliance — cont'd

Rating scale	Author(s), date	Brief description
Eyberg Child Behavior Inventory	Eyberg, 1978	Only tool developed to assess conduct disorders per se. Completed by parents, 36 items, for use with children 2-15 years of age. Screens and measures treatment outcome.
New York— London survey	Thomas and Chess, 1977 Chess and Thomas, 1986	Measures nine dimensions of temperament, activity level, rhythms, approach to or withdrawal from new stimuli, adaptability to new situations, intensity of reactions, threshold of responses, quality of mood, distractibility, attention span, parental evaluation within a developmental framework. To be used with caution with younger age-groups directly and to establish adolescent's developmental history.
Self-Control Rating scale	Kendall and others, 1985	Consists of 33-item self-control scale focusing on adolescent's ability to inhibit behavior, follow rules, control impulsive behavior. Its construct of "self-control" useful for clinicians, parents, and teachers evaluating ADDH deficits. This scale takes into account treatment effects and self-control training.

assessment is particularly valuable. Techniques for behavioral change depend on specific items in various scales that assess and evaluate parental training interventions, drug effects, self-control training, and other interventions. Most experts advise the use of the many statistically reliable behavior modification protocols that have been developed (Stollard, 1988).

DEPRESSION

During the assessment interview, adolescents often are vague and uncertain about the precipitating events or reasons for their depression. Depressive symptoms include dysphoric mood, irritability and weeping, low self-esteem, self-deprecation, hopelessness, recent poor academic performance, disturbed concentration, diminished psychomotor behavior, withdrawal, sleep problems, weight loss or gain, and somatic complaints (DSM-III-R). Other interpersonal difficulties may be present, such as conflicts with parents, fighting with peers and siblings, drug abuse, and antisocial behavior that results in involvement with the law and sexual acting out (Carlson and Carlson, 1980; Shafii, 1988).

The assessment task is to identify transitory depressed moods that are within the limits of normal, shifting moods; periods of sadness that are related to the adolescent's attempts to progress through developmental stages of helplessness and hopelessness that often accompany hormonal changes and physical growth; and social changes that influence the adolescent's adaptation to physiological and environmental changes (Miller, 1986).

CHEMICAL DEPENDENCE

Because the defense mechanisms of denial, projection, and rationalization are associated with chemical dependence, assessment is very difficult. Furthermore, 80% of adolescents abuse alcohol as a part of their social life. All adolescents referred for counseling or inpatient treatment should be screened for chemical dependence; in some cases a complete assessment may be indicated. A chemical dependence assessment must include information from the adolescent, family members (including siblings, teachers or other school personnel), and juvenile court or police records. Before chemical dependence can be ruled out as a primary condition or secondary to another diagnosis, the adolescent should participate in several interviews based on various tools that measure chemical use.

The assessment should include specific questions about what drugs are used, the amounts, frequency of use and effects, how long each drug has been used, and the date of the last use. A careful history must be obtained for events such as blackouts, seizures, drinking and using drugs to the point of unconsciousness, or withdrawal symptoms; accidents, arrests, fights, and family violence; and stealing, skipping school, and patterns of use at school. Money or goods missing from home, changing groups of friends, mysterious telephone calls, and changes in mood and behavior with a deterioration in morals and values may be noted by the family if mentioned by the nurse; the family may not otherwise connect these events with the teenager's drug use. Several adolescent chemical dependence assessment tools have been designed to measure various aspects of use (see boxes on pp. 176-181).

Adolescent Chemical History Assessment

The questions that follow are not definitive; they can be reduced in number, altered, expanded, or rearranged. This is a data-gathering, educational, diagnostic, and awareness-building tool.

1. What do you or have you used (including inhalants)?
2. How long have you used (beginning from experimentation)?
3. Do your parents know you use? What happened when they found out (if they did)? How did you feel about that?
4. How often are you high in a week (or significant period of time)? Drunk? What do "high" and "drunk" mean to you?
5. How many of your friends use? Acquaintances?
6. Are you close to someone you are convinced has a chemical problem? Have you told them about your concern, if you are concerned?
7. Are you taking medication?
8. Do you owe money for chemicals? How much?
9. How much do you spend for chemicals in a month (if you were to pay for all your chemicals)?
10. Who provides if you are broke?
11. Have you received any negative feedback about your use? How did it make you feel?
12. Have you ever lost a friend because of your use? Boyfriends/girlfriends? What happened? How did you feel?
13. Have you lost a job because of your use? What happened? How did you feel?
14. Have you ever been "busted" (police, school, home, DWIs)? What happened? How did you feel?
15. What time of day do you use?
16. Do you use on the job or in school (during school)?
17. How is school going for you? Grades, skips, fails, absences? How do you feel about that?
18. Does it take more, less, or about the same amount to get you high?
19. Have you ever "shot up"? With what? Where on your body?
20. What is a blackout? Ever had one? Pass outs? What happened? How did it make you feel?
21. Are you sexually active?
22. Do you sneak using? How do you do it? How do you feel when you do it?
23. Do you hide stuff? How? How does it make you feel?
24. Do you have rules for using? What are they? How did they come about?
25. Did you break them? What happened? How did it make you feel?
26. Do you use alone? Isolate?
27. Have you ever tried to quit? What made you try? How did it work?
28. Have you had any withdrawal symptoms?
29. Have you lost your "good-time highs"?
30. Have you ever thought about suicide? Tried it? What happened? Were you using or high? How did you feel afterward?
31. Do you mix your chemicals when using?
32. Do you deal?

From Hazelden Foundation, Center City, Minn.

Continued.

Adolescent Chemical History Assessment — cont'd

33. Did you ever shift from one chemical to another? What happened that made you decide to shift?
34. Do you avoid people who don't use?
35. Do you avoid talking about chemical dependency?
36. Have you ever needed help when you were high? What happened? How did you feel afterward?
37. Have you done things you are ashamed of when using? What happened?
38. Who is the most important person in your life, including yourself?
39. How are you taking care of him/her?
40. On a scale of 1 to 10 (can't use 5) how is your life going?
41. Are there any harmful consequences you are aware of in your chemical use other than those touched upon?
42. Do you think your chemical use is harmful to you? Do you think you have a chemical problem?

Adolescent Self-Evaluation of Drinking Behavior

1. Are you male or female? _____
2. How old are you? _____

Nondrinking (cut-off score = 3)

	Yes	No
3. Do you use or have you ever used drugs?	1	0
4. Have you ever been "busted" for possession of an illegal drug?	1	0
5. Have you had a drink of beer, wine, or liquor more than two or three times in your life?	1	0
6. Do you consider yourself as a person who drinks?	1	0
7. Do you favor pot over alcohol?	1	0
8. Do you and your friends think sex and drinking go together?	1	0

Life-Style (cut-off score = 5)

	Yes	No
9. Do you sometimes "hang out" with kids who drink?	1	0
10. Do you prefer to be with friends who drink?	1	0
11. Do you sometimes drink because it makes you feel more at ease on a date?	1	0
12. Do you sometimes drink because it makes you feel more relaxed with the opposite sex?	1	0
13. Do you sometimes drink because it makes you feel better around people?	1	0
14. Do you sometimes drink because it helps you forget your worries?	1	0
15. Do you sometimes drink because it helps to cheer you up when you're in a bad mood?	1	0
16. Do you sometimes drink to change the way you feel?	1	0
17. Do you sometimes drink because it makes you feel stronger?	1	0
18. Have you ever borrowed money or done without other things to buy alcohol?	1	0
19. Have you ever skipped meals while drinking?	1	0
20. Do you sometimes gulp down a drink rather than drink it slowly?	1	0
21. Do you sometimes drink before going to a party?	1	0
22. Do you ever notice that your hands shake when you wake up in the morning?	1	0
23. Have you ever taken a drink in the morning?	1	0
24. Have you ever felt guilty or "bummed out" after drinking?	1	0
25. Do you ever have times when you cannot remember some of what happened while drinking?	2	0
26. Have you ever stayed "high" drinking for a whole day?	2	0
27. Do you ever get mad or get into a heated argument when you drink?	1	0
28. Have you ever gotten into a fight when drinking?	1	0

From Hazelden Foundation, Center City, Minn.

Continued.

Adolescent Self-Evaluation of Drinking Behavior — cont'd

	Yes	No
Consumption (cut-off score = 4)		
29. Do you sometimes drink until there's nothing left to drink?	2	0
30. Would you say that you get "high" when you drink more than half the time?	2	0
31. Would you say that you get "drunk" or "bombed" at least once a month or more?	2	0
32. When you drink, do you usually end up having more than four of whatever you're drinking?	2	0
33. Have you had anything to drink in the last week?	1	0
34. Would you say that you have a drink of beer, wine, or liquor at least once a week or more?	2	0
35. Do you sometimes get drunk when you didn't start out to?	2	0
36. Do you sometimes try to cut down on your drinking?	2	0
Consequences (cut-off score = 2)		
37. Have you ever missed school or missed a class because of drinking?	2	0
38. Have you ever gotten into trouble at home because of your drinking?	1	0
39. Have you ever gotten into trouble outside your home because of your drinking?	1	0
40. Have you ever gotten into trouble with the police because of drinking?	1	0

Interpretation

No problem: Score does not exceed cut-off point in any of the four categories.

Potential problem drinker: Score three or more on nondrinking category plus exceeds cut-off score on one of the remaining categories.

Problem drinker: Score three or more on nondrinking categories plus exceeds cut-off score on two of the remaining categories.

Alcoholic: Score three or more on nondrinking category plus exceeds cut-off score on all three of the remaining categories.

Interview Techniques Checklist

Name of interviewer: _____ Date of interview: _____

Name of interviewee: _____ Rater's name: _____

Rating key: 1 = Excellent demonstration of this skill
2 = Good demonstration of this skill
3 = Fair demonstration of this skill
4 = Poor demonstration of this skill
5 = Very poor demonstration of this skill
NA = Not applicable

Item		Rating				
1. Created a positive interview climate	1	2	3	4	5	NA
2. Showed respect for and attention to interviewee	1	2	3	4	5	NA
3. Used good diction	1	2	3	4	5	NA
4. Used vocabulary understandable to interviewee	1	2	3	4	5	NA
5. Formulated appropriate general questions	1	2	3	4	5	NA
6. Formulated appropriate open-ended questions	1	2	3	4	5	NA
7. Formulated appropriate follow-up questions	1	2	3	4	5	NA
8. Used appropriate structuring statements	1	2	3	4	5	NA
9. Encouraged appropriate replies	1	2	3	4	5	NA
10. Used probes effectively	1	2	3	4	5	NA
11. Allowed interviewee to express feelings and thoughts in his or her own way	1	2	3	4	5	NA
12. Was alert to interviewee's nonverbal behavior	1	2	3	4	5	NA
13. Conveyed to interviewee a desire to understand him or her	1	2	3	4	5	NA
14. Rephrased questions appropriately	1	2	3	4	5	NA
15. Used reflection appropriately	1	2	3	4	5	NA
16. Used feedback appropriately	1	2	3	4	5	NA
17. Handled minimally communicative interviewee appropriately	1	2	3	4	5	NA
18. Handled interviewee's resistance and anxiety appropriately	1	2	3	4	5	NA
19. Clarified areas of confusion in interviewee's statements	1	2	3	4	5	NA
20. Intervened appropriately when interviewee had difficulty expressing thoughts	1	2	3	4	5	NA
21. Handled rambling communications appropriately	1	2	3	4	5	NA

From Sattler JM (1988) Assessment of children, ed 3, San Diego, Jerome M Sattler, Publisher, p. 429.

Continued.

Interview Techniques Checklist — cont'd

Item		Rating				
22. Tolerated difficult behavior in interview	1	2	3	4	5	NA
23. Used props, crayons, clay, or toys appropriately	1	2	3	4	5	NA
24. Timed questions appropriately	1	2	3	4	5	NA
25. Handled silences appropriately	1	2	3	4	5	NA
26. Used periodic summaries appropriately	1	2	3	4	5	NA
27. Made clear transitions	1	2	3	4	5	NA
28. Paced interview appropriately	1	2	3	4	5	NA
29. Maintained appropriate eye contact	1	2	3	4	5	NA
30. Used own nonverbal behavior appropriately	1	2	3	4	5	NA
31. Responded in nonjudgmental manner	1	2	3	4	5	NA
32. Handled interviewee's questions and concerns appropriately	1	2	3	4	5	NA
33. Allowed interviewee to express remaining thoughts and questions at close of interview	1	2	3	4	5	NA
34. Arranged for post-assessment interview	1	2	3	4	5	NA
35. Used appropriate closing statements	1	2	3	4	5	NA
36. Conducted an appropriate interview overall	1	2	3	4	5	NA

37. Comments: _____

_____

_____

REFERENCES AND SUGGESTED READINGS

Achenbach TM and Edelbrock CS (1986) Behavioral problems and competencies reported by parents of normal and disturbed children aged four through sixteen, Monographs of the Society for Research in Child Development, 46 (1, Serial No. 188).

Achenbach TM and Edelbrock CS (1981) Child behavior checklist and youth self-report, Burlington, Vt, Author.

Achenbach TM and Edelbrock CS (1979) The child behavior profile II: boys aged 12-16 and girls aged 6-11 and 12-16, Journal of Consulting and Clinical Psychology 47:232-233.

Achenbach TM and Edelbrock CS (1987) Manual for the youth self-report and profile, Burlington, Vt, University of Vermont, Department of Psychiatry.

Achenbach TM and Edelbrock CS (1986) Manual for teacher's report form and teacher version of the child behavior profile. Burlington, Vt, University of Vermont, Department of Psychiatry.

Adams P and Fras I (1988) Beginning child psychiatry, New York, Brunner/Mazel , Inc.

American Nurses' Association (1985) Council on Psychiatric and Mental Health Nursing, Standards of child and adolescent psychiatric and mental health nursing practice, Kansas City, Mo, The Association.

American Psychiatric Association (1987) Desk reference to the diagnostic criteria from the diagnostic and statistical manual of mental disorders, 3 revised (DSM-III-R), Washington, DC, The Association.

American Psychiatric Association (1980) Diagnostic and statistical manual of mental disorders. 3, Washington DC, American Psychiatric Association.

American Psychiatric Association (1987) Diagnostic and statistical manual of mental disorders. ed 3, revised (DSM-III-R), Washington, DC, American Psychiatric Association.

Barker P (1990) Clinical interviews with children and adolescents, New York, WW Norton Co.

Barkley RA and Edelbrock CS (1987) Assessing situational variations in child behavior problems: the home and school situation questionnaires. In Prinz R, editor: Advances in behavioral assessment of children and families, vol 3, pp. 157-176, Greenwich, Conn, JAI Press.

Beck AT, Weissman A, Lester D, and Trexler L (1974) The measurement of pessimism: the hoplessness scale, Journal of Consulting Clinical Psychology 42:861.

Behar D, Rapoport JL, Berg CJ and others (1984) Computerized tomography and neuropsychological test measures in adolescents with obsessive-compulsive disorder, American Journal of Psychiatry 141:363-369.

Bierman KL and Schwartz LA (1986) Clinical child interviews: approaches and developmental considerations, Journal of Child and Adolescent Psychotherapy 3:267-278.

Blatt S (1987) The Wechsler scales and acting out. In Abt LE and Weissman SL, editors: Acting out, ed 2, Northvale, New Jersey, Jason Aronson, Inc.

Brent DA, Zelenak JP, Bukstein O, and Brown RV (1990) Reliability and validity of the structured interview for personality disorders in adolescents, Journal of the American Academy of Child and Adolescent Psychiatry 29:349-351.

Call JD (1985) Psychiatric evaluation of the infant and child. In Kaplan HI and Sadock SJ, editors, Comprehensive textbook of psychiatry/IV, vol 2, ed 4, Baltimore, Williams & Wilkins.

Callaway E, Halliday R, and Naylor H (1983) Hyperactive children's ERPs fail to support underarousal and maturational lag theories, Archives of General Psychiatry 40:1243-1248.

Carlson GA and Cantwell DP (1980) Unmasking depression in children and adolescents, Am J Psychiatry 26: 645-648.

Chambers WJ, Puig-Antich J, Hirsh M, and others (1985) The assessment of affective disorders in children and adolescents by semi-structured interview: test-retest liability of the K-SADS-P. Archives of General Psychiatry 42:669-674.

Chess S and Thomas A (1986) Temperament in clinical practice, New York, The Guilford Press.

Conners CK (1985) The Conners Rating Scales: instruments for the assessment of childhood psychopathology. Unpublished manuscript. Children's Hospital, National Medical Center, Washington, DC.

Costello A, Edelbrock C, Kalas R, Kessler M, and Klaric SA (1982) Diagnostic Interview Schedule for Children (DISC), Contract No RFP-DB-81-0027, Bethesda, Md, National Institute of Mental Health.

Dodds JB (1985) A child psychotherapy primer, New York, Human Sciences Press.

Dumas JE and Wahler RG (1983) Predictors of treatment outcomes in parent training. Mother insularity and socioeconomic disadvantage, Behavioral Assessment 5:301-313.

Edelbrock C and Costello AJ (1984) Structured psychiatric interviews for children and adolescents. In Goldstein G and Hersen M, Handbook of psychological assessment, New York, Pergamon Press.

Edlebrock CS, Costello AJ, Dulcan MK, Conover NC and Kalas B (1986) Parent child agreement on child psychiatric symptoms assessed via structured interview, Journal of Child Psychology and Psychiatry 27:181-190.

Ehrenberg MF, Cox DN, and Koopman RF (1990) The Millon Adolescent Personality Inventory profiles of depressed adolescents, Adolescence 25:415-420.

Esman AH (1988) Assessment of the adolescent. In Kestsenbaum CJ and Williams DT, editors, Handbook of clinical assessment of children and adolescents, vol 1, New York, 1988, New York, Universities Press.

Eyberg SM and Ross AW (1978) Assessment of child behavior problems: the validation of a new inventory, Journal of Clinical Child Psychology 7:113-116.

Folstein MF, Folstein SW and McHugh PR (1975) Mini-mental state: a practical method of gathering the cognitive state of patients for the clinician, Journal of Psychiatric Research 12: 189-198.

Friedman AM, Kaplan HI, and Sadock BJ, editors (1980) Comprehensive textbook of psychiatry, ed 3, Baltimore, Williams & Wilkins Co.

Gerson R (1984) The family recorder: computer-generated genograms, Atlanta, Humanware Software [61 8th St, 30309].

Gerson R and McGoldrick M (1985) Genograms gathered and displayed by the computer. In Zimmer J, editor, Clinics of primary care: computers in family medicine, Philadelphia, WB Saunders Co.

Gilberg C and Svendsen P (1983) Childhood psychosis and computed tomographic brain scan finding, Journal of Autism and Developmental Disorders 13:19-26.

Goldman J, L'Engle Stein CL, and Guerry S (1983) Psychological methods of child assessment, New York, Brunner/Mazel, Inc.

Hazelden Foundation, Center City, Minnesota.

Hogarth C (1989) Families and family therapy. In Johnson BS, editor, Psychiatric mental health nursing, Philadelphia, JB Lippincott Co.

Hurt SW, Hylker SE, Frances A and Clark JF (1984) Assessing boderline personality disorder with self-report, clinical interview or semi structured interview, American Journal of Psychiatry 141:1228-1231.

Kendall PC, Padawer W, Zupan B, and Braswell L (1985) Developing self-control in children: the manual, Psychology Department, Temple University, Philadelphia.

Kernberg O (1975) Borderline conditions and pathological narcissisn, New York, Jason Aronson, Inc.

Kovacs M (1985) The children's depression inventory (CDI) Psychopharmacological Bulletin 21:995-998.

Kuperman S, Gaffney GR, Hamdan-Allen G, Preston DF, and Venkatesh L (1990) Neuroimaging in child and adolescent psychiatry, Journal of the American Academy of Child and Adolescent Psychiatry 2:159-172.

Leckman JF and Pauls DL (1990) Genetics and child psychiatry: introduction, Journal of the American Academy of Child and Adolescent Psychiatry 29:2-4.

Levi J (1987) Acting out indicators on the Rorschach test. In Abt, LE and Weissman SL editors: Acting out, ed 2, Northvale, New Jersey, Jason Aronson, Inc.

Lyndon B. Johnson School of Public Affairs, University of Texas at Austin (1987) Community analysis research project. In Lyon L, editor, The community in urban society, Chicago, Dorsey Press.

McEnany GW (1990) Psychological indices of bipolar mood disorders: future trends in nursing care, Archives of Psychiatric Nursing 4:29-42.

McGoldrick M and Gerson R (1985) Genograms in family assessment, New York, WW Norton Co.

Miller D (1986) Attack on the self: adolescent behavioral disturbances and their treatment, Northvale, New Jersey, Jason Aronson, Inc.

Millon T, Green C, and Meagher RB (1982) Millon Adolescent Personality Inventory manual, Minneapolis, Interpretive Scoring Systems.

Moos R and Moos B (1981) Family environment scale manual, Palo Alto, Calif, Consulting Psychologists Press.

Morrison E, Fisher LY, Wilson HS et al (1985) NSGAE: Nursing Adaptation Evaluation: a proposed Axis VI of DSM-III, Journal of Psychosocial Nursing and Mental Health Services, 23:(8)10-13.

Nezu AM and Nezu CM, editors (1989) Clinical decision making in behavior therapy, Champaign, Ill, Research Press.

Patterson GB (1976) The aggressive child: victim and architect of a coercive system. In Mash EJ, Hamerlynek JA and Handy LC editors: Behavior modification and families. New York, Brunner/Mazel, Inc.

Patterson GB (1982) Coercive family process, Eugene, Ore, Castalina.

Patterson GB and Stouthamer-Locher M (1982) The correlation of family management practices and delinquency. Child Develoment 55:1299-1304.

Puig-Antich J and Chambers WJ (1983) Schedule for affective disorders and schizophrenia for school-aged children, Unpublished interview schedule, Western Psychiatric Institute and Clinic, Pittsburgh, Penn.

Quay HC and Peterson DR (1987) Manual for the revised behavior problem checklist, Department of Psychology, University of Miami, Coral Gables, Florida.

Rumsey JM, Dorwart R, Vermess M, Denckla MB, Markus JP, Kruesi JP, and Rapoport JL (1986) Magnetic resonance imaging of brain anatomy in severe developmental dyslexia, Archives of Neurology 43:1045-1046.

Rutter M and Cox (1981) Psychiatric interviewing techniques. I. methods and measures, British Journal of Psychiatry 138:273-282.

Ryan ND, Puig-Antich J, Ambrosini P, et al (1987) The clinical picture of major depression in children and adolescents, Archives of General Psychiatry 44:584-561.

Sattler JM (1988) Assessment of children, ed 3, San Diego, Jerome M Sattler, Publisher.

Schulz S, Koller M, Kishore PR, Hamer RM, Gehl JJ, and Friedel RO (1983) Ventricular enlargement in teen-age patients with schizophrenia spectrum disorder, American Journal of Psychiatry 140:1592-1595.

Sedgewick R (1988) The adolescent. In Beck CK, Rawlins RP, and Williams SR, editors, Mental health — psychiatric nursing, St Louis, The CV Mosby Co.

Shafii M, Stelz-Lenarsky J, Derrick AM et al (1988) Co-morbidity of mental disorders in post-mortem diagnosis of completed suicide in children and adolescents, Journal of Affective Disorders 15:227-233.

Shea SC (1988) Psychiatric interviewing: the art of understanding, Philadelphia, WB Saunders Co.

Skodol AE (1989) Problems in differential diagnosis: from DSM-III to DSM-III-R in clinical practice, Washington, DC, American Psychiatric Press.

Slenkowich JE (1983) PL 94-142 as applied to DSM-III diagnoses, Cupertino, Calif, Kinghorn.

Spirito A, Faustr D, Myers B, and Bechtell D (1988) Clinical utility of the MMPI in the evaluation of adolescent suicide attempters, Journal of Personality Assessment 52:204.

Spitzer RL, Williams JBW, and Gibbon M (1987) The structured clinical interview for DSM-III-R (SCID), New York, Biometrics Reserach Department.

Sullivan HS (1953) The interpersonal theory of psychiatry, New York, WW Norton Co.

Tarter RE (1990) Evaluation and treatment of adolescent substance abuse: a decision tree method, American Journal of Drug and Alcohol Abuse 16:1.

Teri L (1982) The use of the Beck Depression Inventory with adolescents, Journal of Abnormal Child Psychology 2:277.

Thomas A and Chess S (1976) Evolution of behavior disorders into adolescence, American Journal of Psychiatry 133:5-9.

Thomas A and Chess S (1980) Dynamics of psychological development, New York, Brunner/Mazel, Inc.

Thomas MD, Sanger E, and Whitsney JD (1986) Nursing diagnosis of depression: clinical identification on an inpatient unit, Journal of Psychosocial Nursing and Mental Health Services 24:6-12.

Volkow ND, Brodie JD, Wolf AP, and others (1986) Brain organization in schizophrenia, Journal of Cerebral Blood Flow and Metabolism 6:441-446.

Wallace ER (1983) Dynamic psychiatry in theory and practice, Philadelphia, Lea & Febiger.

Welner Z, Reich W, Herjanic B, Jung K, and Amado K (1987) Reliability, validity, and parent-child agreement studies of the Diagnostic Interview for Children and Adolescents (DICA), Journal of the American Academy of Child and Adolescent Psychiatry 26:649-654.

Westermeyer J (1985) Psychiatric diagnosis across cultural boundaries, American Journal of Psychiatry 142:798-805.

Wodrich D (1984) Children's psychological testing, A guide for nonpsychologists, Baltimore, MD, Brooke.

Wolff S (1984) The concept of personality disorder in children, Journal of Child Psychology and Psychiatry 25:5-13.

Woolf VV (1983) Family network systems in transgenerational psychotherapy: the theory, advantages and expanded application of the genogram, Family Therapy 10:119-137.

Chapter 7

A System of Care for Emotionally Disturbed Children and Adolescents

Cary Hatton

STANDARD IX. *Interdisciplinary Collaboration*

THE NURSE COLLABORATES WITH OTHER HEALTH CARE PROVIDERS IN ASSESSING, PLANNING, IMPLEMENTING AND EVALUATING PROGRAMS AND OTHER ACTIVITIES RELATED TO CHILD AND ADOLESCENT PSYCHIATRIC AND MENTAL HEALTH NURSING.

STANDARD X. *Use of Community Health Systems*

THE NURSE PARTICIPATES WITH OTHER MEMBERS OF THE COMMUNITY IN ASSESSING, PLANNING, IMPLEMENTING, AND EVALUATING MENTAL HEALTH SERVICES AND COMMUNITY SYSTEMS THAT ATTEND TO PRIMARY, SECONDARY, AND TERTIARY PREVENTION OF MENTAL DISORDERS IN CHILDREN AND ADOLESCENTS.

Historical Context

More than 80 years has passed since the first White House Conference on Children in 1909. One of the recommendations resulting from that early look at the needs of youth was to develop new programs to care for emotionally disturbed children. The nation has barely begun to address that recommendation.

To understand the concept of a "system of care," the development of a variety of systems must be explored. In the late 1800s and early 1900s interests emerged that gave rise to that White House Conference. During that time the various states were enacting compulsory school attendance legislation. Because the laws required all children to attend school, the need arose for programs that could handle "special" children. The development of child labor laws limited the amount of time and the type of job a youngster could work. This contributed to an increased awareness of the need to do something with youth who did not fit into the mainstream. Meanwhile, the juvenile court system was created to help cities deal with the "deviant" behavior of youth. A special emphasis was put on children from lower socioeconomic classes and immigrant families.

Between World Wars I and II the federal bureaus concerned with health, education, corrections, and social services began to develop structural frameworks to address the challenge of providing services for children who were "different." The first studies on psychosis in children were published, and a realization grew that mental health problems in children were not the same as those in adults and that treatment approaches might have to be different. Educational systems began to develop special tracks for youngsters who were mentally retarded, had serious behavior problems, or were "exceptionalities." In 1930 a second White House Conference on Children concluded that emotionally disturbed children had the same right to develop to their fullest potential that other children did. Once again the development of new treatment programs to care for these youth was recommended.

Within the last 60 years a large number of federal, state, and private commissions, panels, projects, and surveys have dealt with the problem of treating children who are emotionally disturbed. They have consistently sent the same message: services to this population are inadequate, fragmented, uncoordinated, and overly dependent on institutionalization. During the 1970s priorities and values began shifting away from the placement of children into large, residential-type institutions that isolated youth and separated them from their families and communities; the focus moved to the development of alternatives. Stimulated by research, legislation, and litigation, mental health service providers attempted to address the need for treatment in the least restrictive, most normative environment that was therapeutically appropriate. There were also advocacy efforts directed at "delabeling" youth and protecting their civil rights. Community mental health centers began programing in the areas of outreach, prevention, consultation, and education. Family therapy and the concept of using natural and community support systems became more widely accepted as helpful interventions for children and adolescents assessed as emotionally disturbed.

Despite this long process of identifying the problem and calling for solutions, far too many of the nation's most vulnerable youth still do not receive any mental health services. Of those who do get care, a large percentage are served inappropriately in overly restrictive settings—frequently in institutions—because of a lack of alternatives. Although recent years have seen a decline in the number of children treated in state- or county-run mental hospitals, this trend has been accompanied by an almost identical increase in admissions to private psychiatric facilities (Saxe and others, 1987). Until sufficient and effective services are developed and implemented within a comprehensive system of care that can meet the needs of emotionally disturbed youth and their families, these children will continue to be underserved and overinstitutionalized.

A System of Care

Although there has long been a notion of a continuum of services within the mental health field, the concept of a system of care encompasses more than a variety of therapy services. Stroul and Friedman (1986) offer the following definition:

> A system of care is a comprehensive spectrum of mental health and other necessary services which are organized into a coordinated network to meet the multiple and changing needs of severely emotionally disturbed children and adolescents.

There are four key elements to the definition. First is the call for a range of mental health services. For many years, severely emotionally disturbed children could be divided into three categories: those who received no services, those who received outpatient care once per week, and those who were hospitalized for months or sometimes years. Children and their families with a wide variety of diagnoses and symptoms, strengths, and resources seek help. They need an equally wide variety of approaches to treatment. A truly comprehensive spectrum allows the unique needs of youth to be met while empowering the available family and community systems to continue their support.

Second, the definition refers to other necessary services. These youth do not live in a vacuum, and their needs are rarely confined solely to the mental health area. They usually require assistance from a large number of agencies and organizations. All youth need education of one kind or another, and federal law mandates a "free and appropriate" education for all handicapped youth, including the severely emotionally disturbed. Some children carry the additional handicapping condition of mental retardation or developmental disabilities. These "dually diagnosed" young people need extensive services that address all their needs, but they are frequently shunted from one system to another because no single entity can provide all that they require. Many families with severely emotionally disturbed youth also are involved with "protective" or "family support" services from welfare or human services departments. Particularly if custody of the child is an issue, this system may be a frightening but necessary imposition on the family. Often emotionally disturbed youth are caught up in the juvenile justice system. Confronting and controlling inappropriate behavior and treating the underlying emotional problems demand a delicate balance. Sadly, some emotionally disturbed children and adolescents have physical illnesses or handicaps that further stretch the resources available and compound the difficulty of providing appropriate treatment. All children, even those experiencing emotional problems, need social and recreational outlets. This is seldom a priority but may be essential to promote healthful functioning.

The third key element of the definition of a system of care states that all these services should be "organized into a coordinated network." The brief descriptions already presented only hint at the challenge inherent in this requirement. It asks an extremely diverse set of helpers to work together to ensure that the youth and family neither fall through the cracks between systems nor become overwhelmed by the numerous and sometimes conflicting demands of the individuals and organizations whose services they need. Collaboration like this almost always requires a component of systems management, and few state or local service systems provide such a superstructure. Although some parents have the time, skills, energy, and determination to maneuver through the tangled web of providers and over the gaps where there are no providers, usually a case manager is needed to maximize the use of available resources and minimize risks for the youth and family.

Finally, because of the diversity of children and families and the developmental changes inherent in them, their needs are multiple, changing, and situationally unique. Thus it is not enough to have a coordinated range of services. A true system of care requires flexibility for adaptation to specific individuals at a given moment and the ability to alter as the individual or the times change.

One way of envisioning a system of care is shown in Figure 7-1. The child and family are the center of the system; everything else should revolve around them rather than demand that they change to meet the needs of the various providers. A "layer" of case management connects the provider agencies to each other and to the family. The ring of services is community based; the resort to more restrictive placements comes only after the network of local resources is judged inappropriate.

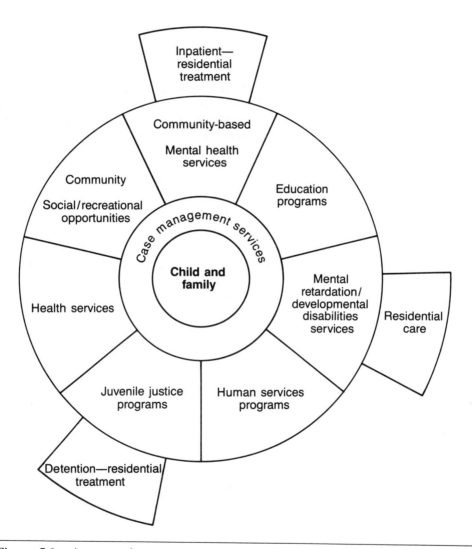

Figure   7-1   A system of care.

BASIC ASSUMPTIONS

Underlying the concept of a system of care is a philosophy encompassing the kinds of services that should be available and how these services should be delivered. Although there are differences—both pragmatic and theoretical—regarding specific programs and structural organization, general agreement exists about the most important values embodied in the philosophy. The box outlines eight basic assumptions.

1. A system of care should be child centered and family focused, with the unique needs of the family guiding all decisions.

No two children or families are alike. Often one or two types of services are locally available, and if they do not happen to meet the child's needs, then the child and family "make do" or do without. A system of care requires a commitment to make the services fit the needs—not the other way around. The commitment includes responsiveness to the needs of the family, which is seen as the primary support system for the child.

An autistic 8 year-old, a suicidal pre-teen, and a schizophrenic adolescent all need therapeutic mental health care, but would not all benefit from the same kinds of services. Similarly, an upper–middle class family with a large, supportive extended

---

Basic Assumptions About a System of Care

1. A system of care should be child centered and family focused, with the unique needs of the family guiding all decisions.
2. A system of care should ensure that whenever possible and appropriate, the child and family are actively involved in planning strategies and making decisions related to the delivery of treatment and services.
3. A system of care should promote early identification of and interventions for children at risk of developing severe emotional disturbance to maximize the possibility of preventing or reducing chronic distress and dysfunction.
4. A system of care should provide a wide range of services to meet the emotional, physical, educational, and social needs of emotionally disturbed youth and families so that they may function as well as possible within their community.
5. Within a system of care, services should be individualized and organized through a coordinated, integrated plan that includes ongoing case management and allows for smooth transitions as needs change.
6. A system of care should ensure that the planning and management of treatment occur in the community and that services are provided in the least restrictive environment that is therapeutically appropriate and as close to the youth's home and family as possible.
7. A system of care should promote advocacy for the needs and rights of emotionally disturbed youth and their families and should always be respectful of those needs and rights.
8. A system of care should ensure that children and families receive services without regard to race, religion, national origin, sex, ability to pay, or other handicaps or characteristics, and that services are responsive to cultural and other differences.

network brings different problems and resources to an emotionally disturbed child than does a single parent on public assistance. Age, diagnosis, level of functioning, special problems, emotional and financial resources, and many other factors influence treatment choices.

Additionally, neither children nor families are unchanging. As they pass through developmental phases and cycles, both their needs and their resources evolve. Remaining child centered and family focused means that assessments must be ongoing and done within the context of an ever-changing environment.

 2. *A system of care should ensure that whenever possible and appropriate, the child and family are actively involved in planning strategies and making decisions related to the delivery of treatment and services.*

No one has more at stake in the planning and decision-making process than the clients. If they are not encouraged to become active partners in the treatment, they are less likely to be committed to making the treatment successful and more likely either to resist or to sabotage even the most inspired service plans. The child and family are the treatment providers' best and most significant source of information about historical and current aspects of the problem.

In the vast majority of cases professionals will come and go, but the child and family will be dealing with each other and their problems for a lifetime. A system of care should provide support and empowerment to families with the goal of maximizing their abilities to function well. The system must, however, be flexible enough so that when families refuse involvement or cannot be safely involved at the time, children are not excluded from services or from nurturing, stable environments.

 3. *A system of care should promote early identification of and interventions for children at risk of developing severe emotional disturbance to maximize the possibility of preventing or reducing chronic distress and dysfunction.*

The earlier a problem is identified, the easier it is to develop means to ameliorate it. In many cases early treatment programs can resolve issues before an individual or family becomes dysfunctional. The "savings" in terms of suffering, as well as in dollars, are difficult to measure in objective ways, but they are nonetheless significant. The current reality, however, is that the extreme limits on resources for emotionally disturbed youth usually mean that the focus of assistance is on those classified as most in need. A system of care seeks to find a reasonable middle ground that through early interventions will reduce the severity of symptoms and the number of youth who become chronically mentally disturbed, and still provide services for those who are already experiencing serious problems.

 4. *A system of care should provide a wide range of services to meet the emotional, physical, educational, and social needs of emotionally disturbed youth and families so that they may function as well as possible within their community.*

Children and families should have access to a continuum of mental health services, from occasional crisis intervention or outpatient therapy to hospitalization or residential treatment. However, many experts (Behar, 1986; Joint Commission on Mental Health of Children, 1969; Knitzer, 1982; President's Commission on Mental Health, 1978; Stroul and Friedman, 1986) have forcefully stated that mental health services alone, even if expansive in nature, are not able to provide effectively for the multidimensional needs of severely emotionally disturbed youth. It is unusual and becoming even more so for youths to be permanently institutionalized. Shipping children away to be "cured" and then returning them to families and neighborhoods that have not been prepared to meet their ongoing needs is an expensive and futile effort.

5. *Within a system of care, services should be individualized and organized through a coordinated, integrated plan that includes ongoing case management and allows for smooth transitions as needs change.*

Even when the appropriate range of services is available, a family is often completely overwhelmed by the number of systems, agencies, and individuals that must be negotiated with to gain access to those services. In long-term cases the family may find it difficult to shift services as its needs change. The creation of a single plan, designed by the entire team of service providers with input from the client and family, helps avoid duplication of efforts, gaps in services, conflicting demands on the family, and general confusion. The plan should identify problems, resources, goals, and interventions across all areas of need. It should include a frequent review and revision process to adjust for changing needs and circumstances. It should be particularly attentive to the problems a youth and family may anticipate when the youth "outgrows" the various components of the child-serving system.

In most cases the key to pulling together such a plan is the case manager. A single individual must maintain the responsibility and authority to provide ongoing coordination, planning, monitoring, and advocacy. Without this leader, the system is unlikely to remain focused and flexible enough to meet the evolving needs of the youth and family. This role is discussed in detail later in the chapter.

6. *A system of care should ensure that the planning and management of treatment occur in the community and that services are provided in the least restrictive environment that is therapeutically appropriate and as close to the youth's home and family as possible.*

Treatment that is planned and managed locally is more apt to be consistent and holistic and to provide continuity of care over a long-term illness. All available community resources and natural support systems can be considered during the decision-making process. The family and community providers who are most likely to be involved with the child into adulthood should be the primary "stakeholders" in treatment.

The concept of least restrictive environment is not only a clinical principle; it is also a legal one. Federal legislation and judicial decisions have made it clear that services should be provided in the most natural and normal setting possible. The trauma and long-term negative effects of removing a child from home and family are factors that must be weighed against the potential benefits of inpatient or residential treatment. If the placement is in or near the child's community, the opportunity for ongoing family involvement in treatment and preparation for discharge is greatly enhanced. This not only minimizes the impact of removal but also improves the odds of successful aftercare. The family will be more able to provide what the child needs, and the community-based mental health services can be mobilized and ready to offer support.

7. *A system of care should promote advocacy for the needs and rights of emotionally disturbed youth and their families and should always be respectful of those needs and rights.*

There are two types of advocacy. *Case advocacy* refers to efforts on behalf of an individual youth to guarantee that services are appropriate and rights are protected. *Class advocacy* is the term for efforts to improve services, benefits, and rights for the whole group of emotionally disturbed youth (Knitzer, 1982). There are widespread data that this population is ineffectively served and that the available services are fragmented. Advocacy to change the system is urgently needed. National and local consumer groups such as the National Alliance for the Mentally Ill (NAMI) are beginning to develop efforts to help emotionally disturbed children and their families.

A system of care should ensure that the rights of youth are protected. These rights include treatment in the least restrictive and most appropriate setting, as well as the assurance that any removal from home will occur only when absolutely necessary for protection of the child or family. Rights within hospitals and residential treatment settings should be clearly outlined to the child and family and must be carefully guarded. The issue of complications when the rights of the child conflict with those of other family members should be carefully addressed.

8. *A system of care should ensure that children and families receive services without regard to race, religion, national origin, sex, ability to pay, or other handicaps or characteristics, and that services are responsive to cultural and other differences.*

That a system of care should not discriminate against youth for any of these reasons seems obvious. The President's Commission on Mental Health (1978) was very clear on this principle. The reality, however, is that youth and their families are not legally "entitled" to mental health care, and a wide discrepancy exists in the amount and type of treatment accessible to families. This is without a doubt an area of challenge for the developers of truly child-centered services. Minorities, the physically or mentally handicapped, the poor, and others out of the mainstream should have equal access to quality treatment that is adapted to meet their needs.

Systems and Services

As shown in Figure 7-1, seven components must be involved if a system of care is to be truly comprehensive in its response to emotionally disturbed youth and their families. Although particular cases that necessitate the entire range of services are rare, it is equally unusual to find a severely emotionally disturbed youth whose needs did not span several systems. Few communities have the capabilities to develop all the services described here, and no two communities are likely to identify the need for the same specific array of services. This section outlines and discusses a broad menu of options. Generalized information is provided on criteria for access to and interventions provided by mental health services.

MENTAL HEALTH

Mental health services can be separated into three broad categories, with an understanding that the continuum has several overlapping features. First, there are the general mental health clinic services, including prevention, outreach, assessment, outpatient therapies, and emergency or crisis interventions. Most of these services are addressed elsewhere in the text and are briefly reviewed here. Second are the community-based alternatives for more severely disturbed youth, including day treatment, partial hospitalization, home-based interventions, therapeutic foster care, group care, and respite care. These are described here in more depth. Finally, for those who need the most intensive treatment settings, there are psychiatric hospitals and residential treatment centers. These are reviewed here and explored thoroughly in subsequent chapters.

Prevention services are usually provided in non–mental-health settings in the community, frequently in conjunction with other resources such as schools, churches, or day-care centers. The goal is to provide families and other child-serving entities with information and skills that maximize their abilities to provide healthful, nurturing, and empowering environments. In this way the likelihood of emotional disturbances is reduced and the severity of distress, when it does occur, may be lessened. Prevention services also frequently train non–mental-health providers in the identification of those youth at risk for or already needing treatment. These services may be provided through written materials, media presentations, in-services, or classes for youth and family members.

Outreach is another indirect service. Its purpose is to identify youth and families in need of mental health services and to make those services accessible. Outreach involves networking and collaboration among mental health providers and between those providers and other child-serving entities. It also requires the ability to reach out to those people experiencing emotional disturbances who may not be aware of the need for or availability of mental health services, or who may be resistant to them.

Assessment includes both preliminary and ongoing services. It is a challenging and complex task that may involve clinical interviews of the child and other family members; discussions with other professionals and extended support system people; construction of a social history; assessment of family functions; evaluation of intelligence; assessment of academic, vocational, and recreational needs; determination of chemical use, abuse, and dependence; developmental and neurological work-ups; physical and psychiatric examinations; and other reviews of specific needs or conditions. The purpose of a multifactored assessment is to enable the youth, family, and providers to make good decisions about the best possible mix of services to meet the needs. Although more extensive assessments provide more information, it is important to avoid overwhelming the family with duplications of procedures and to minimize the strains on them in terms of time, emotional energy, and financial resources. One of the roles of a case manager is to ensure this balance.

Outpatient services are most often provided in a mental health clinic or office setting on a regularly scheduled basis. They include individual, family, and group therapy; medication prescription and monitoring; educational training; support services; and consultation. These are available as a single service or as part of an individualized service delivery plan using a combination of mental health treatment strategies and other components of the system of care.

One of the potential assets of outpatient services is flexibility. These services are normally provided on a 50-minute, once per week basis, but they can be adapted to the varied needs of clients. They are appropriate for the whole range of emotional disturbances, from situational emotional discomfort to psychosis. For emotionally disturbed youth, a mix of these services is often optimal. Individual counseling or play therapy provides one-to-one assessment and intervention, and group therapy can address issues related to skill building, peer relationships, and adaptive behaviors. Simultaneously, family members can garner support, parenting skills, or assistance with their own emotional problems. Family therapy often restructures relationships and communication, improves behavior patterns, and teaches new ways of interacting that can benefit all family members. Most medication needs for youth can be managed on an outpatient basis with careful monitoring by a psychiatrist.

Education, support, and consultation services can be vital for the family, natural support system, and other community providers as they attempt to meet the needs of an emotionally disturbed child. Even if more intensive treatment must be prescribed for the youth, outpatient services can be a tremendous adjunct to treatment and preparation for the return of a child placed outside the home.

The boundaries of outpatient services also tend to be the entry and exit points of the mental health system. As the least restrictive of all treatments, outpatient services are a crucial first line of offense in the continuum. On the other end of the treatment process, they can provide a gradual weaning from professional care as the youth and family recover and go on with their lives.

Emergency services are the interventions required when an individual or family experiences a crisis. They may be precipitated by a sudden deterioration in overall functioning, suicidal or homicidal urges, a situational trauma, or other events that trigger acute distress.

Within the category of emergency services are two types of interventions. Hot line services allow the patient or a member of the support system to access a crisis worker, therapist, or case manager by telephone when an emergency arises. Typically this service is available 24 hours per day, 7 days per week. Ambulatory emergency services are provided on a face-to-face basis, either in an office or in the natural or community environment. Available interventions can include assessment, counseling, case management, and referral to more restrictive or ongoing services if appropriate.

Day treatment is one of the most intensive of nonresidential services. It is designed for youth whose mental health needs cannot be met on an outpatient basis and who require more intense, daily therapeutic intervention. Many youth would require psychiatric hospitalization or residential treatment if day treatment were not available. It can serve as an excellent transition for youth coming out of these environments and may allow for a shorter length of stay in the more restrictive settings. Some programs may target a specific subset of emotionally disturbed youth—for example, substance abusers.

Day treatment programs are typically run by hospitals or mental health agencies. They follow a regular schedule, although the length and times may vary. Some programs provide after school and early evening hours; others are held during the school day. The programs operate usually between 3 and 8 hours per day, most often 5 days per week. The staff/client ratio is high, between 1:2 and 1:6, including support personnel.

Different programs have varying areas of focus and emphasis, but all tend to have eight key components. *Group counseling* is provided one or more times daily. Patients may set goals and discuss their progress; share thoughts, ideas, and feelings; learn from group leaders and each other more effective ways of interacting with adults and peers; and deal with common issues and interests. *Individual counseling* occurs on both scheduled and as needed bases. With the therapist the youth explores those issues not appropriate for group processing or individualizes concerns arising from group or family therapy. This may take the form of play therapy, informal chats with staff, or traditional insight-oriented intervention. *Family therapy* and other forms of parent education and support assist those with whom the youth lives in carrying over the gains made in treatment to the natural environment. When the family situation is unhealthful, this component seeks to improve the functioning of the natural system so that the youth can remain in the family. If the youth is living in an out-of-home setting, therapy should occur with both the birth family (if reunification is planned) and the current caretakers of the child. *Skill-building* provides training and practice in problematic areas of functioning. Usually there are programs in the areas of problem solving, decision making, appropriate handling of anger and other emotions, substance abuse, social skills, sex education, and other age-appropriate topics. *Behavior modification* programs are designed to extinguish inappropriate or unhealthy activities and increase more adaptive and positive behaviors. Goals and objectives are set, and reinforcement is provided through interventions such as token economies, point or level systems, participation in field trips, and other pleasurable activities. *Recreational, art, and music therapies* allow for a range of therapeutic approaches and outlets for physical, mental, and emotional energies. They can sometimes reach a youth and provide a release when more traditional therapies are unsuccessful or insufficient. *Special education* services are usually provided in collaboration with the youth's home school and based on an Individualized Education Plan (IEP) developed with or by them. The classes or tutoring allow the youth to obtain education while receiving day treatment care. Finally, the *therapeutic milieu* encompasses the total program environment. This is usually highly structured but flexible enough to meet different needs. The milieu should nurture and empower the youth with a sense of independence, responsibility, and competence. It should also be pervasive, including support and educational staff, as well as the clinical team.

    Partial hospitalization programs have the same components, but they include psychiatric services, the administration of psychotropic medications as needed, and usually a more highly trained staff. Essentially, the youth is in a hospital-like environment without the beds. Some programs have an acute, short-term focus, but most have lengths of stay of at least 3 to 6 months.

    Home-based services provide extremely intensive, crisis-oriented services to a family when out-of-home placement is an imminent likelihood. A new concept in the mental health field, home-based programs have emerged as an alternative to hospitalization or residential treatment in many cases. Several models have been developed since the mid-1970s, but there are common characteristics across most programs. Services are typically provided in the family's home by staff, who frequently work in teams, on a flexible schedule with 24-hour availability. Usually a crisis precipitates the referral, and most programs do not carry a waiting list. If a slot is not immediately available, alternative means of handling the situation must be accessed to ensure that no child or family member is in danger. Services are intensive, frequently requiring up to 20 or more hours per week at the outset. The focus is on improving family functioning and often includes assistance with accessing necessary resources. Staff caseloads must be quite small, usually including no more than three to six families at a time. Length of stay varies; some programs focus on short-term (4 to 6 weeks) interventions, whereas others may work with families for as long as several years.

Six types of interventions are most often found in home-based programs. *Crisis intervention* strategies, which are used at the time of intake, include assessing the immediate and long-term needs, stabilizing the family, and reducing acute distress. These strategies may also be used at various points during the family's involvement with the program. *Counseling* is provided to any and all family members individually, as a family unit, and in whatever combinations seem appropriate. Counseling tends to occur as problems arise and are dealt with, as opposed to the scheduled appointments found in a clinic setting. *Skill building* is provided to family members with the use of strategies from modeling to direct teaching. Whatever deficits are found, whether related to interpersonal functioning, emotional distress, or behavioral inadequacies, the home-based worker assists with addressing the problem. Assistance is also provided with *home management,* which helps parents learn to make wise use of time, money, and energy. Home-based staff members also do *advocacy,* networking with other providers in the system of care to ensure that the rights and needs of the child and family are being met. Finally, there is initial assistance with *accessing needed resources* (including "hard" services such as food and clothing if necessary); family members are then taught more effective ways of doing this for themselves.

Whatever the length of involvement with the family, home-based programs tend to phase out gradually as families stabilize. Families must also be connected with other ongoing services before they are actually discharged from the program.

Therapeutic foster care and group home services are designed to provide a safe, supportive milieu for those youth whose emotional disturbances are exacerbated by their natural environments. These are the least restrictive options available for youth who cannot remain in their own homes. Both types of programs are typically provided as part of a continuum of services by a mental health agency or residential treatment facility. The organization recruits staff and provides extensive screening and training to find those adults who have the desire and skills to work intensively with any youth experiencing severe emotional problems. The agency provides staff for supervision, assistance, and support services. Ideally, a case manager works to integrate the child and "family providers" with the other mental health services and community services that are needed. There is also a focus on maintaining relationships with peers and other natural support systems. When reunification with the natural family is a goal, ongoing treatment occurs with the parents to promote a favorable outcome. At other times the focus is on preparing the youth for transition into independent living and appropriate adult services.

In therapeutic foster care, providers offer support and structure in a home environment. There is usually only one child (or at the most two) placed in the home at any time. The foster parents serve as "lay therapists" and are considered part of a treatment team with the other mental health workers assigned to the child. This may include outpatient therapist(s), day treatment staff, and a case manager, as well as personnel who specifically support the therapeutic foster care program. Ideally, the program consists of a network of foster homes that form an extended family and will work together for training, support, and respite. This allows for flexibility in matching children who have special needs or characteristics with families who can best provide for them. Frequently it can include crisis-oriented, acute options for youth who might otherwise be hospitalized but who do not require a medical setting. It also reduces burn-out and turnover for providers. The interventions in this environment are primarily the ones used in a healthy family (see Chapter 3).

Some children with severe emotional problems are unable to handle the level of family-like involvement in a treatment foster care environment. *Therapeutic group homes,* which typically serve 5 to 10 youth, are another option. Some group homes are operated by a 24-hour-per-day live-in couple with staff support; others use a shift rotation model. Although the focus is still on providing a homelike atmosphere within a community setting, there is more of a treatment orientation. Typically, the group home would provide behavior modification programing, formal and informal group interactions, and individual counseling. The youth may also be involved with other treatment programs, and usually a case manager is assigned to facilitate coordination of services.

Respite care allows families (either natural or foster) who are caring for a severely emotionally disturbed youth time away from the daily challenges they face. *Emergency respite care* provides an escape for the youth or family in crisis when longer-term removal is not needed. It is designed for situations in which a youth has acute symptoms that are aggravated by the current environment and requires a very short-term period of 24-hour care and supervision outside the current home. The interventions provided are essentially those found in emergency services; in this case they are provided in an out-of-home setting, typically for up to 72 hours. *Planned respite* is, as the name implies, a scheduled "break" for the youth and family. It is usually brief, sometimes no more than a few hours on a regular basis, or may allow for a longer "vacation." This service may be provided in or out of the home and can be provided by extended family or community volunteers with appropriate case management and professional support. This service can be a powerful resource, especially when attempts are being made to maintain a severely emotionally disturbed youth in a natural, nonresidential setting.

Psychiatric hospitalization, which typically follows a medical model, is one of the most restrictive alternatives in the system of care. It is reserved for the youth experiencing the most severe disturbances—those who are at imminent risk of self-harm or harm to others or who are in need of intensive therapy and monitoring 24 hours per day. There has been a long-standing tendency to overuse inpatient services, primarily because of a lack of appropriate alternatives. Hospitalization is, however, a very important component of a system of care, and access to this service should be guaranteed to all youth who need it.

There are three primary uses of hospitalization. The first is for *acute stabilization* and *intensive treatment.* When a youth is in severe distress and a less restrictive environment may be unsafe, a short-term stay (from a few days to a few weeks) may provide the best option. The focus of an inpatient stay is to take advantage of the readiness of the adolescent and family in crisis to identify problems, develop improved communication and coping skills, renew hope, and connect the family and adolescent with the appropriate services to maintain the progress of the inpatient interventions.

A second reason for hospitalizing a youth is for a *comprehensive evaluation,* particularly when there are indications of a need for physical, neuropsychological, or chemotherapy work-ups that may not safely be done on an outpatient basis. This should also be seen as a short-term stay, again with the goal of reintegration into community-based treatment as quickly as possible.

Finally, there is a small percentage of severely emotionally disturbed youth who require *long-term treatment* in an inpatient facility. Sometimes long-term treatment is chosen because of a lack of appropriate discharge or aftercare placements. When long-term hospitalization is actually required, it most often is because of the difficulty of stabilizing a youth on appropriate and therapeutically safe medication or because of aggression that cannot otherwise be controlled.

Inpatient treatment is discussed at length in subsequent chapters, which explore therapies, intervention strategies, and use of medications.

Residential treatment is the final category of mental health services, and is perhaps the most difficult to describe. A complete continuum is built into the group of facilities that have only one common characteristic: treatment of youth with an identified mental health problem in a 24-hour-per-day setting. Some residential treatment centers have more traits in common with therapeutic group homes, whereas others look remarkably like hospital units. In some cases a single facility may actually provide the entire range of care options.

The concept of therapeutic milieu (see Chapter 11) is basic to most residential treatment centers. Another widely implemented model that is based on Project Re-Ed (Hobbs, 1979) focuses on building competencies in the present. Intrinsic to all approaches are the three components of clinical treatment, educational programing, and facilitative living arrangements.

The major drawback to residential treatment is that in most cases the youth is removed not only from home but also from the community. Placements far from the family reduce the chances for their ongoing involvement in the youth's treatment and often result in difficult reintegration. This problem can be compounded when the youth reaches the upper age limit of the facility and requires further care. Continuity of care in these situations becomes extremely problematic because often there is no one to guarantee it. As communities actually develop systems of care that can incorporate residential treatment as a component, the number of youth needing the resource is expected to drop. The therapeutic benefits can be made available to those who need them without the disruption that occurs when a youth is placed far from home (Figure 7-2).

EDUCATION

No other system in our country serves more adolescents than education does. *All* children are entitled to free and appropriate services, and federal legislation guarantees this right to severely emotionally disturbed children under the Education for All Handicapped Children Act (PL 94-142) passed in 1975. This law specifies that schools not only must provide an education but also must offer those related services, such as counseling, that a child might need to benefit from special education. Sadly,

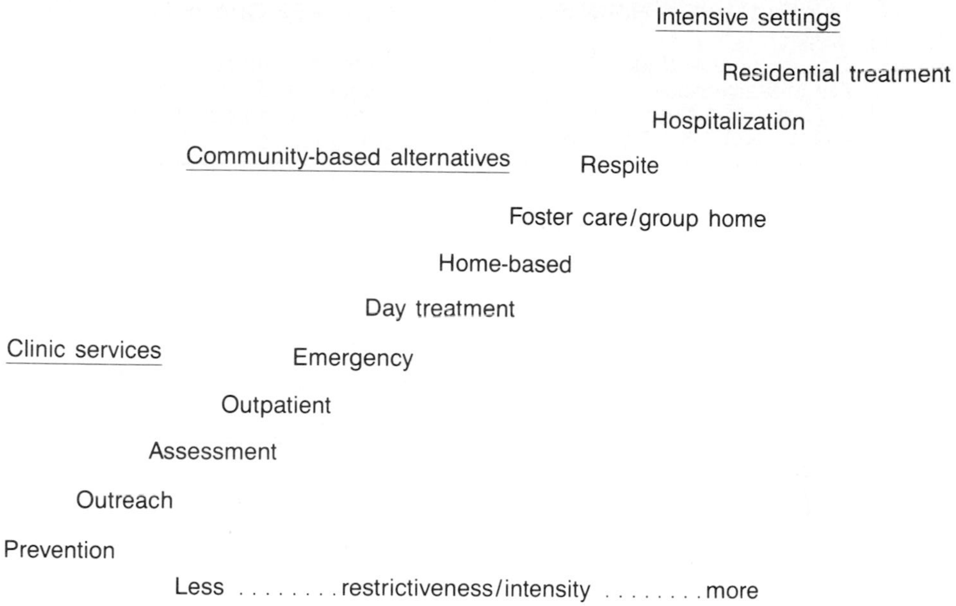

```
                                              Intensive settings

                                                 Residential treatment

                                              Hospitalization

              Community-based alternatives      Respite

                                         Foster care/group home

                               Home-based

                         Day treatment

  Clinic services            Emergency

                  Outpatient

            Assessment

       Outreach

  Prevention

          Less  . . . . . . . . restrictiveness/intensity  . . . . . . . . more
```

Figure 7-2   The continuum of mental health services.

there is still no consensus regarding exactly what schools are obligated to provide or pay for concerning the services that an emotionally disturbed youth might need.

Each state education agency has developed policies used by local school systems to determine program guidelines under PL 94-142. There are regulations that delineate who is to be certified as severely emotionally disturbed, how to make the identification (Figure 7-3 on p. 202), and how to determine the appropriate educational placement. By law, these policies stringently require service in the least restrictive environment. Counseling and career and vocational services, when available, are provided without necessarily being a part of the educational continuum. The six general categories of educational services are listed here in order of restrictiveness and briefly described.

Counseling services are generally available through the schools. The primary focus in most cases is on screening and evaluation, career and academic guidance, and personal counseling relating to school problems. The guidance counselor is usually the primary link from the school to the family and other community resources.

Assessment services for identification and placement in a special education program are conducted by a multidisciplinary team. Informed consent must be obtained before the evaluation is done, and an explanation of the child's due process rights must be included. A typical multifactored assessment includes evaluation in the areas of physical health, vision, hearing, motor abilities, communication skills, intelligence, academic performance, educational and family history, behavioral observations, and personality. The results of the assessment should be the development of an Individualized Education Plan that addresses how the child's

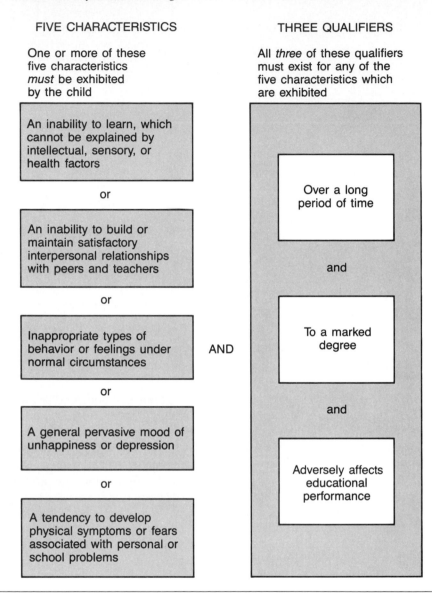

FIVE CHARACTERISTICS

One or more of these
five characteristics
must be exhibited
by the child

An inability to learn, which
cannot be explained by
intellectual, sensory, or
health factors

or

An inability to build or
maintain satisfactory
interpersonal relationships
with peers and teachers

or

Inappropriate types of
behavior or feelings under
normal circumstances

or

A general pervasive mood of
unhappiness or depression

or

A tendency to develop
physical symptoms or fears
associated with personal or
school problems

AND

THREE QUALIFIERS

All *three* of these qualifiers
must exist for any of the
five characteristics which
are exhibited

Over a long
period of time

and

To a marked
degree

and

Adversely affects
educational
performance

Figure 7-3   P.L. 94-142 Definition of seriously emotionally disturbed. (From Ohio Department of Education (1987) Ohio handbook for the identification of children with
severe behavior handicaps, Columbus, Ohio Department of Education.)

academic and special needs will be met.

Resource rooms can be used as an augmentation of the school program for children
who can be maintained in the regular classroom, with support. A variety of
organizational structures is used for this service, but typically a youth is assigned to
this classroom or teacher for assistance and individualized or small group instruction
for one to three periods of the school day.

Special education classrooms or units provide academic and supportive services to students who cannot be maintained in a normal classroom environment. The following three types of youth may be placed in these units: students in the normal range of intelligence who have learning disabilities and deficiencies in one or more academic areas or skills; the developmentally handicapped; those with mental retardation or another pervasive developmental problem; and youth who are experiencing severe emotional or behavioral problems, identified as severely behaviorally handicapped (SBH) or severely emotionally disturbed (SED). Special education classrooms offer small class sizes and support services to provide intensive supervision and specialized assistance to maximize the child's educational progress and minimize the identified handicap(s). For multihandicapped students, it is crucial that the teacher work collaboratively with the family and other service providers if the youth is to make consistent gains and be able to generalize improvement in skills and behaviors to areas outside the special education classroom.

Home-bound instruction can be arranged by the school for students who are unable to attend any part of the school program, even with support. A tutor provides instruction, usually in the youth's home on a one-to-one basis for approximately 5 hours per week. Too often this option is used to exclude those whose behavior is difficult to manage, rather than developing special programs to meet their needs.

Career and vocational services range from assessment and counseling related to job aptitudes and abilities to training that helps prepare for direct entry into a skilled field of work. This area has been overlooked for most handicapped youth, and this gap creates real and ongoing problems for adolescents attempting to make the transition into successful adulthood. The Carl Perkins Vocational Education Act (P.L. 98-524) was passed in 1985 to assist states in the development and improvement of vocational education programs; there is a focus on handicapped students in the bill. Services needed in this area include career education; assessment of skills, interests, and work adjustment capability; job survival training; vocational skills training; and assistance with seeking and retaining employment.

MENTAL RETARDATION AND DEVELOPMENTAL DISABILITIES

Services for children and adolescents who are both emotionally disturbed and mentally retarded or developmentally disabled are difficult to find in most areas. To be eligible for the services of an MR/DD agency, a child must usually have general intellectual functioning that is significantly below average and have observable deficiencies in adaptive behavior or a long-term disability that handicaps normal functioning and is attributable to mental retardation or a similar condition. Some services are available only to those determined to be moderately, severely, or profoundly retarded (an IQ below 54, as measured by the Wechsler Intelligence Scale for Children — Revised). These services include the following:

Assessment services are provided to determine eligibility for other services and as a basis for the development of an individual habilitation plan. A comprehensive evaluation includes observation, testing, and interviews by a multidisciplinary team including professionals from medicine, education, psychology, and social work. Again, the system mandates that services be provided in the least restrictive setting available.

Family resource services are provided to families who are caring for an individual with an MR/DD handicap. They are designed to improve the living environment and provide relief and practical assistance to the natural support system. This includes respite care, family education and training, special equipment or adaptive structural modifications, and some reimbursement for costs of direct services.

Educational and vocational training includes activities designed to maintain or increase the competence of the mentally retarded. For school-age children these are provided through the educational system, but these services are also available through sheltered workshop facilities.

Intermediate care facilities are licensed nursing homes or residential care centers whose focus is on the development of skills, habits, and attitudes for adapting to community-based living.

HUMAN SERVICES

The social services provided by departments of human services are frequently required by families who have a child with severe emotional problems. Children who are or have been maltreated are clearly at risk for needing mental health services. On the other hand, families coping with a severely emotionally disturbed child face multiple problems and stresses and often need extensive support to avoid the risk of maltreatment under such trying conditions. Brief descriptions of the four categories of services generally provided by this system follow:

Protective services are initiated following a referral and determination that a child or children are being maltreated in the home. The purpose is to prevent the occurrence or continuation of abuse (emotional, physical, or sexual); neglect (emotional or physical); or dependence. The goal is twofold: to keep the child(ren) safe and to preserve and strengthen the family unit whenever possible. Supervision and ongoing monitoring of the family occurs, along with—if absolutely necessary—removal of the child(ren) and development of a reunification plan to be implemented before the return.

Supportive casework services are provided to ameliorate family problems that contribute to risk for the children. These services include counseling with parents and children, assistance in accessing financial support and other welfare and human services interventions, and referrals to other service providers such as mental health therapists or physicians.

Homemaker services include direct, hands-on assistance to families, including help with home management chores, child care responsibilities, and respite care. These are often provided by volunteers or nonprofessionals, but it is important that they be recruited, trained, and supervised appropriately.

Substitute care occurs when there is no safe way to maintain the child in the family home. Ideally it should be provided within the community so that the child's support system is minimally disrupted and so that ongoing contact with family members can occur as appropriate. Reunification of the family is less likely if members have no opportunity to work on problems together. *Shelter* refers to a temporary placement in a foster or group home setting, typically for no more than a few days. This is a crisis-oriented service intended to occur for very brief periods of time; unfortunately the absence of suitable placements often mandates that a child remain in shelter care, and thus in "limbo," longer than is appropriate. Foster care and related placements are used when a child has been removed from the home because of abuse, neglect, or dependence, or when a family voluntarily relinquishes custody. Placement may actually be in a foster home, a group home, a child care facility, or a residential treatment center. Again, this is designed to be a temporary arrangement with a goal of working with the family toward reunification. State laws vary regarding the amount of time children may spend in foster placements with no permanent legal or familial status. Adoption is the preferred option for children who cannot return to the biological family. This requires termination of all parental rights, which judges are frequently reluctant to impose. Permanent placement of severely emotionally disturbed children, as well as those with other handicaps, is often difficult and requires extensive and ongoing support for the adoptive family and child.

JUVENILE JUSTICE

Although the juvenile justice system provides several services to youth and families who come under its jurisdiction, its primary role is that of a correctional system with a duty to protect the community from dangerous and illegal activity. This dual nature compounds the difficulty of assuring that the rights and needs of young people, their families, and society are all served.

The system usually includes local juvenile and family courts; probation departments; correctional facilities; and often an agency that provides prevention, diversion, and related services. In many states another component of the system, at a regional or state level, deals with those convicted of more serious crimes. The following are brief descriptions of typical services:

Prevention and *diversion* services are designed to reduce the number of youth who move into the correctional system. Included are outreach programs in schools, community awareness efforts, and counseling for children who are status offenders or who are involved in misdemeanor charges on a first-time basis. Many who "act out" their emotional problems may be first identified as disturbed through these services, and referral to other child-serving systems is an important consequence.

Probation officers may provide much more than legal supervision to youth adjudicated by the court. Support for the child and family; referral, assistance, and follow-through on other services; and a back-up to appropriate disciplinary measures may all be a part of the duties a probation officer performs.

Detention facilities provide evaluation and assessment services, as well as short-term correctional placements. Youth workers may provide individual and group counseling, behavior management programs, academic tutoring, and emotional support during the time the adolescent is being detained. Longer-term facilities for those convicted of more serious crimes are usually separate, but may provide many similar services.

Residential placements are provided for juvenile offenders who are identified as severely emotionally disturbed. Depending on the severity of the offense and the level of adjudication, placements may be made in general treatment centers or in secure correctional facilities.

HEALTH

Just as all children are entitled to appropriate educational services, they must receive needed medical care. A strong relationship exists between physical health and mental health, making these services even more important for those experiencing emotional problems. Severely emotionally disturbed youth are also at a particularly high risk for health and health-related problems such as sexually transmitted diseases, substance abuse, and pregnancy.

Health care services are provided in a variety of settings ranging from school-based clinics to nursing homes that specialize in chronic medical conditions. Services are usually accessed through private practitioners, public health clinics, ambulatory care clinics, and hospital emergency rooms or outpatient clinics. A system of care is not complete without assuring necessary preventive and clinical services. A great deal of advocacy may be needed to develop a responsive, systematic approach to accessing appropriate care for the severely emotionally disturbed. Some of the services that should be included follow:

Education and prevention services are most often used in conjunction with other systems including the media and schools. Local United Way agencies or the local health department may provide leadership in this area.

Screening and assessment designed to identify health problems should be an integral part of a multifactored assessment of youth being referred for mental health treatment. These may be provided by the family physician, a local clinic, or occasionally through school-based clinics.

Primary care encompasses routine medical examinations and checks on growth and developmental milestones, vision and hearing care, dental care, reproductive health services, and assessment and follow-up on chemical use and abuse issues. Particularly if the family is unable or unwilling to access this care for children, other professionals involved should ensure that these physical needs are being addressed.

Long-term medical care is often unnecessary; however, some children have chronic medical needs. These conditions are frequently a trigger for or are exacerbated by serious emotional problems, and closer attention must be given to the interplay of medical and mental health treatment.

SOCIAL AND RECREATIONAL NEEDS

Every model of child development stresses the importance of social interaction and play for healthful growth. All too often severely emotionally disturbed children become isolated from natural and community support systems. The lack of opportunities to be involved with peers and adults in recreational situations deprives these youth of an important element in the total treatment package. Whether activities are structured around a group of severely emotionally disturbed youth, or individuals are integrated into existing settings, the following types of services should be made available:

Healthy interaction with adults provides a vital means of social growth. Helping parents and extended family members to provide this may involve teaching them how to better relate to their severely emotionally disturbed child or focusing on the importance of making the time to do so. For youth without appropriate adult family resources, other organizations may provide volunteers. Possibilities include Big

Brother or Big Sister programs, church or civic groups, or Parent-Teacher organizations.

Structured recreation time allows play in a supervised setting. Scouting, 4-H Clubs, after-school clubs, and local recreation centers all have programs that might be open to, or adaptable for, children with emotional and other handicaps.

Residential or day camps that serve the handicapped offer a truly therapeutic program component that can be especially valuable during the summer months when school-based programs may not be available. Not only do they provide structure and recreation for the child, but also they provide a respite for the family striving to maintain the severely emotionally disturbed youth in the home environment. Some potential resources may be nearby residential programs, charitable organizations, mental health associations or agencies, or the YMCA or YWCA.

Case Management

A system of care does not become a system without a means of coordinating all of the various helpers and programs. Because no state has an approach to children's services that is truly systematic, this management function must be accomplished at the local level in most cases. The crucial component is usually identified as the children's case manager (Behar, 1985; Stroul and Friedman, 1986). Although this role has become more widely recognized in recent years, it is still a theoretical option in most areas. Experts are not in accord about how or where to position the case manager for maximal effectiveness, nor is there widespread agreement concerning what qualifications a case manager should have or who should receive case manager services. Based on those few areas that have implemented this service, however, there is some agreement about the tasks case managers perform.

Nine activities have been identified as services that can be provided by a children's case manager. A brief description of each follows:

Assessment refers to a review of the needs of the child and family from their perspective, combined with a review of the evaluations conducted by mental health professionals and other providers. This review may point to a need for further evaluation, or — if the assessment is complete — provides the basis for the development of a plan.

Planning and coordinating services involves pulling together the youth, family, and all service providers and formulating a single, overall "blueprint" of care. By working with all concerned parties, the case manager can help clarify the needs and goals of the family and minimize the confusion resulting from having a number of people and agencies involved. This also reduces misunderstandings and conflicting assumptions about who is responsible for which functions. For this reason the plan must be written out and everyone must sign it. A sample plan is shown in the box on the following pages. It is important to review such plans on a regular basis or as the needs of the youth and family change.

Linking the child and family to all appropriate services is a vital component of case management. Families may not be aware of or know how to access resources, programs, or people that could be helpful to them.

Monitoring the care and services provided ensures continuity. Severely emotionally

Youth Service Coordination Plan

Name _____

Parent(s) _____

Address _____

_____

Date _____

Client number _____

Home Phone _____

Work Phone(s) _____

_____

Agency-required information

Client/family strengths and resources:

_____

_____

_____

Client/family needs (check all that apply and specify as needed):

___ Mental health: _____

___ Health: _____

___ Education: _____

___ In-home: _____

___ Out-of-home placement:_____

___ Financial: _____

___ Employment/training: _____

___ Recreation: _____

___ Housing: _____

___ Legal: _____

___ Other: _____

_____

Goals and objectives

For each goal listed below, indicate specific system objectives, services/strategies needed, provider, and target date.

I. _____

_____

_____

II. _____

_____

_____

III. _____

_____

_____

IV. _____

_____

_____

V. _____

_____

_____

Continued.

Youth Service Coordination Plan — cont'd

Additional services

Services needed	Strategy for development of options	Agency/Individual responsible for strategy

Providers

Lead agency _____

Service provider _____ Phone _____

Other providers involved:

Name	Agency	Phone

Signatures

Name	Agency	Date
	Client	
	Parent/guardian	
	Parent/guardian	

---

disturbed youth are frequently apt to "fall between the cracks." If the case manager maintains a careful watch over family, community supports, and agency providers, this is not likely to be a problem.

Supportive counseling is a service most case managers provide. Although the role is separate from that of therapist, the case manager is usually perceived by the youth and family as someone who is on their side. Being involved in a therapeutic relationship with the case manager gives the family an additional line of defense during the day-to-day efforts of meeting the many needs of the child.

Crisis intervention activities are often performed by the case manager because of the intensity of involvement and the frequency of contact. In fact, families may be very comfortable reaching out to the case manager in a particularly stressful situation. The case manager can assist them in reaching other emergency service providers if appropriate.

Transportation may be provided by the case manager to some services as part of an overall plan to make treatment accessible. Although case managers should not be viewed as providers of free transportation, helping clients keep necessary appointments may be the only means of ensuring access to them.

Advocacy occurs on two levels. Primarily, case managers work on behalf of a specific client to push for all the rights and services to which the client is entitled. Through knowledge of systems, regulations, programs, and individuals, an assertive case manager can usually improve the care clients receive. The second level of advocacy focuses on improving the systems and their responsiveness to this population as a group.

Outreach, consultation, and education efforts allow case managers to identify unserved or underserved youth by getting out into the community and helping other providers be more aware of the needs of and programs for severely emotionally disturbed children.

Clearly, a case manager must be a multitalented individual. The ability to communicate clearly and effectively with seriously disturbed youth, their families, and the broad range of professional and nonprofessional people across the system of care is essential. A case manager must have enormous reserves of creativity, enthusiasm, and perseverance. The person in this role needs a wide knowledge base that includes child development, family functioning, mental health assessment and treatment issues, and the rights of clients within all systems or agencies. Finally, because a case manager's authority is usually informal, the role requires strong networking and persuasiveness.

A system of care such as the one just described requires substantial funding for services, as well as training for personnel. Normally, considerable lobbying is necessary to obtain the legislation and appropriations for such a wide-ranging effort. Furthermore, mental health workers need both education in the field's methodologies and persuasion to try new and unusual treatment strategies.

REFERENCES AND SUGGESTED READINGS

Behar L (1985) Changing patterns of state responsibility: a case study of North Carolina, Journal of Clinical Child Psychology 14:188-195.

Behar L (1986) A model for child mental health services: the North Carolina experience, Children Today 15(3):16-21.

Hobbs N (1979) Helping disturbed children: psychological and ecological strategies. II. Project Re-Ed twenty years later. Nashville, Tenn, Center for the Study of Families and Children, Vanderbilt University.

Joint Commission on Mental Health of Children (1969) Crisis in child mental health, New York, Harper & Row Publishers, Inc.

Knitzer J (1982) Unclaimed children, Washington, DC, Children's Defense Fund.

Ohio Department of Education (1987) Ohio handbook for the identification of children with severe behavior handicaps, Columbus, Ohio, Ohio Department of Education.

President's Commission on Mental Health (1978) Report of the sub-task panel on infants, children, and adolescents, Washington, DC, US Government Printing Office.

Saxe L, Cross TP, and Silverman N, with Dougherty D (1987) Children's mental health: problems and services, Durham, NC, Duke University Press.

Stroul BA and Friedman RM (1986) A system of care for severely emotionally disturbed children and youth, Washington, DC, Child and Adolescent Service System Program (CASSP) Technical Assistance Center, Georgetown University Child Development Center.

Part II

Strategies for Adolescent Psychiatric Nursing

Part VI

Chapter 8

Intervention Strategies for Adolescent Psychiatric Nurses: an Overview

In this chapter the major categories of adolescent psychiatric nursing interventions are described. These actions are the basic strategies used for adolescents and their families by nurses who are generalists or staff nurses. Clinical specialists also use these strategies, along with consultation and individual, group, family, and multifamily group therapy.

Therapeutic Relationships

Peplau (1952) states that nursing is "an educative instrument, a maturing force that aims to promote forward movement of the personality in the direction of creative, constructive, productive personal and community living." The therapeutic relationship is what allows the adolescent to assimilate the maturing force; it is the nurse's basis for helping people to change. In this relationship the nurse uses communication and counseling techniques to assist the adolescent and family to identify problem areas, to develop insight into the origin of the problems, and to change the unsatisfactory patterns of behavior.

The nurse's ability to form therapeutic relationships depends on his or her self-awareness, empathy, and communication skills. *Self-awareness* is the identification of and acceptance of one's feelings, insight into the meaning of one's behavior patterns, and a clear understanding of one's value system and how one is perceived by others. The nurse who does not possess self-awareness will not be able to understand others and determine which issues originated with the patient. Nurses can develop self-awareness by participating in activities that require introspection and feedback from others. Individual and group psychotherapy or counseling are excellent means of developing self-awareness, particularly if the nurse is uncomfortable about some personal issues. Several organizations sponsor seminars of varying lengths, including weekend experiences, that are geared to developing self-awareness. There are growth experiences for helping professionals such as nurses, teachers, and counselors. Gestalt institutes are good resources, as are the crisis intervention training programs provided for school systems.

Empathy — the ability to be subjective, to lose separateness and become the other person for a while, to feel how the adolescent feels, to view the world from the adolescent's perspective, and to value this perception — is essential for establishing therapeutic relationships. With empathy the nurse can help the adolescent attain self-understanding and solve problems. The most successful therapists are those whose adolescents "felt understood" (Whitehorn and Betz, 1975). If an adolescent and family believe that the nurse understands their situation both emotionally and intellectually and cares about them and the outcomes of the relationship, they can progress in their treatment.

Empathy can be developed in nurses. A wide variety of life experiences is invaluable for developing empathy. Exposure to people of different cultures, religions, and socioeconomic groups helps the nurse to understand others better. Another way of developing empathy is to be exposed to the arts, media, and literature. For instance, viewing the film *Ordinary People* will help a nurse understand the pain and anxiety of a depressed teen and his family. Reading *The Catcher in the Rye* (Salinger, 1951) or *Walking Across Egypt* (Edgerton, 1987) can sensitize nurses to the experience of adolescence. Kalisch (1971, 1973) developed an empathy training program for nurses.

Therapeutic communication techniques are used in therapeutic relationships, particularly in structured one-to-one sessions. Therapeutic communication involves talking with adolescents in a way that promotes self-disclosure, self-understanding, and the problem-solving abilities of adolescents and their families. The basic techniques used in a therapeutic relationship include listening; providing broad openings; restating; clarifying; reflecting; focusing; sharing perceptions, silence, and humor; giving information; and suggesting and identifying themes. See the box on pp. 217-218 for a brief description of these techniques. Communicating with adolescents requires additional techniques. Teenagers are very self-conscious, and considerable tact and respect for their privacy are needed to establish trust. Because adolescents, especially younger teenagers, vary in their cognitive development, the nurse must adjust vocabulary and use of abstract concepts to the adolescent's level. Nonverbal techniques, including writing, doing activity sheets, drawing, or other artistic expressions, are helpful in facilitating expression. Some adolescents may share more freely if they are participating in an activity with the nurse.

Developing therapeutic communication skills entails conscious practice, preferably with audiotaping or videotaping of one-to-one sessions. Written process recordings can be used but are tedious and less reliable. Tapes, process recordings, or sessions repeated from memory should be reviewed regularly with a clinical supervisor or with experienced peers. Clinical supervision, that is, reviewing one's practice with a clinical specialist or other experienced masters' level therapist, psychiatrist, or psychologist, is the best way to develop and improve communication and other counseling skills.

Surveillance

Surveillance is the process of watching over adolescents and their environment to determine if they are safe, keeping their rules, making good decisions, or if they need

Therapeutic Communication Techniques

Technique: LISTENING

Definition: An active process of receiving information and examining one's reaction to the messages received

Example: Maintaining eye contact and receptive nonverbal communication

Therapeutic value: Nonverbally communicates to the patient the nurse's interest and acceptance

Nontherapeutic threat: Failure to listen

Technique: BROAD OPENINGS

Definition: Encouraging the patient to select topics for discussion

Example: "What are you thinking about?"

Therapeutic value: Indicates acceptance by the nurse and the value of the patient's initiative

Nontherapeutic threat: Domination of the interaction by the nurse; rejecting responses

Technique: RESTATING

Definition: Repeating to the patient the main thought he has expressed

Example: "You say that your mother left you when you were five years old."

Therapeutic value: Indicates that the nurse is listening and validates, reinforces, or calls attention to something important that has been said

Nontherapeutic threat: Lack of validation of the nurse's interpretation of the message; being judgmental; reassuring; defending

Technique: CLARIFICATION

Definition: Attempting to put into words vague ideas or unclear thoughts of the patient to enhance the nurse's understanding or asking the patient to explain what he means

Example: "I'm not sure what you mean. Could you tell me about that again?"

Therapeutic value: Helps to clarify feelings, ideas, and perceptions of the patient and provide an explicit correlation between them and the patient's actions

Nontherapeutic threat: Failure to probe; assumed understanding

Technique: REFLECTION

Definition: Directing back to the patient his ideas, feelings, questions, and content

Example: "You're feeling tense and anxious and it's related to a conversation you had with your husband last night?"

Therapeutic value: Validates the nurse's understanding of what the patient is saying and signifies empathy, interest, and respect for the patient

Nontherapeutic threat: Stereotyping the patient's responses; inappropriate timing of reflections; inappropriate depth of feeling of the reflections; inappropriate to the cultural experience and educational level of the patient

Technique: FOCUSING

Definition: Questions or statements that help the patient expand on a topic of importance

Example: "I think that we should talk more about your relationship with your father."

Therapeutic value: Allows the patient to discuss central issues related to his problem and keeps the communication process goal-directed

Nontherapeutic threat: Allowing abstractions and generalizations; changing topics

From Stuart GW and Sundeen CJ (1991) Principles and practice of psychiatric nursing, ed 3, St. Louis, Mosby–Year Book, Inc.

Continued.

Therapeutic Communication Techniques — cont'd

Technique: SHARING PERCEPTIONS
Definition: Asking the patient to verify the nurse's understanding of what he is thinking or feeling
Example: "You're smiling but I sense that you are really very angry with me."
Therapeutic value: Conveys the nurse's understanding to the patient and has the potential for clearing up confusing communication
Nontherapeutic threat: Challenging the patient; accepting literal responses; reassuring; testing; defending

Technique: THEME IDENTIFICATION
Definition: Underlying issues or problems experienced by the patient that emerge repeatedly during the course of the nurse-patient relationship
Example: "I've noticed that in all of the relationships that you have described, you've been hurt or rejected by the man. Do you think this is an underlying issue?"
Therapeutic value: Allows the nurse to best promote the patient's exploration and understanding of important problems
Nontherapeutic threat: Giving advice; reassuring; disapproving

Technique: SILENCE
Definition: Lack of verbal communication for a therapeutic reason
Example: Sitting with a patient and nonverbally communicating interest and involvement
Therapeutic value: Allows the patient time to think and gain insights, slows the pace of the interaction and encourages the patient to initiate conversation, while conveying the nurse's support, understanding, and acceptance
Nontherapeutic threat: Questioning the patient; asking for "why" responses, failure to break a nontherapeutic silence

Technique: HUMOR
Definition: The discharge of energy through the comic enjoyment of the imperfect
Example: "That gives a whole new meaning to the word 'nervous,'" said with shared kidding between the nurse and patient
Therapeutic value: Can promote insight by making conscious repressed material, resolve paradoxes, temper aggression, reveal new options, and is a socially acceptable form of sublimation
Nontherapeutic threat: Indiscriminate use; belittling patient; screen to avoid therapeutic intimacy

Technique: INFORMING
Definition: The skill of information giving
Example: "I think you need to know more about how your medication works."
Therapeutic value: Helpful in health teaching or patient education about relevant aspects of patient's well-being and self-care
Nontherapeutic threat: Giving advice

Technique: SUGGESTING
Definition: Presentation of alternative ideas for the patient's consideration relative to his problem solving
Example: "Have you thought about responding to your boss in a different way when he raises that issue with you? For example, you could ask him if a specific problem has occurred."
Therapeutic value: Increases the patient's perceived options or choices
Nontherapeutic threat: Giving advice; inappropriate timing; being judgmental

adult intervention. Watching over involves actively observing, listening, interacting, and monitoring for signs and symptoms of difficulties in all aspects of the adolescent's life. The intensity of the surveillance depends on the risks to the adolescent and the setting in which the nurse practices. A school nurse may need to coordinate with teachers and counselors to monitor a particular student's well-being. In an inpatient unit one nurse provides surveillance for four adolescents. The ultimate goal of surveillance is to find opportunities to assist adolescents with building skills and developing self-esteem. Those opportunities will not be noticed if the nurse is not watching; crisis situations will develop instead.

Building Self-Esteem

Every interaction with adolescents is directed toward raising their self-esteem. Giving eye contact, using the teenager's name, and starting with a friendly greeting (with a touch on the shoulder or a hug if appropriate) make a teenager feel accepted and valued. Lecturing and giving advice do not enhance communication. Interactions with adolescents should be directed so that the teenager assumes as much responsibility as possible for problem solving. Praising the adolescent for day-to-day efforts, as well as for special accomplishments, teaches that successes are recognized and encourages continued progress. Thanking teens for their help and requesting assistance rather than ordering it are ways to show respect and consideration. If the adolescent needs correcting or limit setting, or if consequences must be applied, the process should be done so that the adolescent is not shamed or embarrassed and so that the young person can assume responsibility for behavior as soon as possible. The nurse assumes that the family of the adolescent wants to do well and is frightened and discouraged about the child's problems. The family is treated in the same friendly, respectful way, with praise given when appropriate.

Role Modeling

The adolescent psychiatric nurse serves as a role model of a healthy adult. The nurse demonstrates excellent communication skills, good manners, and good health habits and personal grooming. A positive, hopeful, professional demeanor reassures adolescents and families that the nurse is a professional who can help. Smoking, eating, chewing gum, or wearing casual clothing in the family's presence may cause the family to doubt the nurse's ability.

Teaching

Nurses use formal and informal teaching methods to provide information to adolescents and their families about growth and development, sexuality, parenting, medications, and physical and mental health problems such as substance abuse. There are numerous teaching programs available for various areas of concern for adolescents; however, these programs can be very expensive. A good teaching plan includes clear objectives that describe what teaching methods the nurse will use and what the learner's outcome will be, as well as an evaluation to determine if the objectives were met. The subject matter should be presented in short, interesting segments that are directed to the learner's cognitive level. Visual aids and experiential exercises such as role playing help improve learning.

Limit Setting

An important strategy in adolescent psychiatric nursing is effective limit setting, especially in the therapeutic milieu. The nurse must approach the process of limit setting with several basic premises:
1. Adolescents need limits to test as a part of normal growth and development.
2. The focus of control should shift from external sources to the adolescent's own resources as quickly as possible with each episode.
3. Each attempt to exceed limits of acceptable behavior is a learning experience.

Reality therapy is an excellent approach to use with adolescents (Jones and Jones, 1981; Wubbolding, 1988; Glasser, 1980). Steps to be used when the adolescent is testing a limit, breaking a rule, or not meeting an expectation or goal are presented in the box below.

Restraint, seclusion, and medication are used in inpatient, partial hospitalization, or severe behavior disorder classroom situations to control aggressive behavior. See Chapters 11 and 14 for a more detailed discussion of limit setting in these situations.

Because limit setting is often used with adolescents who are angry or aggressive, the *problem solving* approach using reality therapy is usually supplemented with other behavior management techniques. Training in the management of anger is a strategy discussed in the next section of this chapter. *Contingency management* is the use of natural or contrived outcomes to influence the adolescent's behavior. Some contingency management techniques that increase positive behavior are reinforcement, differential reinforcement, contingency contracting, and token reinforcement (Milan and Kolko, 1985).

Steps of Limit Setting Using Principles of Reality Therapy

1. Establish a therapeutic relationship
2. Ask the adolescent:
   A. What are you doing?
   B. What are you feeling?
   C. Is what you are doing helping you get what you want?
   D. Make a plan for getting what you want (or dealing with your feelings).
3. Follow through with obtaining the plan.
4. Follow through with the outcome of the plan.
5. If adolescent cannot make a plan or follow through, start again and coach the adolescent.
6. Remind the adolescent of consequences.
7. If the adolescent will not make an alternative plan, apply consequences.
8. Remediate after the consequences by repeating steps.

Reinforcement is the praising or rewarding of expected behavior. *Differential reinforcement* is the positive reinforcement of positive behaviors without addressing negative behaviors. This method alone is effective over long periods of time but is not effective in changing the severe problems seen in treatment situations. In *contingency contracting,* the adolescent and significant others combine with the nurse to develop a written set of target behaviors and their contingent reinforcers (Rimm and Masters, 1979). The privilege system of an inpatient program is an example of a type of contingency contract. This technique is very useful for families. *Token reinforcement* is the reward of specific positive behaviors with tangible tokens, which may then be used to "purchase" another reward. For instance, a young adolescent with attention deficit disorder who stays seated for an unbroken 30 minutes in school or in a group receives a gold sticker. After accumulating four stickers, 15 minutes of Nintendo can be purchased. Point systems used in inpatient treatment are a type of token reinforcement.

Contingency management techniques that decrease undesirable behavior are time out, response cost, and punishment through aversive stimulation. The latter is not used in mental health treatment. (The practice of room isolation for days at a time, used in some treatment centers, should be considered aversive treatment and is not an acceptable practice.) *Time out* is a commonly used technique wherein the adolescent removes himself or is assisted to leave the disrupted situation for a quiet place to regain control or prevent loss of control. This technique is very effective in controlling aggressive behavior (Milan and Kolko, 1985). *Response cost* contingency management occurs when the adolescent loses positive reinforcement for negative behavior. An example of response cost management occurs when the adolescent is grounded one weekend day if he stays out past his curfew.

Nurses often work with families who do not set limits or who are having difficulty setting limits. Relatively healthy families can be assisted to establish rules and consequences and can be taught the processes described in this section. Parents' participation in behavior management schemes ensures a more positive outcome (Patterson and Gullion, 1976). For more disturbed families a referral to family therapy is appropriate.

Skill Development and Goal Setting

Helping families and adolescents ". . . develop, improve or regain their adaptive functioning . . . " is a goal of adolescent psychiatric nursing (American Nurses Association, 1985). Adaptive functioning includes cognitive, social, and psychological skills. The nurse helps the teenager identify areas needing change and then assists the adolescent to set goals and follow steps to achieve them. This process can be done individually, in groups, or with families.

Generally, skill development techniques have their roots in behavior therapy and cognitive therapy. Behavior therapy consists of (1) a *teaching* component, which may include *modeling* (demonstration), *shaping* (assisting and coaching the adolescent in the desired behavior and then *fading* the amount of prompting; (2) an *incentive* component, such as a behavioral contract or privilege system to motivate the adolescent; and (3) the delivery of the incentive in step 2 contingent on the desired behavior (Braukmann and others, 1976). Cognitive therapy consists of identifying attitudes, ideas, and self-talk that are nonproductive and using cognitive skills such as decision-making, problem-solving, and self-talk or instruction to change the attitude, thought, or behavior (Meichenbaum, 1979; Hobb and others, 1980; Urbain and Kendall, 1980; Kendall, 1981; Yule, 1984). The behavior therapies are more effective with the addition of cognitive approaches; both of these approaches need reinforcement in the social context outside of the treatment setting, especially in the family. (Pellegrini and Urbain, 1984; Patterson, 1982; Patterson and Gullion, 1976).

Skill development and goal setting take place in the context of a therapeutic relationship wherein the adolescent feels comfortable, cared for, and understood. Discussing problem areas and behaviors is especially difficult and embarrassing, so patience and considerable coaching are required. Goal setting in groups is very effective because the group provides pressure and support to achieve goals, and peers contribute their ideas and experiences to the development of activities to meet the goals. Daily goal setting in inpatient or partial hospitalization is effective for ensuring progress toward achieving overall treatment goals.

With adolescents, goals should be based on the need for development of specific cognitive, psychological (coping), and social skills, beginning with the basic and progressing to the more complex. Goals and skills must be developed to identify the problem itself, identify the feelings, thoughts and situations associated with it, identify alternative behaviors (new skills), and then practice the alternatives. Identifying a problem (skill deficit) and discovering the feelings, thoughts, and situations associated with it are ways of developing self-awareness, and self-awareness is essential to changing behavior. Brigham (1989) describes several components of behavioral analysis or self- and other-awareness:

Self-observation of behavior: What do I do?
Self-environment observation: What do others do?
                                     What do I do in response to the environment?
Self-observation, private events: What do I think?
                                     What do I feel?
                                     How do I talk to myself inside myself?

Once these questions are answered about a behavior, then alternative behaviors can be chosen and practiced:

Modification   What can I do differently?
    Change behavior
        Social skills training
        Anger management
    Change attitude/perception
        Problem-solve
        Positive self-talk
        Think out loud
    Restructure environment
Practice, practice, practice   Practice it!

There are a variety of tools for nurses and therapists to assess skill deficits in adolescents. Goldstein and others (1980) offer a structured learning skill checklist and a skill checklist summary for tracking progress. Brigham (1989) provides a youth behavior inventory for the student/patient, the parent and peers. These tools are easy to use and do not require strict interrater reliability or other research techniques. See Chapter 6 for other behavior rating scales. Goldstein and others (1980) propose four cognitive skills development activities that assist adolescents in determining their needs: (1) setting a goal, (2) deciding on their abilities, (3) gathering information, and (4) deciding what caused a problem. Similar activities are available in Dupont and Dupont (1979); two books by Bingham and others (1984); and Brigham (1988).

Once the problem or skill deficit is identified, then the nurse and the adolescent set out to develop the skill by taking very specific steps. A series of steps or goals may be devised to meet a larger goal. For instance, if the nurse and adolescent want to work on improving relations with the parents, then the adolescent must develop listening skills and basic clear communication ("I" statements). If the adolescent is a good communicator but needs to learn temper control, then a series of goals can be worked out to teach the adolescent to identify early signs of angry feelings, identify trigger situations, and then identify and practice new ways to handle the anger-causing situations.

The steps toward the goals should be action oriented and involve others. The teenager can do structured written exercises, make lists, contact others for feedback, and role play a variety of situations with the nurse and finally practice these new behaviors with others.

Social Skills Development

Social skills training consists of teaching the steps of the desired goal, modeling them, and then demonstrating the steps, having the adolescent role play the behavior before practicing it with the nurse, peers, and adults on the unit or at school or with parents and siblings at home. Social skills training programs are usually designed for groups but can be easily adapted to the adolescent and nurse, or other dyads (Shaw and others, 1980). There are many social skills that an adolescent needs to be a successful adult. Goldstein and others (1980) name 50 skills in their program; several of them are listed in this book as cognitive and coping skills (see box on p. 224). Suggestions for developing the social skills necessary for competence in adolescence (described in Chapter 1) are discussed below.

FRIENDLINESS

For adolescents to act in a friendly manner, they must be able to perform a variety of skills (see boxes on pp. 225-226). These include nine skills listed by Goldstein and others (1980): (1) listening, (2) starting a conversation, (3) having a conversation, (4) asking a question, (5) saying thank you, (6) introducing yourself, (7) introducing other people, (8) giving a compliment, and (9) joining in. Deficits in these areas may be brought to the adolescent's attention by using assessment tools or nurse, teacher, peer, or family observation. After the adolescent identifies a difficulty in one area, specific steps can be taught by written instructions and by demonstration of the behaviors needed. For instance, the steps suggested by Goldstein and others (1980)

Beginning Social Skills: Asking a Question

Steps	Trainer Notes
1. Decide what you'd like to know more about.	Ask about something you don't understand, something you didn't hear, or something confusing.
2. Decide whom to ask.	Think about who has the best information on a topic; consider asking several people.
3. Think about different ways to ask your question and pick one way.	Think about wording; raise your hand; ask nonchallengingly.
4. Pick the right time and place to ask your question.	Wait for a pause; wait for privacy.
5. Ask your question.	

Suggested Content for Modeling Displays

A. School or neighborhood: Main actor asks teacher to explain something he/she finds unclear.
B. Home: Main actor asks mother to explain new curfew decision.
C. Peer group: Main actor asks classmate about missed schoolwork.

Comments

Trainers are advised to model only single, answerable questions. In role play, trainees should be instructed to do likewise.

From Goldstein A, Sprafkin R, Gershaw J, and Klein P (1980) Skillstreaming the adolescent, Champaign, Ill, Research Press.

for listening are the following:
1. Look at the person who is talking.
2. Think about what is being said (nod your head, say "hmmm").
3. Wait your turn to talk (don't fidget).
4. Say what you want to say (ask questions, express feelings and ideas).

Have the adolescent practice these steps with the nurse and in other situations. In inpatient units the adolescent should practice these steps about three times each shift with a variety of people, peers as well as adults. In a therapeutic milieu the practice behaviors can be recorded in a journal and initialed by the person who has listened to the adolescent, who then gets credit or points toward making progress in the privilege system. The behavior gets reinforced in the contingency contract. In outpatient settings the adolescent practices the behavior in a less structured setting, but validation (by signing off or verbal reports) by parents and teachers can be used. The adolescent can keep a journal for recording successes or failures each day and might have a contingency contract for reinforcing the behavior. For instance, if Mary is able to listen once each day for a week, she may have an extra hour of Nintendo on Saturday. Considerable coaching may be needed initially or if the skill is difficult

Text continued on p. 226.

Skills for Adolescents

Group I. Beginning Social Skills

1. Listening
2. Starting a conversation
3. Having a conversation
4. Asking a question
5. Saying thank you
6. Introducing yourself
7. Introducing other people
8. Giving a compliment

Group II. Advanced Social Skills

9. Asking for help
10. Joining in
11. Giving instructions
12. Following instructions
13. Apologizing
14. Convincing others

Group III. Skills for Dealing with Feelings

15. Knowing your feelings
16. Expressing your feelings
17. Understanding the feelings of others
18. Dealing with someone else's anger
19. Expressing affection
20. Dealing with fear
21. Rewarding yourself

Group IV. Skill Alternatives to Aggression

22. Asking permission
23. Sharing something
24. Helping others
25. Negotiation
26. Using self-control
27. Standing up for your rights
28. Responding to teasing
29. Avoiding trouble with others
30. Keeping out of fights

From Goldstein A, Sprafkin R, Gershaw J, and Klein P (1980) Skillstreaming the adolescent, Champaign, Ill, Research Press.

Continued.

Skills for Adolescents — cont'd

Group V. Skills for Dealing with Stress

31. Making a complaint
32. Answering a complaint
33. Sportsmanship after the game
34. Dealing with embarrassment
35. Dealing with being left out
36. Standing up for a friend
37. Responding to persuasion
38. Responding to failure
39. Dealing with contradictory messages
40. Dealing with an accusation
41. Getting ready for a difficult conversation
42. Dealing with group pressure

Group VI. Planning Skills

43. Deciding on something to do
44. Deciding what caused a problem
45. Setting a goal
46. Deciding on your abilities
47. Gathering information
48. Arranging problems by importance
49. Making a decision
50. Concentrating on a task

---

for the adolescent. With all of the nine skills needed to develop friendliness, Goldstein and others provide the steps, trainer notes, and suggested scenarios for role playing. Another program, developed by Gazda and others (1980; 1980; 1985) provides a similar approach. A collection of activity sheets for getting along with others is provided in Brewner and others (1984). There are also some units in Brigham (1988) that apply to developing friendliness.

INTERPERSONAL SENSITIVITY

To develop sensitivity to others and to know the effect of one's behavior on others requires several abilities. Goldstein and others list (1) understanding the feelings of others, (2) dealing with someone else's anger, and (3) apologizing. Dupont and Dupont (1979) give components on encouraging openness and trust. Brigham (1988) provides activities for (1) dealing with impatience (unit 27) and (2) reciprocity and equity, or fairness (unit 19). Developing sensitivity in interpersonal situations requires the recognition of verbal and nonverbal communication, which is taught in the Dupont book (program component No. 3). Interpersonal sensitivity may also be enhanced by introducing adolescents to other cultures through school programs or media and through values-clarification exercises. Values-clarification exercises are available in the two books by Bingham and others (1984), in Dupont and Dupont (1979; program component 5), and in Simon and others (1978).

COOPERATIVENESS

Assisting an adolescent to become more cooperative requires several other skills suggested by Goldstein and others (1980). They are (1) asking for help, (2) following instructions, (3) asking permission, (4) sharing something, and (5) helping others. Many adolescents, especially those with low self-esteem and a history of rejection or abuse, have difficulty asking for help. These adolescents may benefit from training in dealing with fear or anxiety before attempting to ask for help. Goldstein and others provide activities for these skills, as do Brewner and others (1984). In addition to specific social skills training, adolescents can learn cooperativeness during group activities in school and the community, and in treatment. Community service projects are useful in developing cooperativeness and interpersonal sensitivity. In one inpatient adolescent program, the teen patients made favors, dressed in costumes, and visited the pediatrics and extended care units in the hospital on Haloween. Even the most aggressive and uncooperative adolescents were able to participate.

CURIOSITY

Adolescents from socially, culturally, or economically deprived families or communities have not been exposed to a variety of people, ideas and sources of information. In spite of—or because of—electronic media, many adolescents do not seek or have information. Infants, toddlers and preschoolers are naturally curious, but by adolescence teenagers may be preoccupied with their own lives. Exposing adolescents to a variety of ideas, peoples, cultures, arts, and current events can stimulate the natural curiosity that has been diminished. Field trips, extracurricular activities, and exercises in critical thinking boost curiosity. The United Learning program (1983) stimulates thinking and curiosity.

CAPACITY TO WORK AND TO ENGAGE IN ALTERNATE ROLES

Adolescents must be prepared to work and maintain themselves independently as adults. Besides the cognitive or manual abilities needed for a job or career, competent people have social skills that enable them to obtain a job and remain at it. The social skills needed for work may include (1) listening, (2) asking a question, (3) introducing oneself, (4) giving instructions, (5) following directions, (6) convincing others, (7) asking permission, (8) negotiating, (9) using self-control, (10) making a complaint, (11) answering a complaint, (12) responding to failure, (13) having a difficult conversation, (14) gathering information, and (15) concentrating on a task (Goldstein and others, 1980). Most of these skills must be mastered before an adolescent can be successful at work. The Goldstein book provides activities for each of these skills. Activities for making decisions about work and future roles are provided in the Bingham books. There are a variety of materials available on job interviewing.

Teenagers need to observe and try out various roles to develop self-confidence and determine the fitness of the role for him or her. The recent trends of business and local government "adopting" schools to provide experiences for youth are promising. Adolescents who are performing poorly do not typically engage in these programs. Troubled or deprived adolescents can become involved in Big Brother or Big Sister programs. Field trips or visits from various persons in different work roles in the community help adolescents in treatment programs learn about various careers.

Therapeutic communities provide jobs and activities in the milieu to encourage adolescents to practice leadership behaviors and work skills such as kitchen chores, developing a newsletter, and community meals. Career-development activities are available in the Bingham books and in high school career-development curriculums.

Cognitive Skill Development

INTELLIGENCE AND THE ABILITY TO ABSTRACT

In today's complex, technological society, intelligence is an important factor in becoming a competent adult. Although intelligence levels are influenced heavily by heredity, culturally deprived children and adolescents have deficits in many areas of cognitive functioning. These adolescents benefit from treatment for anxiety, depression, and other disorders, and the capabilities they do have can be stimulated through academic tutoring, exposure to information in situations that are conducive to learning, and social and cognitive skill training.

The ability to think abstractly develops from early adolescence to middle adolescence. Abstract thinking allows the adolescent to think about possibilities that are not connected to a concrete idea or perception. Because adolescents vary widely in their ability to abstract, it is important to assess that ability and to use concrete events as starting points for skill training. This is why it is so important for adolescents to determine what the problem is and what their experience of it is before they can change their behavior. Younger adolescents are preoccupied with themselves and their own experience and tend not to differentiate their ideas from others, even though they do have the ability to discriminate their own thoughts and feelings from those of others. Interventions that assist adolescents to develop critical thinking skills include those in United Learning (1983); skill training proposed by Goldstein and others (1980) for (1) deciding what caused a problem, (2) arranging problems by importance, (3) gathering information, and (4) making a decision; and component 1 in Dupont and Dupont (1979).

PROBLEM SOLVING AND DECISION MAKING

The ability to problem solve and make good decisions are so important for success that they are discussed separately from intelligence and abstract thinking. Behavior therapy and cognitive therapies, including reality therapy, are based on a problem-solving approach: What am I doing (thinking, feeling)? What is the effect of the other person or situation? What can I do to change myself or the situation? The adolescent may not know the solutions but must learn how to find them. Until adolescents learn effective solutions, the nurse models solutions, coaches the teens, or provides learning materials. A number of problem solving/decision-making skill training programs are available for developing the general skill and for problem solving in certain situations (such as the pressure to use chemicals or participate in sex). The Goldstein training modules are listed in the previous section. The Transition program (Dupont and Dupont, 1979) has a model for problem-solving. A skills program for chemically dependent adolescents is provided by Monti and others (1989). Another program, by Hazel and others (1981), contains a component for problem solving. These and other programs provide the educational and modeling components for building these skills—but adolescents must practice them with the assistance and supervision of a nurse, especially in inpatient or day treatment programs.

VERBAL COMMUNICATION

Competent adolescents verbally express themselves appropriately for the situation, with correct grammar and word usage and accompanying congruent nonverbal communication. Correct grammar and vocabulary are generally taught in school. However, word lists for feelings can be helpful to the adolescent in treatment settings. Teaching "I" statements and having the adolescent practice them is a simple and effective beginning method. The following is an example of an "I" statement:

I feel _____

because _____

and I want _____ .

Effective or active listening is a basic and important aspect of good communication. Goldstein and others (1980) provide several activities for listening and communicating, as do the Duponts. The Goldstein program proposes (1) listening, (2) starting a conversation, (3) having a conversation, (4) asking a question, (5) asking for help, (6) convincing others, (7) expressing feelings, (8) expressing affection, (9) responding to persuasion, (10) dealing with contradictory messages, and (11) dealing with group pressure. Bell (1977) has a program that provides opportunities for improving verbal communication skills. Hazel and others (1981) have a component on giving and receiving feedback for adolescents.

RESPONSIBILITY

Many times an adolescent is given too much responsibility with too little preparation. For instance, a teenager may be told to clean the house but not shown how or what exactly to do. The adolescent then does the cleaning, and the parent is distressed at the results and criticizes or punishes the teen. The adolescent then avoids the chore and becomes resistant.

Chemically dependent adolescents are usually irresponsible. Treating the addiction is necessary for a change in this area. Contingency management contracts are very helpful in assisting the adolescent to produce responsible behavior contingent on rewards or consequences. Learning the right or responsible thing to do can be accomplished by role modeling, discussions in groups or in dyads about moral decision-making, or formal training.

Brewner and others (1984) provide some activity sheets for very basic responsibilities such as being on time. The Bingham (1984) books provide several activities for preparing for adult responsibilities. Arbuthnot and Gordon (1986) provide a program for the development of moral reasoning for behavior-disordered adolescents.

ACHIEVEMENT BASED ON CONFORMITY TO COMMUNITY STANDARDS

For adolescents to become competent, they must demonstrate achievement in areas acceptable to the community. Adolescents are expected to attend school, complete assignments, and pass courses. They are also expected to make positive contributions to the family and to the community through service activities, sports, or the arts. Adolescents need structure and support to achieve. Positive reinforcement over time from at least one adult is vital. Programs to encourage parent involvement at school and in the adolescent's academic progress are helpful. Nurses should encourage parental contact with school while their teenager is in inpatient treatment; others should not have to provide it for the parents. Being successful in goal setting and achievement in groups and activities related to treatment start the process of achieving.

PSYCHOLOGICAL AND COPING SKILL DEVELOPMENT

SELF-AWARENESS

Self-awareness is a prerequisite to developing coping skills. A cognitive approach to developing self-awareness is described earlier in the chapter. Other techniques used to develop an awareness of feelings, especially painful ones, are more psychotherapeutic in nature. Gestalt therapy techniques are useful for developing self-awareness, particularly if resistance is a factor. Gestalt therapy focuses on the adolescent's experience here and now. The nurse or therapist helps the teen focus on his physical experience at the moment and gradually encourages him to experience the sensation more fully—to exaggerate it, to act it out—until the sensation becomes connected to its source. For instance, the adolescent can be guided through a progressive relaxation exercise until he feels tingling in his arms. As he focuses on the sensation in his arms, he becomes aware that he would like to strike out in anger. With coaching, the adolescent can enact a striking and be asked to name all the possibilities of that position or what else that pose might represent: anger, a reaching-out for acceptance, love, and so forth (Zinker, 1977).

Art and other media, music, and movement help an adolescent discover and express his feelings, problems, and other therapeutic issues. They are especially helpful with an adolescent who has verbal communication problems. Nurses may learn some of these techniques, but consultation with an occupational art, music, or dance therapist may be very helpful.

SELF-ESTEEM

Having positive thoughts and feelings about oneself is a prerequisite to most coping skills. Adolescents need positive feelings about school and their performance in it, their relationship with peers, and their physical selves. Raising self-esteem can begin with having the adolescent list positive aspects of himself; he can obtain this information from parents, peers, siblings, and others. When the adolescent cannot find one acceptable thing about himself, the nurse or adolescent can start with some of the negative behaviors he performs very well. For instance, a 15-year-old boy who was in his third inpatient program had felony charges, failed two grades in school, and decided that he really was an excellent con artist. He and the nurse were then able to identify his ability to negotiate and persuade as a positive trait. Adolescents sometimes have an inflated sense of self-esteem, which prevents them from making realistic plans or accepting criticism and feedback. Nurses interact with adolescents in ways that promote self-esteem: by being friendly, being supportive, and using problem-solving approaches to inappropriate behavior. Cognitive approaches to building self-esteem are very helpful. Adolescents can be taught ways to "talk" to themselves about themselves. Criticizing and "shoulding" are common kinds of self-talk that people with low self-esteem use. Adolescents can be given or can choose new self-talks. For instance, instead of telling themselves, "You're so stupid, you got a C on the test," they can learn to say, "I got a C on this test—that's an average grade." "You're so fat and ugly" can become "I look nice in these colors." A self-esteem assessment can help an adolescent get his self-worth into perspective. Many books and programs have been designed to help teenagers develop self-esteem. Stuart and Sundeen (1991) provide an excellent discussion of alterations in self-concept and a nursing care plan that uses a counseling approach. Some other programs are *Developing Self-Respect* (Learning Tree Filmstrips), *Overcoming Inferiority* (Human Relations Media), and books by Rowe and others (1983) and McKay and Fanning (1987).

INTERNAL LOCUS OF CONTROL AND IMPULSE CONTROL

These two areas of competence are discussed together because impulse control is maintained by an internal locus of control in a competent adolescent. Poor impulse control is a major focus of intervention with adolescents. Developmentally, adolescents normally engage in some risk-taking behavior, usually associated with peer pressure. Disturbed adolescents act out pain and depression, and many adolescents seen in treatment have attention deficit hyperactivity disorder (ADHD) and bipolar disorder (mania and hypomania). Aggression is common with disturbed adolescents. The discussion of impulse control is divided into hyperactivity control and anger and aggression control. Problems with control require creating a structured environment and setting up contingency contracts.

Techniques for assisting adolescents with ADHD include referral for medication, teaching parents about the disorder and the management techniques, and developing a behavior management plan with the adolescent that gradually increases the amount of quiet and concentration time. "Thinking out loud"—saying "Stop and think!"—helps a younger adolescent begin to manage overactivity. This progresses to internal self-talk, including a miniproblem-solving process such as "Stop and think: what am I supposed to be doing? I can do this for 15 minutes." A token economy can be set up for 15 minutes to 1- or 2-hour periods until medications take effect. Manic and hypomanic adolescents may be managed in this way while medications are building to therapeutic levels. Stimulation should be reduced when concentration is needed.

Anger and aggression management respond well to behavioral and cognitive techniques, as well as to social skills training. Many adolescents have problems with anger and aggression but do not possess the social skills necessary for appropriate expressions of anger (see box on p. 232). Goldstein and others (1980) suggest several skill alternatives to aggression that may be helpful. They are (1) asking permission, (2) sharing something, (3) helping others, (4) negotiating, (5) using self-control, (6) standing up for one's rights, (7) responding to teasing, (8) avoiding trouble with others, (9) keeping out of fights, (10) dealing with embarrassment, and (11) dealing with an accusation.

Skill Alternatives to Aggression: Responding to Teasing

Steps	Trainer Notes
Decide if you are being teased.	Are others making jokes or whispering?
Think about ways to deal with the teasing.	Gracefully accept it; make a joke of it; ignore it.
Choose the best way and do it.	When possible, avoid alternatives that foster aggression, malicious counter-teasing, and withdrawal.

Suggested Content for Modeling Displays

School or neighborhood: main actor ignores classmate's comments when volunteering to help teacher after class.
Home: main actor tells sibling to stop teasing about new haircut.
Peer group: main actor deals with peer's teasing about a girlfriend or boyfriend by making a joke of it.

From Goldstein A, Sprafkin R, Gershon NJ, and Klein P (1980) Skillstreaming the adolescent, Champaign, Ill, Research Press.

Another approach involves making an anger chart. This is a project with which the adolescent describes his levels of anger—from a little angry to out of control—in his own words and prints them on a section of the chart. In the next column he describes what his body feels like (nonverbals), and in the next column what his behavior is. A fourth column may be added for alternative behaviors. See Chapter 11 for a sample chart. The chart is an excellent self-awareness exercise. The adolescent must be coached through this process. Another technique for managing anger is to take one or two deep breaths and then to stop and think. Full relaxation training is helpful. Exercise is very important in reducing tension and anger and should be structured in the adolescent's daily routine.

As a comprehensive approach to self-control, anger management consists of self-awareness, problem solving, self-instruction, stress inoculation, and contingency management that includes time-out and response cost (Milan and Kolko, 1985; Varley, 1984). Combining these strategies provides better results than any individual strategy (Novaco, 1975, 1978; Kolko and others, 1981). The adolescent with significant anger or aggression problems should do the following:

1. The adolescent has a clear structure of expectations for each day, whether at home or in a program at school or a treatment facility.
2. The adolescent has a contingency management contract, including home and school, and treatment expectations with contingencies for meeting or not meeting them; a supplemental contract may be developed for aggressive behavior separately (contingency management).

3. The adolescent is talked through the reality therapy processing approach (described earlier in this chapter) at early signs of agitation (problem solving/coaching).
4. The adolescent is taught to take himself through this process by saying it out loud and then silently instructing himself (problem solving/self-instruction, self-talk).
5. Time out is used whenever appropriate for *short* periods of time (5 to 15 minutes); this may be selected by the adolescent (neutral reinforcement).
6. The adolescent is trained in various alternatives to losing control through the social skills training activities already noted (social skill training).
7. After control is established, the adolescent is subjected to stress in role playing and in increasing expectations, so that he may practice maintaining control under stressful conditions (stress inoculation).
8. Medication is used to treat underlying disorders; sedation and benzodiazepines are to be avoided.

Several programs develop self-control: Goldstein and others (1980), Novako (1975, 1978), Kolko and others (1981), *Understanding and Accepting Yourself* (Learning Tree Filmstrips) and Monti and others (1989).

Personal Power and Control over Environment

The sense of personal power comes from having the skills listed in this chapter. The adolescent who is successful in school, is friendly and cooperative, and has an internal locus of control will feel able to handle most situations. Highly competent adolescents can manage their lives on short- and long-term bases in spite of stunting environments. They can find ways to structure their environments and to prevent negative elements from controlling them. Nurses can assist adolescents to gain personal power by helping them to develop these skills.

Coping with Stress

Adolescents may be taught stress management techniques to add to their repertoire of coping skills. Relaxation training and exercise are helpful for teenagers. Adolescents experiencing severe stress may be taught visualization and imagery to replace traumatic memories and images. Self-soothing activities may be explored with the adolescent to relieve pain—for example, singing to self, playing tapes recorded by kind and supportive people when they are not available, even regressing to childhood activities for a time. There are many stress management programs available. One for high school-aged adolescents is by Emery (1987).

Skill Development with Families

Since the adolescent's focus for learning ranges from treatment centers to the home, the family should be involved in the training process, especially with aggressive adolescents (Patterson and Gullion, 1976; Patterson, 1982). Several packages are available for developing parenting skills. The STEP-Teen Program (Dinkmeyer, 1983) and *Active Parenting* (Popkin, 1987) are two programs for motivated verbal parents. Paterson and Gullion's program (1976) and one by Robin (1980) are better suited to troubled families. *Raising Children for Success* (Glenn and Nelsen, 1987) is useful for motivated families. Kline and others (1990) provide a workbook for parents, teachers, and others to improve family life.

Crisis Intervention

The adolescent psychiatric nurse "uses crisis intervention to promote growth and aid the personal and social integration of the . . . adolescent and family in developmental or situational crisis and suicidal crisis" (American Nurses Association, 1985). When an adolescent and family are unable to cope because of an event or series of events, they are said to be in a crisis state; at this point they are very amenable to assistance. Crisis intervention is a widely used technique in nursing and mental health services and is increasingly used in schools. Crisis intervention techniques are also used in crisis centers, suicide and teen hot lines, police departments, and emergency rooms. The steps in crisis intervention are discussed in Chapter 10.

The growth of drug and alcohol problems has led to the use of a variation of traditional crisis intervention called an "intervention" (Johnson, 1986). An intervention is a process wherein the nurse or helping professional and significant others gather assessment information about an adolescent whose substance abuse is affecting all their lives. The adolescent is then confronted by family members, friends, and the counselor in a caring way to encourage the adolescent to obtain help for the problem. Because denial is so strong in chemical dependence, the dependent person rarely seeks help; therefore a crisis is created for the dependent person by the intervention. All types of crisis intervention require training and supervised practice.

Case Management

Case management has been an informal nursing activity for many years. Recently, however, case management has become structured in response to the complexity and expense of health care systems and other services, especially the ones provided for children and adolescents. Case management is not a treatment modality. In the community it is the providing of *coordination* of services for individuals and families (including transportation to those services), *advocacy* for adolescents with those systems and services, and the arranging of *crisis intervention* when needed. The ultimate purposes of case management are to save money (by reducing use of inpatient services) and to prevent adolescents from dropping out of treatment and decompensating (Forchuk, 1989; Pittman, 1989). Normally, the severely emotionally disturbed adolescents qualify for case management. Nurses with baccalaureate degrees in nursing and experience in adolescent psychiatric nursing make excellent case managers. However, the public sector's funding for these positions provides lower salaries than those from hospitals. Reimbursement by third parties is spotty for this service.

Primary nursing includes case management in the hospital setting. Sometimes hospitals assign case managers to coordinate inpatient services with outpatient service providers and referral sources. Some programs assign various multidisciplinary staff members as case managers to coordinate information flow about an adolescent.

Collaboration

Collaboration is a strategy used to improve the care and services provided for adolescents. The nurse works with other disciplines so that the "different abilities of health care providers are used to communicate, plan, solve problems, and offer a variety of treatment problems" (American Nurses Association, 1985). Nurses should articulate the knowledge they have regarding patients and programs and seek input from others. Nurses must be present at the meetings at which information is shared and decisions are made about care and programs.

Advocacy

Nurses serve as advocates for adolescents by representing their cause. An adolescent does not always have the power to advocate for himself in the hospital, community, or family system. The nurse can assist the adolescent to be assertive, or the nurse may make the case for whatever is needed on the adolescent's behalf (Kohnke, 1982).

Referral

Psychiatric nurses make referrals within the systems in which they work and to people and agencies in the community. A referral is the process of identifying the need, locating a service to fill the need, discussing it with the adolescent and family, then making the arrangement for the contact to occur. Simply telling someone what services are available is insufficient (Wolfe, 1962). Making referrals is an integral part of discharge planning and case management.

Community Action

Adolescent psychiatric nurses have a responsibility to take part in community activities that relate to the well-being of adolescents. This participation can be accomplished by joining community task forces, being on school committees, writing letters to newspaper editors or public officials, working for political candidates who are concerned about youth problems, or running for political office. State and local nurses' associations have political action committees. The Advocates for Child Psychiatric Nursing represent child and adolescent issues at the regional and national levels. See Chapter 9 for a list of organizations relevant to adolescent issues.

Consultation

Consultation is the process of giving expert advice to groups or organizations who request it. The advice may include diagnosing problems, developing solutions, and assisting in implementation of those solutions, and it often includes training. Usually the clinical specialist is in the consulting role, but the generalist staff or school nurse may serve as an informal consultant for peers and some community groups. Consultation can be provided on a free basis, but normally consultation is provided for a fee.

Somatic Therapies

Nurses are responsible for administering medications, monitoring their effects, and teaching adolescents and their parents and teachers about the medications. Adolescent psychiatric nurses also educate teachers, school nurses, and therapists about the results and about the side effects and dosage of medications. The following boxes on pp. 237-241 list publishers and sources for additional materials that may be useful in working with adolescents. Chapter 13 discusses these therapies in detail.

Individual, Family, and Group Therapy

Psychotherapy and family therapy are provided by nurses who have graduate education in these modalities. This area of practice is reserved for the clinical specialist in psychiatric nursing. See Chapter 12 for a discussion of these strategies.

Listing of Publishers

Advanced Learning Concepts
211 W. Wisconsin Avenue
Milwaukee, WI 53203

Animal Town Game Co.
P.O. Box 2002
Santa Barbara, CA 93120

Argus Communications
7440 Natchez Avenue
Niles, IL 60658

ATC Publishing Corp.
J.S. Latta, Inc.
P.O. Box 1276
Huntington, WV 25715

Constructive Playthings
1040 East 85th Street
Kansas City, MO 64131

The Council for Exceptional Children
1920 Association Drive
Reston, VA 22901

Creative Therapeutics
155 County Road
Cresskill, NJ 07626

DLM Teaching Resources
One DLM Park
Allen, TX 75002

EBSCO Curriculum Materials
Division EBSCO Industries, Inc.
Box 11521
Birmingham, AL 35202

Educational Activities, Inc.
P.O. Box 392
Freeport, NY 11520

Educational Design, Inc.
47 W. 13th St.
New York, NY 10011

Films Incorporated
733 Green Bay Road
Wilmette, IL 60091

Gamco Industries, Inc.
P.O. Box 1862 K
Big Spring, TX 79720

Guidance Associates
Communications Park
Box 3000
Mount Kisco, NY 10549

Human Development Training
   Institute, Inc.
7574 University Avenue
La Mesa, CA 92041
800-854-2166

Human Science Press
72 Fifth Avenue
New York, NY 10011

Institute for Rational Living
45 East 65th Street
New York, NY 10021

J. Weston Walch, Publisher
Portland, ME 04104

Kimbo Educational Activities
P.O. Box 477
Long Branch, NJ 07740

Kino Publications
P.O. Box 43584
Tucson, AZ 85733

Life Skills Training Associates, Inc.
1211 W. 22nd St.
Oak Brook, IL 60521
213-986-0070

Love Publishing Company
1777 South Bellaire St.
Denver, CO 80222

From Cartledge G and Milburn JF (1986) Teaching social skills to children: innovative approaches, ed 2, appendix B, New York, Pergamon Press.

Continued.

Listing of Publishers — cont'd

Lyons
5030 Riverview Avenue
Elkhart, IN 46514

McGraw-Hill
Cedar Hollow & Matthews Hill Rd.
Paoli, PA 19301

Nasco Learning Fun
901 Janesville Avenue
Fort Atkinson, WI 53538

Opportunities for Learning, Inc.
8950 Lurline Avenue
Department 9AB
Chatsworth, CA 91311

Pro-Ed
5341 Industrial Oaks Blvd.
Austin, TX 78735

Prentice-Hall
Englewood Cliffs, NJ 07632

Scholastic Instructional Materials
904 Sylvan Avenue
Englewood Cliffs, NJ 07632

Scott Foresman and Company
1900 East Lake Avenue
Glenview, IL 60025

Social Effectiveness Training
P.O. Box 6664
Reno, NV 89513-6664

Society for Visual Education
1345 Diversey Parkway
Chicago, IL 60614

Teacher's College Press
Teachers College
Columbia University
New York, NY

Teaching Resources Corp.
100 Boylston Street
Boston, MA 02116

Troll Associates
320 Route 17
Mahwah, NJ 07430

Walker Educational Book Corp.
720 Fifth Avenue
New York, NY 10019

Word Books
Word Incorporated
P.O. Box 1790
Waco, TX 76703

Sources for Skill Development

Sensitivity

Junior and Senior High. Set of 46 cards containing scenarios for various social situations. Students are encouraged to think out appropriate responses to these problems. (DLM Teaching Resources)

Activities for Exploring Conflict and Aggression

Secondary. Instructional activities focused on means for conflict resolution. Can be used as separate unit or integrated into regular curriculum. (J Weston Walch, Publisher)

Essential Social Skills

Secondary. A variety of exercises and activities addressing social situations typically experienced by most teenagers, for example, dating, sex-roles. Spirit duplicating masters. (EBSCO Curriculum Materials)

Peace, Harmony, Awareness

All ages. Audio program that teaches relaxation, self-confidence and control, and helps improve relationships. Can be used with individuals, groups, and children with special needs. Consists of a manual, six audio cassettes, and seven $8'' \times 10''$ color photographs. (Teaching Resources Corporation)

Transition

Elementary and junior high. Emphasizes social and emotional growth of middle school and junior high school student. Appreciation of human differences is stressed by presenting a wide range of racial, ethnic, and economic groups and physical handicaps. Students write out and act out scenarios about personal conflicts and decision making; simulated encounters; directed observation and analysis of human behavior; and large and small group discussions. Program consists of five units entitled: (a) Communication and Problem Solving Skills; (b) Encouraging Openness and Trust; (c) Verbal and Nonverbal Communication of Feelings; (d) Needs, Goals, and Expectations; and (e) Increasing Awareness of Values. (American Guidance Service)

Asset: A Social Skills Program for Adolescents

Adolescents. A social skills training program that addresses giving and receiving feedback, resisting peer pressure, problem solving, negotiating, following instructions, and conversing. The program consists of 8 films or videocassettes, leader's guide, and program materials. (Research Press)

Coping with Series (Revised)

Secondary. Twenty-three books dealing with serious ethical and personal problems and everyday problems of school, home, and friendship. Attention is given to many different kinds of relationships. Titles include "Easing the Scene," "To Like and Be Liked," "You Always Communicate Something," "Can You Talk with Someone Else?" Includes manual. (American Guidance Service)

Healthy Feelings

Filmstrip series about four teenagers helps students learn that certain feelings can cause other feelings, that feeling can be related to physical health, and that a behavior change can affect the way they feel. Titles include: "Feelings: Ours and Others," "Feelings Are Made," "Feelings: What We Do," and "Feeling Good." Set of four sound filmstrips and four cassettes. (BFA Educational Media)

Understanding and Accepting Yourself

Ungraded. Four color filmstrips with four cassettes and teacher guide. Titles include: "Health and Behavior," "Feelings and Behavior," "Experience and Behavior," "Controlling Your Behavior." (Learning Tree Filmstrips)

From Curtledge G and Milburn J (1986) Teaching social skills to children: innovative approaches, ed 2, appendix A, New York, Pergamon Press.

Continued.

Sources for Skill Development — cont'd

Arbuthnot J and Gordon DA (1986) Behavioral and cognitive effects of a moral reasoning development intervention for high risk behavior disordered adolescents, Journal of Department of Psychology, Ohio University, Athens, OH 45701-2979

Attitudes in Everyday Living
Brewner MN, McMahon WC, Roche MP
Paris, KA Educational Design, Inc.

Bingham M, Edmondsdon J, and Stryker S (1984) Challenges: a young man's journal for self-awareness and planning, Santa Barbara, CA, Advocacy Press

Bingham M, Edmondson J, and Stryker S (1984) Choices: a teen woman's journal for self-awareness and personal planning, Santa Barbara, CA, Advocacy Press

Brigham TA (1988) Managing everyday problems, New York, NY, Guilford Press

Developing self-respect, and Understanding and accepting yourself,
Learning Tree
Filmstrips, audio, tapes, filmstrips
P.O. Box 4116
Englewood, CO 80115

Dinkmeyer DM (1983) STEP-Teen (systematic training for effective parenting), Circle Pines, MN, American Guidance Service

Gazda GM, Walters RP, and Childers WC (1980) Realtalk: exercises in friendship and helping skills, Atlanta, GA, Humanics

Goldstein A, Sprafkin R, Gershaw J, and Klein P (1980) Skillstreaming the adolescent, Champaign, IL, Research Press

Improving Your Thinking Skills
United Learning
6633 W. Howard St.
Niles, IL 60648

Innerchange a Journey in Self Learning Through Group Interaction
(Magic Circle) Human Development Training Institute, Inc.
La Mesa, CA

Kline BE, Kline KE, and Overholt M (1990) Awareness and change: relationship building between children, youth and adults,
McPherson, KS, McPherson Family Life Center, Inc.
224 S. Maple
McPherson, KS 67460

Monti PM, Abrams DB, Kadden RM, and Cooney NL (1989) Treating alcohol dependence: a coping skills training guide, New York, The Guilford Press

Overcoming Inferiority
Human Relations Media
105 Tompkins Ave.
Pleasantville, NY 10570

Patterson G and Gullion M (1976) Living with children: new methods for parents and teachers, Champaign, IL, Research Press

Continued.

Sources for Skill Development — cont'd

Robin A (1980) Parent-adolescent conflict: a skill training approach. In Rathjen DP and Foreyt JP, editors: Social competence interventions for children and adults, New York, NY Pergamon Press

Simon SB, Howe CW, and Kirschen-baum H (1978) Values clarification: a handbook of strategies for teachers and students, New York, NY Dodd & Mead Co.

Stress Free Center,
Association for Advanced Training
3456 Olympic Blvd.
Los Angeles, CA 90019
800-472-1931

Stress Free Program Therapist Manual
Gary Emery, Ph.D.

REFERENCES AND SUGGESTED READINGS

Aguilera D and Messick J (1990) Crisis intervention: theory and methodology, ed 6, St Louis, Mosby–Year Book, Inc.

American Nurses Association (1985) Standards of child and adolescent psychiatric and mental health nursing practice, Kansas City, Mo, The Association.

Bell G (1977) Innerchange: a journey into self-learning through group interaction (Magic Circle) [senior high kit and junior high kit], La Mesa, Calif, Human Development Training Institute, Inc.

Bingham M, Edmondson J, and Stryker S (1984) Challenges: a young man's journal for self-awareness and planning, Santa Barbara, Calif, Advocacy Press.

Bingham M, Edmondson J, and Stryker S (1984) Choices: a teen woman's journal for self-awareness and personal planning, Santa Barbara, Calif, Advocacy Press.

Braukmann CL and Fixsen DL (1976) Behavior modification with delinquents. In Huson M, Fisler RM, and Miller PM, editors, Progress in behavior modification, New York, Academic Press.

Brewner MM, McMahon WC, Paris KA, and Roche MP (1984) Attitudes in everyday living, New York, Educational Design, Inc.

Brigham TA (1988) Managing everyday problems, New York, Guilford Press.

Brigham TA (1989) Self-management for adolescents: a skills training program, New York, Guilford Press.

Dinkmeyer DM (1983) STEP-Teen (systematic training for effective parenting), Circle Pines, Minn, American Guidance Service.

Dixon SL (1987) Working with people in crisis, Columbus, Ohio, Merrill Publishing Co.

Dupont H and Dupont C (1979) Transition: a program to help students through the difficult transition from childhood to middle adolescence, Circle Pines, Minn, American Guidance Service.

Edgerton C (1987) Walking across Egypt, New York, Ballantine/Del Rey/Fawcett Books.

Emery G (1987) Stress-free program therapist manual, Los Angeles, Stress Free Center, Association for Advanced Training.

Forchuk C, Beaton S, Crawford L, Ide L, Voorberg N, and Bethune T (1989) Incorporating Peplau's theory and case management, Journal of Psychosocial Nursing 27:35-38.

Gazda GM and Brooks DK (1980) A comprehensive approach to developmental interventions, Journal for Specialists in Group Work 5:120-126.

Gazda GM and Brooks DK (1985) Life skills training. In L'Abate L and Milan M, editors: Handbook of social skills training and research, New York, John Wiley & Sons.

Gazda GM, Walters RP, and Childers WC (1980) Realtalk: exercises in friendship and helping skills, Atlanta, Humanics.

Glasser N (1980) What are you doing? New York, Harper & Row Publishers, Inc.

Glenn S and Nelsen J (1987) Raising children for success: blueprints and building blocks for developing capable people, Fair Oaks, Calif, Sunrise Press.

Goldstein A, Sprafkin R, Gershaw J, and Klein P (1980) Skillstreaming the adolescent, Champaign, Ill, Research Press.

Guest J (1976) Ordinary people, New York, Ballantine/Del Rey/Fawcett Books.

Hazel J, Bragg-Schumaker J, Sherman J, and Sheldon-Wildgen J (1981) Asset: a social skills program for adolescents, Champaign, Ill, Research Press.

Hobbs SA, Moquin LE, Typoler M, and Lahey BB (1980) Cognitive behavior therapy with children: has clinical utility been demonstrated? Psychological Bulletin 87:147-165.

Johnson V (1986) Intervention, Minneapolis, Johnson Books.

Jones V and Jones L (1981) Responsible classroom discipline, Boston, Allyn & Bacon, Inc.

Kalisch BJ (1971) An experiment in the development of empathy in nursing students, Nursing Research 20:11-20.

Kalisch BJ (1973) What is empathy? American Journal of Nursing 73:1548.

Kendall PC (1981) Cognitive behavioral interventions with children. In Lahey BB and Kazdin AE, editors: Advances in clinical child psychology, vol 4, New York, Plenum Press.

Kohnke MF (1982) Advocacy: what is it? Nursing and Health Care 3:314.

Kolko D, Dorsett P, and Milan M (1981) A total assessment approach in the evaluation of social skills training: the effectiveness of an anger control program for adolescent psychiatric patients, Behavior Assessment 3:382-402.

McKay M and Fanning P (1987) Self-esteem: a proven program of cognitive techniques for assessing, improving, and maintaining self-esteem, Oakland, Calif, New Harbinger Publications.

Meichenbaum D (1977) Cognitive-behavior modification, New York, Plenum Press.

Meichenbaum D (1979) Teaching children self-control. In Lahey BB and Kazdin AE, editors, Advances in clinical child psychology, vol 2, New York, Plenum Press.

Milan MA and Kolko DJ (1985) Social skills training and complementary strategies in anger control and the treatment of aggressive behavior. In L'Abate L and Milan MA, editors, Handbook of social skills training and research, New York, John Wiley & Sons.

Monti PM, Abrams DB, Kadden RM, and Cooney NC (1989) Treating alcohol dependence: a coping skills training guide, New York, The Guilford Press.

Novaco R (1975) Anger control: the development and evaluation of an experimental treatment, Lexington, Mass, Heath.

Novaco R (1978) Anger and coping with stress: cognitive behavioral interventions. In Foreyt J and Rathjen D, editors, Cognitive behavior therapy: research and application, New York, Plenum Press.

Patterson GR (1982) Coercive family process, Eugene, Ore, Castalia Publishing Co.

Patterson G and Gullion M (1976) Living with children: new methods for parents and teachers, Champaign, Ill, Research Press.

Peplau H (1952) Interpersonal relations in nursing, New York, Putnam Publishing Group, Inc.

Pittman DC (1989) Nursing case management: holistic care for the deinstitutionalized mentally ill, Journal of Psychosocial Nursing 27(11):23-27.

Popkin M (1987) Active parenting: teaching cooperation, courage, and responsibility, New York, Harper & Row Publishers, Inc.

Rimm D and Masters D (1979) Behavior therapy: techniques and findings, New York, Academic Press.

Robin A (1980) Parent-adolescent conflict: a skill training approach. In Rathjen DP and Foreyt JP, editors, Social competence interventions for children and adults, New York, Pergamon Press.

Rowe JL, Pasch M, and Hamilton WF (1983) The new model me, ed 2, New York, Teachers College Press.

Salinger JD (1951) The catcher in the rye, New York, Bantam Books.

Shaw ME, Corsini RJ, Blake RR, and Mouton SS (1980) Role playing, San Diego, University Associates.

Simon SB, Howe CW, and Kirschenbaum H (1978) Values clarification: a handbook of strategies for teachers and students, New York, Dodd & Mead Co.

Stuart GW and Sundeen SJ (1991) Principles and practice of psychiatric nursing, St Louis, Mosby–Year Book, Inc.

United Learning (1983) Improving your thinking skills, Niles, Ill, United Learning.

Urbain ES and Kendall PC (1980) Review of social-cognitive problem-solving interventions with children, Psychology Bulletin 88:109-143.

Varley WH (1984) Behavior modification approaches to the aggressive adolescent. In Keith CR, editor, The aggressive adolescent: clinical perspectives, New York, The Free Press.

Whitehorn J and Betz B (1975) Effective psychotherapy with the schizophrenic patient, New York, Jason Aronson, Inc.

Wolfe I (1962) Referral: a process and a skill, Nursing Outlook 10:253-256.

Wubbolding RE (1988) Using reality therapy, New York, Harper & Row Publishers, Inc.

Yule W (1984) Behavioral treatments. In Taylor E, editor, The overactive child, [Clinics in developmental medicine], London, Heinemann Medical/Spastics International Medical Publications.

Zinker J (1977) Creative process in gestalt therapy, New York, Random House.

Chapter 9

Strategies for Prevention

STANDARD V-C. *Intervention: Psychotherapeutic Interventions*

THE NURSE USES PSYCHOTHERAPEUTIC INTERVENTIONS TO ASSIST CHILDREN OR ADOLESCENTS AND FAMILIES TO DEVELOP, IMPROVE THEIR ADAPTIVE FUNCTIONING, PROMOTE HEALTH, AND PREVENT ILLNESS.

STANDARD V-E. *Intervention: Health Teaching and Anticipatory Guidance*

THE NURSE ASSISTS THE CHILD OR ADOLESCENT AND FAMILY TO ACHIEVE MORE SATISFYING AND PRODUCTIVE PATTERNS OF LIVING THROUGH HEALTH TEACHING AND ANTICIPATORY GUIDANCE.

STANDARD X. *Use of Community Health Systems*

THE NURSE PARTICIPATES WITH OTHER MEMBERS OF THE COMMUNITY IN ASSESSING, PLANNING, IMPLEMENTING, AND EVALUATING MENTAL HEALTH SERVICES AND COMMUNITY SYSTEMS THAT ATTEND TO PRIMARY, SECONDARY, AND TERTIARY PREVENTION OF MENTAL DISORDERS IN CHILDREN AND ADOLESCENTS.

Prevention of mental health problems has been a concern for many years. Caplan (1964) described three levels of preventive intervention. Primary prevention attempts to lower the incidence of mental disorders, secondary prevention is aimed at reducing the duration of a disorder, and tertiary prevention attempts to reduce the severity of a disorder. In this chapter primary prevention activities are discussed.

Primary prevention consists of efforts either to prevent problems from developing (anticipating a disorder) or to promote emotional health (Goldston, 1977). Several categories of interventions are used to prevent mental health problems: (1) interventions (consultation and community action) in community organizations and systems; (2) education for health promotion and anticipatory guidance (teaching); (3) competence building (skill development); and (4) natural caregiving or social support (Gullotta, 1987; Heller, 1984). Almost all interventions for children and teenagers require considerable interaction with community organizations. The community itself or a community system may be the focus of prevention as well.

Educational programs for health promotion have been successful with many health problems, such as reducing heart disease. However, education for prevention of teenage pregnancy, substance abuse and the like has been remarkably unsuccessful for adolescents. Their propensity for believing they are invincible, the denial associated with substance abuse, and the attractiveness of the risky behavior outweigh any benefit of education. Studies have shown, however, that adolescents do benefit from education about transition periods, such as the entry into high school (Felner and others, 1982).

Children and adolescents also benefit from training in social skills and social problem solving (Spivak and Shure, 1974; Hawkins and Weis, 1983; Ladd and Mize, 1983; Goldstein and others, 1980; Weissberg, 1985). Adequate social supports such as friends and supportive persons who are not family (for instance, teachers and neighbors) are associated with well-being (Gottlieb, 1987). However, efforts to develop or improve networking among supportive people have had little effect. Peer counseling programs in high schools are an example of such a support that has been helpful. Students Against Drunk Driving (SADD) is a mutual aid–preventive program provided by students for each other (Students Against Drunk Driving, 1983).

All programs require people, time, and money, and their effectiveness should be evaluated over time. Various organizations—including the National Institute on Mental Health (NIMH), nursing organizations, foundations, and universities—award grant money for implementation and evaluation of prevention projects. Prevention programs and projects require careful planning, much persuasion, working through resistance, and sufficient intensity over time. Some studies have shown that urban lower socioeconomic groups need longer and more intensive interventions. Nurses should study the literature relevant to the desired intervention to prevent failure. Fortunately, nurses can take many actions to promote adolescent mental health and prevent problems that do not require sophisticated techniques.

Adolescent psychiatric nurses can engage in preventive activities in their roles as private citizens or as professional nurses working in schools, community mental health centers, clinics, and physicians' offices. Strategies aimed at reducing the incidence of adolescent problems are *community action, teaching, advocacy, skill development,* and *consultation.*

Community Action

Community action can be directed at a number of community institutions and organizations:
1. Government-related agencies
   a. City or county government
   b. Police departments
   c. Park and recreation departments and boards
   d. School boards
2. Churches and ministerial associations
3. Community social groups
   a. Service clubs such as Kiwanis, Optimist, Soroptimist, Jaycees, and Junior League

    b. Mothers Against Drunk Driving (MADD)
4. Youth organizations
    a. Scouts
    b. 4-H clubs
    c. Youth groups affiliated with churches
    d. School clubs
5. Schools
    a. Parent-teacher organizations
    b. Teachers
    c. Parents
    d. Coaches

Community action involving governmental bodies can encompass the following variety of activities:

1. Campaigning for candidates who have interest in and influence on legislation for adolescent issues
2. Speaking at city council or school board meetings to urge action or present a plan for services and legislation
3. Submitting letters to the editor or writing guest editorials in the community newspaper
4. Monitoring juvenile arrests (or lack thereof) and disposition of these cases
5. Expressing concern directly to the Chief of Police
6. Assembling or participating in community task forces that deal with preventing adolescent problems
7. Reporting liquor violations (sales to teenagers)
8. Reporting adolescent liquor violations — public consumption and drunkenness — and filing charges if appropriate
9. Insisting that the school system have prevention and intervention programs for substance abuse
10. Demanding firm discipline in schools
11. Speaking to the park board and insisting on provisions for adolescent drug-free "hangouts" and programs for younger and older teens
12. Lobbying for key ordinances
13. Encouraging the district nurses association to become active in adolescent health problems

Churches are excellent places to launch preventive efforts. Most churches have youth programs and family life programs. The church clerical and lay leaders are interested in promoting programs to help families with adolescents. Furthermore, the individual churches, represented by the pastors, usually form local organizations called ministerial associations. These groups can be very influential in initiating prevention programs and dealing with subjects such as parenting and alcohol education for parents. They can also encourage community leaders to endorse programs or legislation for preventing adolescent problems.

Community *social* or *service groups* can be persuaded to assist prevention programs through financial support or other services. Many service clubs focus their efforts on youth projects. For instance, the Optimist clubs sponsor Just Say No Clubs in the schools in Kettering, Ohio. Boy Scouts of America provide training for Students

Against Drunk Driving. These service groups are always looking for speakers for their weekly meetings and seeking causes to sponsor, and their members will serve on task force committees that address adolescent problems. These are excellent forums for inspiring concern for teenagers' problems.

Youth groups can be a focus of community action. Scout troops and 4-H Clubs can participate in many community activities geared toward preventing adolescent substance abuse and other problems. Youth groups also provide supervised drug- and alcohol-free social activities, which are prevention strategies in themselves.

Schools are institutions where adolescents, parents, and youth leaders are easily accessed. Parent-teacher organizations can be influential in raising money and demanding preventive programs in the schools, including supervised activities and firm discipline. All schools have a school nurse who is in a key position to promote prevention activities, as well as to provide crisis intervention. School nurses can provide leadership by educating families and the administration about the need for various programs related to adolescents' learning and emotional needs, substance abuse, and sexuality. Coaches and student club faculty advisors need support, education, and encouragement to discourage substance abuse and other dangerous activities. The parent booster groups for student activities can be a fertile source of support for preventive programs and appropriate social activities.

The local and regional *media* play an important role in enhancing community action on behalf of teenagers' needs. It is useful to develop relationships with newspaper, television, radio, and magazine staff. To be interested in a topic or group, media people must believe that their story is newsworthy. Often the media have their own agendas. If the newspaper, television, or radio station is not interested in a story, a public service announcement (PSA) is another way to get a message to the community.

Teaching

Another strategy for preventing adolescent problems is *teaching* adolescents, their parents, and other adults including teachers, coaches, youth leaders, and clergy. Adults need to know the incidence and symptoms of adolescent substance use and abuse, suicide, depression, and sexual activity. They also need to know how to talk to teenagers about these issues, how to set limits, where to get information and assistance, and how to obtain support from other parents. Adolescents should be educated about drugs and alcohol, sexuality, and suicide without sensationalism but with value clarification, self-esteem building, and social skills training included in the program (DiCicco and others, 1984).

Although the obvious forum for teaching both parents and adolescents is the school system, it is actually very difficult to interest parents in talking about problems in the school setting. Parents often fear that if they call attention to adolescent problems their children will suffer. Ideally, the leadership in this area should come from the school system administration. However, principals who deal daily with serious teen problems often hide this fact from the public, fearing that a bad image might result in reduced taxes for school support. So before the public can be educated, community leaders must be trained and a lot of community action must take place. However, there is greater general knowledge of adolescent problems than there has been in the past. Educational mass mailings and speakers at parent-teacher organization meetings can be effective sources of information. There are many excellent packaged educational programs available as bases for adolescent school curricula, for training teachers and other youth leaders, and for educating parents and professionals. The boxes on pp. 250-251 are representative lists of available programs and resources.

Nurses who work in *doctors' offices, clinics,* and *HMOs* have excellent opportunities to teach. All offices that serve adolescents should have attractive, easy-to-read literature to give to teenagers and their parents. An extensive referral list of qualified professionals should be available as well.

Skill Development

Adolescents can develop problems because they have inadequate problem-solving and decision-making and social skills or because their self-esteem is not high enough to permit them to overrule the dictates of their peer group. Every adult who has responsibility for teenagers should provide opportunities to discuss problems or concerns and then guide the adolescents through the problem-solving process or use the Reality Therapy steps described in Chapter 8. "Preaching" to adolescents is a sure way to lose their attention. Learning to make good decisions in the presence of caring adults is critical in preventing poor choices. Adolescents must be taught to consider the payoffs and consequences of decisions. Although this process is time consuming and requires patience, spending this kind of time and feeling real concern for the young person is the best investment an adult can make. Unfortunately, busy and ambitious parents, guidance counselors, and nurses bogged down with paper work, discouraged or uncommitted teachers, and coaches charged with winning often claim they do not have the time.

Many programs exist for teaching children and adolescents skills in structured settings, especially in schools. Some of these are discussed in Chapter 8. A representative list is shown in the box on p. 252-254.

A leadership training program, Teenage Institute, is outlined and described in the case study and box on pp. 255-256.

Focus and Strategies for Prevention

Problem	Client	Helper	Locations	Interventions
Suicide/ depression	Adolescents	School nurse Psychiatric nurses	School	Teaching
		Mental health center staff Suicide prevention service Office Nurses Pediatric Nurse Practitioners (PNPs)	Doctors' offices	Skill development
Suicide/ depression	Parents	School nurse Psychiatric nurses	School Media	Teaching Skill development
		Mental health center staff Suicide prevention service Office nurses HMO staff	Church Doctor's office HMOs Adult classes	Community action
Substance abuse	Community	Private citizens	City Council	Community action
		School nurses School crisis/ drug coordinator	School Board Park Board	Teaching Consultation
		Teachers	Police department	
		School offices Substance abuse treatment staff Addiction nurses	Service organizations	
Substance abuse	Parents	School nurse Addictions nurse Psychiatric nurse School drug counselor Drug and alcohol counselors Treatment program staff	School PTA Church Social groups Media Adult school	Community action Teaching Skill development

Continued.

Focus and Strategies for Prevention — cont'd

Problem	Client	Helper	Locations	Interventions
Substance abuse	Adolescents	School nurse School drug counselor	School curriculum Activity groups	Skill development
		Teachers and health teachers		Teaching
		School administrators	Leadership	
		Youth group leaders	Training seminars	
		Faculty advisors	Athletics	
		Peer counselors		
Sexual promiscuity/teen pregnancy	Community	School nurses OB nurses	School Board City government	Community action
		Community health nurses Obstetricians	Media Churches	Teaching Consultation
Sexual promiscuity/teen pregnancy	Parents Adolescents	School Nurse Physicians	School PTA	Teaching Skill development
		OB nurses	Physicians office	
		Community health nurses	Clinics — HMOs	
		School administration	Media	

Prevention/Intervention Resources

Schools

Curriculum

Skills for Adolescence (Grades 6-8)
The Quest National Center
6655 Sharon Woods Blvd.
Columbus, OH 43229
1-800-233-7900

From Peer Pressure to Peer Support
   (Grades 7-12)
AUTHORS: Shelley MacKay Freeman
Johnson Institute
7151 Metro Blvd.
Minneapolis, MN 55435

BABES (Beginning Alcohol and
   Addictions Basic Education Studies)
17330 Northland Park Court
Southfield, MI 48075
1-800-54BABES

CASPAR
AUTHOR: Lena Di Cicco
Alcohol Education Program
226 Highland Ave.
Sommerville, MA 02143

Children Are People, Inc.
Barb Naiditch/Rokelle Lerner, Directors
K-8 Group Process Kit
1599 Selby Ave.
St. Paul, MN 55104

Elementary Curriculum Guides for
   Chemical Awareness and Personal
   Development
Planning Development and Evaluation
Minneapolis Public Schools
807 Northeast Broadway
Minneapolis, MN 55413

Student assistance/prevention

Teenage Institute
170 N. High St. 3rd Floor
Columbus, OH 43266
1-614-466-3445

Skillstreaming the Adolescent (1980)
AUTHORS: A.P. Goldstein, and others
Champaign, IL: Research Press Co.

The Rochester Social Problem
   Solving (SPS) Program: a training
   manual for teachers of 2nd to 4th
   grade children
Department of Psychology
University of Rochester
Rochester, NY 14627

The Social Adjustment of Young
   Children: a cognitive approach to
   real-life problems
AUTHORS: G. Spivack and M. Shure
Jossey Bass Publishers
San Francisco (1974)
(includes training manual)

Social Competence Interventions
   for Children and Adults
AUTHORS:D.P. Rathgen and J.P.
   Foreyt
Pergamon Press (New York (1980)
[includes training guides for school,
child, and adolescent. and parent
competency training]

Drug Prevention Program for Athletes
Drug Enforcement Administration
Demand Reduction Station
1405 I. Street NW
Washington, DC 20537

Forest Hills School District
7575 Beechmont Avenue
Cincinnati, C .I 45230
1-513-231-3600

Prevention/Intervention Resources — cont'd

Community and parents

Organizations/programs

PRIDE (National Parents Resource
Institute for Drug Education, Inc.)
100 Edgewood Avenue, Suite 1002
Atlanta, GA 30303
1-800-241-7946

Community Intervention, Inc.
529 South 7th St. Suite 570
Minneapolis, MN 55415
1-800-328-0417

TWIKA (Talking with Kids About
   Alcohol)
Prevention Research Institute
Suite 210
629 N. Broadway
Lexington, KY 40508
1-606-254-9489

Stepfamily Association of America
28 Allegheny Avenue
Towson, MD 21204

Mental Health Association in Ohio
Advocates for Invisible Children
   Project
50 W. Broad Street
Columbus, OH 43215
1-614-221-5383

Family Wellness Kit
Aid Association for Lutherans
Appleton, WI
1-414-734-5721

Videos

Drug-Free Kids (70 min)
Scott Newman Foundation
1987 LCA, A New World Company,
Los Angeles, CA
1-213-469-2029

Choices and Consequences (33 min)
Johnson Institute
7151 Metro Blvd.
Minneapolis, MN 55435
1-800-231-5165

Sons and Daughters: Drugs and Booze
Gerald T. Rogers Productions Inc.
5215 Old Orchard Road Suite 990
Skokie, IL 60077
1-708-967-8080

Books

Glenn HS and Nelsen J (1987) Raising children for success: blue prints and building
   blocks for developing capable people, Fair Oaks, CA, Sunrise Press.
Joan P (1986) Preventing teenage suicide: the living alternative handbook, New
   York, Human Sciences Press, Inc.
Kline BE, Kline K, and Overholt M (1990) Awareness and change: relationship
   building between children, youth, and adults, ed 2, McPherson, KS, McPherson
   Family Life Center, Inc.
Poplin M (1987) Active parenting: teaching cooperation, courage, and responsibility,
   San Francisco, Harper & Row, Publishers, Inc.
Schaefer D (1987) Choices and consequences, Minneapolis, Johnson Institute.
Shure MB and Spivack G (1978) Problem-solving techniques in child-rearing,
   San Francisco, Jossey-Bass.
Wilmes D (1988) Parenting for Prevention. Minneapolis, Johnson Institute.

Continued.

Prevention/Intervention Resources—cont'd

Information sources

The Johnson Institute
510 First Avenue North
Minneapolis, MN 55403-1607
1-800-231-5165

The Alcohol Education Project
National Congress of Parents and
   Teachers
700 North Rush Street
Chicago, IL 60611

American Council for Drug
Education
5820 Hubbard Drive
Rockville, MD 20852
1-312-787-0977

Children's Defense Fund
122 C Street NW
Washington, DC 20001
1-202-628-8787

Drug Enforcement Administration
Public Affairs Office
1405 I Street NW
Washington, DC 20537
1-202-633-1469

National Association for Children
   of Alcoholics
31706 Coast Highway
South Laguna, CA 92677
1-714-499-3889

Drug Abuse Task Force
Boy Scouts of America
1325 Walnut Hill Lane
Irving, TX 75038
1-214-580-2000

National Clearinghouse for
   Alcohol and Drug Information
PO Box 2345
Rockville, MD 20852
1-301-468-2600

National Council on Alcoholism,
   Inc.
12 West 21st St.
New York, NY 10010
1-212-206-6770

National Institute on Alcohol
   Abuse and Alcoholism (NIAAA)
5600 Fishers Ln.
Rockville, MD 20857

National Institute on Drug Abuse
   (NIDA)
5600 Fishers Ln.
Rockville, MD 20857

Planned Parenthood Federation of
   America
810 Seventh Ave.
New York, NY 10019
1-212-541-7800

U.S. Department of Education,
   Alcohol, and Drug Abuse
Education
400 Maryland Ave. SW
Room 4145, MS 6411
Washington, DC 20202
1-202-732-3030

Case Study   *A Teenage Mini-Institute Weekend*

In February of 1988 a Teenage Mini-Institute weekend was held for junior and senior high school students of suburban high schools in a medium-sized Midwestern city. As the chair of a community substance abuse prevention task force, former nurse administrator of inpatient adolescent psychiatric services, and adolescent therapist, I was looking forward to the experience of working with teenagers who were interested in providing student leadership to reduce alcohol use and abuse among their peers.

The Teenage Institute (TI) staff consisted of a dynamic, experienced TI leader and several adults who gave presentations and seminars and served as faculty and "family" group leaders. The TI youth staff performed skits, role-modeled leadership behavior, assisted adult staff, and gave presentations. Several school nurses served as faculty.

The topic for the institute was education about the consequences of alcohol use, chemical dependence, family chemical dependence, alternative to drugs and alcohol, and personal growth and development skills. Recreational activities were held in the evenings. The components were divided into various 1- to 1½-hour segments with lots of skits, singing, cheering, and friendship. The family groups were held two or three times per day and were geared toward self-awareness and growth, usually around a particular relevant issue. My role was family group facilitator.

My group consisted of the editor of a large high school newspaper, a student playwright, student council officers, a recovering teen, a choir member, and other high-achieving students. I was amazed at the maturity, talent, openness, honesty, and positive outlook of these young people. Some of the students had struggled with family or other problems but had overcome their difficulties and were willing to assist others to do the same. The students thoroughly enjoyed the weekend, were excited about its special closeness, and learned new skills for coping and leading. The ultimate outcome of the weekend for students at our high school was the development of a peer counseling program. The ultimate outcome for me was pure joy and reinvigoration for working with youth. I recommend this wonderful experience for all adolescent psychiatric nurses.

Teenage Institute for the Prevention of Alcohol and Other Drug Abuse

GOAL

To provide education and training to Ohio high school students and advisors, assisting them in developing sound habilitative concepts and effective prevention programs that positively impact on alcohol and other drug abuse problems within their communities.

OBJECTIVES

• To provide relevant alcohol and other drug information
• To develop/enhance habilitative skills
• To increase knowledge and appreciation of alternative activities
• To develop/enhance an appreciation of the importance of personal wellness achieved through the practice of holistic health
• To encourage and facilitate post-Institute involvement in prevention and early intervention activities

METHODS

• Major educational presentations, courses and workshops
• Educational materials
• Small "family" group interactions
• Structured and unstructured free time (AA/Al-Anon/EA support group sessions, small gatherings, one-to-one discussions, recreational activities, a picnic, a dance)
• Regional planning meetings
• Involvement of county and local agencies concerned with chemical abuse prevention
• Sustaining efforts of present and former Teenage Institute staff and participants in carrying on the spirit and the teachings of the Institute
• Committed support of parents, educators, civic organizations, businesses, and other community members from throughout the state

Ohio Department of Health (1987) Teenage Institute Participant Handbook, Ohio Department of Health.

REFERENCES AND SUGGESTED READINGS

Abate LL and Milan M (1985) Handbook of social skill training, New York, John Wiley & Sons, Inc.

Caplan G (1964) Principles of preventive psychiatry, New York, Basic Books, Inc, Publishers.

DiCicco L, Biron R, Carifio J, Deutsch C, Mills D, Orenstein A, Unterberger H, Re A, and White R (1984) Evaluation of the CASPAR alcohol education curriculum, Journal of Studies on Alcohol 45:160-189.

Felner RD, Ginter MI, and Primavera J (1982) Primary prevention during school transitions: social support and environmental structure, American Journal of Community Psychology 10:277-290.

Goldstein AP, Sprafkin RP, Gershaw NJ, and Klein P (1980) Skillstreaming the adolescent: a structured learning approach to teaching prosocial skills, Champaign, Ill, Research Press Co.

Goldston S (1977) Defining primary prevention. In Albee GW and Jaffe JM, editors: Primary prevention of psychopathology, vol 1: The issues, Hanover, NH, University of New England Press.

Gottlieb BH (1987) Using social support to promote and protect health, Journal of Primary Prevention 8(1, 2):70.

Gullotta T (1987) Preventions technology, Journal of Primary Prevention 8(1, 2):4-24.

Hawkins JD and Weis JG (1983): The social development model: an integrated approach to delinquency prevention. In Dubel RJ, editor: Juvenile delinquency prevention: emerging perspectives of the 1980s, San Marcos, Tex, Institute of Criminal Justice Studies, Southwest Texas State University.

Heller K (1984) Prevention and health promotion. In Heller K, Price R, Shulamit R, Riger S, and Wandersman A: Psychology and community change: challenges of the future, Homeword, Ill, The Dorsey Press.

Ladd EW and Mize J (1983) A cognitive-social learning model of social skill training, Psychological Review 90:127-157.

Merjus J and Parsms R (1987) Prevention planning in the school system. In Hermalin J and Morell J, editors: Prevention planning in mental health, vol 9, Sage Studies in Community Mental Health, Newbury Park, Sage Publications.

Rathjen DP and Foreyt JP (1980) Social competence interventions for children and families, New York, Pergamon Press.

Spivak G and Shure MB (1974) Social adjustment of young children: a cognitive approach to solving real-life problems, San Francisco, Jossey-Bass.

Students Against Drunk Driving (1983) S.A.D.D. chapter handbook and curriculum, Marlboro, Mass, Students Against Drunk Driving.

Weissberg RP (1985) Developing effective social problem-solving programs for the classroom. In Schnieder B, Rubin KH, and Ledingham J, editors: Peer relationships and social skills in childhood, vol 2, New York, Springer-Verlag, New York, Inc.

Chapter 10

Strategies for Crisis Intervention

STANDARD V-C. *Intervention: Psychotherapeutic Interventions*

THE NURSE USES PSYCHOTHERAPEUTIC INTERVENTIONS TO ASSIST ADOLESCENTS AND THEIR FAMILIES TO DEVELOP, IMPROVE, OR REGAIN THEIR ADAPTIVE FUNCTIONING AND TO PREVENT ILLNESS.

STANDARD X. *Use of Community Health Systems*

THE NURSE PARTICIPATES WITH OTHER MEMBERS OF THE COMMUNITY IN ASSESSING, PLANNING, IMPLEMENTING, AND EVALUATING MENTAL HEALTH SERVICES AND COMMUNITY SYSTEMS THAT ATTEND TO PRIMARY, SECONDARY, AND TERTIARY PREVENTION OF MENTAL DISORDERS IN CHILDREN AND ADOLESCENTS.

Secondary prevention consists of preventing or reducing problems in high-risk groups and in individuals experiencing a crisis. Intervention with groups of adolescents or families at risk consist of *teaching, skill development, crisis intervention, group therapy, referrals* for intensive treatment, or self-help groups.

At-Risk Populations

Identifying adolescents who are at risk for problems or who come from high-risk families is an essential component of intervention. The following are examples of high-risk adolescents:
- Children of chemically dependent families
- Children of emotionally ill parents
- Adolescents with chronic illness, learning disabilities, or attention deficit disorder
- Adolescents who are socially or economically deprived
- Adolescents who have experienced the divorce of their parents
- Adolescents living in blended families

Interventions with high-risk adolescents and their families usually occur in schools and various treatment facilities. School systems often have support groups for children and adolescents at risk. These groups are usually for children with physical illness (Conley and Kendall, 1989), children of chemically dependent parents, or abused children and adolescents. Several models for intervention in schools use consultation (Edelson and Williams, 1985), consultation assessment referral, and treatment (Cauce and others, 1987; Cowen and others, 1980; Weissberg and others, 1981; Kriechman, 1985). Recently student assistance programs, modeled on employee assistance programs, have been implemented in schools — initially to intervene in substance abuse, but now expanded to all student emotional problems.

Crisis theory and crisis intervention evolved from Lindemann's research (1944) on the needs of persons who were grieving the loss of relatives from war, disaster, and natural death. In 1946 Lindemann and Caplan started the first community mental health program based on crisis intervention concepts. Caplan (1951) also developed the idea that crisis periods occur in individual and group life. According to Caplan (1961) a crisis is a time

when a person faces an obstacle to important life goals that is for a time insurmountable through the utilization of customary methods of problem solving. . . . Disorganization ensues, a period of upset, during which many abortive attempts at solution are made.

The person who feels helpless is receptive to assistance; thus if proper assistance is available, the person is able to resolve the crisis, prevent further deterioration, and develop new coping skills.

The three types of crises are situational, maturational, and adventitious (disaster). Situational crises are events that are or are perceived to be threatening and lead to disorganization. Some examples are divorce of parents, abuse incidents, physical illness, deaths, loss of peer relationships, and pregnancy. Maturational crises occur during the "periods of great social, physical, and psychological change experienced by all human beings in the normal growth process" (Aguilera, 1990). Adolescence is a period when those growth processes are rapid and profound. In the absence of adequate support, the opportunity arises for a crisis to develop. Adventitious crises are the result of natural and other disasters.

Crisis intervention is widely used by mental health providers, medical emergency personnel, police departments, and clergy (Table 10-1). In addition, volunteers are trained to staff crisis hot lines and provide peer counseling in schools, factories, and professional organizations (such as the state nurses' association's peer assistance programs). Crisis intervention includes the efforts of a helping person (school nurse, suicide hot line worker) to get a person in crisis to a counselor, as well as the brief therapy process following the emergency intervention.

Steps in Crisis Intervention

The first step in crisis intervention is *to establish a therapeutic relationship rapidly* (see boxes on pp. 261-263). This is done by empathizing and actively listening to the teenager's concerns. Therapeutic communication skills will bring about the second step, which is *to elicit and encourage expression of painful feelings*. The validation of the adolescent's feelings helps to develop rapport and provides information about the cognitive and emotional style of the teenager. The next step is to *discuss the*

Text continued on p. 263.

Table 10–1 Focus and Strategies for Crisis Intervention

Crisis	Client	Location	Helper	Intervention
Contemplated or attempted suicide	Suicidal adolescent and family	School	Teacher Counselor Peer counselor Nurse	Therapeutic relationships
			Crisis coordinator	Referral
		Crisis center/ hot line	Suicide prevention worker	Individual/ family therapy
		Church	Clergy	
		Hospital emergency room	Physician Nurse	Physical care Physical care
		Mental health center	Mental health center staff	
Completed suicide	Survivors	School	Teacher Administrators Counselor	Referral Individual and group therapy
			Nurse Outside therapists	Individual/ group therapy
		Home	Mental health center staff	Individual/ family therapy
Substance abuse	Adolescent and family	School	Nurse	Therapeutic relationship
			Administrators Drug counselor	Referral Limit setting, referral
		Hospital emergency room	Physician Nurse	Physical care Referral Physical care
		Police department	Police officer	Referral Limit setting
		Juvenile court	Juvenile court officer	Limit setting
		Treatment center	Alcohol/drug counselor Addiction nurse	Individual group, family therapy Teaching

Continued.

Table 10–1   Focus and Strategies for Crisis Intervention—cont'd

Crisis	Client	Location	Helper	Intervention
Sexual/physical abuse/neglect	Adolescent and family	School	Nurse	Referral
			Counselor	Therapeutic relationships
		Hospital emergency room	Physician	Physical care
			Nurse	Physical care
		Physician's office	Physician	Physical care
			Nurse	Physical care
		Police department	Police officer	
		Child services board	Counselor	Group/individual/family therapy
			Social worker	Group/individual/family therapy
Pregnancy/sexually transmitted disease	Adolescent	School	Nurse	Case management
			Counselor	
		Women's clinic	Physician	Physical care
			Nurse	Physical care
			Counselor	
			Social worker	
		Physician's office	Physician	Physical care
				Teaching
				Prenatal care
			Nurse	Physical care
				Teaching
				Prenatal care

Resources for Crisis Intervention and At-Risk Adolescents

Alanon/Alateen
PO Box 1872
Madison Square, NY 10159

Children Are People, Inc.
Barb Naidetch/Rokelle Lerner,
   Directors
K-8 Group Process Kit
1599 Selby Avenue
St Paul, MN 55104
(Children of chemically dependent
   parents)

Crisis Line Team Training manual
   (1987)
Lifesave Program Manual (1988)
Suicide Prevention Center
PO Box 1393
Dayton, OH 45401

Families Anonymous
PO Box 528
Van Nuys, CA 91408

From Peer Pressure to Peer Support
AUTHOR: Shelly MacKay Freeman
Johnson Institute
7151 Metro Blvd
Minneapolis, MN 55345

*Intervention: How to Help Someone Who
   Doesn't Want Help*
AUTHOR: Vernon E. Johnson
Johnson Institute
7151 Metro Blvd
Minneapolis, MN

NALSAP (National Association of
   Leadership for Student Assistance
   Programs)
PO Box 21838
Milwaukee, WI 53221

NarAnon Family Groups
PO Box 2562
Palos Verdes, CA 92704

Narcotics Anonymous
NA World Service Office, Inc
Sun Valley, CA 93152

National Institute of Mental Health
Mental Health Emergencies Section
5600 Fishers Ln
Rockville, MD 20852

Parents Anonymous
7120 Franklin Ave
Los Angeles, CA 90046

Students Against Drunk Driving
   (SADD)
*SADD Chapter Handbook and
Curriculum* (1983)
Marlborough, MA

Student Assistance Journal
Performance Resource Press
2145 Crooks Rd, Suite 103
Troy, MI 48084

Toughlove
PO Box 1069
Doylestown, PA 18901

precipitating event that caused the emotional upset. The precipitating event is usually the last in a series of frustrating incidents, so *to determine the hazardous events* is the next step. In the following case study the adolescent became despondent about losing a girlfriend and developed signs of depression, including a drop in grades, irritability, and a feeling of panic at school. With further discussion, it became obvious that the adolescent was vulnerable to crisis because his parents had divorced and his best friend had moved away. These were the hazardous events.

Case Study: *Crisis Intervention*

John, a 15-year-old sophomore at a large suburban high school, became panicky and upset, requesting to go home early from school. On the second occasion of this behavior, John was sent to the school nurse for assessment. John was known to the school nurse because of his unusual athletic ability in football and baseball and his excellent academic progress. John was a quiet young man who had no behavior problems. The nurse expressed her concern about his anxiety and encouraged him to talk about what was bothering him. He said his grades were dropping because he stopped doing his work and could not concentrate. He also was losing weight in spite of his weight-lifting program. After a while he told the nurse about the breakup with his girlfriend. The nurse called John's mother, who promptly came to school. The nurse suggested that they obtain an assessment and counseling immediately. John's mother's place of employment had an employee assistance program (EAP) that provided assessments and short-term counseling. An appointment was arranged for the next day.

The EAP counselor, who was a psychiatric nurse clinical specialist, determined that John was experiencing significant depressive symptoms: irritability, prolonged sleep, loss of appetite, loss of weight, crying spells, and dropping grades. These symptoms began when his girlfriend broke up with him. Further assessment revealed that John's parents had divorced 1 year ago, and 6 months ago his father had moved several states away. Moreover, his best friend had moved to another state. His friend had visited last weekend and got drunk at a party; this was a disappointment to John, who does not drink. Another problematic aspect of John's life was that his father was dependent on prescription medication and possibly other drugs. John and his mother were discouraged because they had argued lately, and a younger brother who is hyperactive was recently troublesome to John.

John's mother was very concerned about him but had minimized her perception of the effect of all these losses on John. She was so relieved to have her husband out of her life that she did not consider the effect his leaving might have on her son. She also was accustomed to a stellar performance from her son and did not understand that irritability and falling grades are signs of emotional trouble and not necessarily rebellion. John and his mother were relieved to hear that there were plausible reasons for John's crisis and that counseling should help. If John did not improve in 4 weeks, a psychiatric consultation would be sought.

John was seen twice weekly for 2 weeks and once a week for 3 more weeks. His mother joined the sessions on two occasions. John and his mother were able to see that they expected John to continue his usual pursuits and behaviors without talking about the pain he felt because of his losses. He did tell her a little about his girlfriend's leaving but not about the other problems. His mother became more empathic, and John talked more to her and to the therapist. His mother received information about gifted children, and they both were given information about the college athlete recruiting process. The concept of codependence and John's tendency to play the "hero" role was discussed. John's mother could see this but John did not, in part because he denied his father's addiction even though his father had undergone treatment for it.

All of John's symptoms lifted; he began a plan for catching up on his school work, and his relationship with his mother improved. He expressed some anger about his girlfriend's mixed messages and decided he did not deserve that kind of treatment. He expressed some interest in another girl but not as intensely.

After learning what the precipitating and hazardous events are, the nurse must *assess the balancing factors:* perception of the event, coping skills, and situational supports. It must be determined whether the adolescent has a realistic or distorted view of the magnitude of the event. In this case the adolescent experienced great pain at the loss of his girlfriend; this is a normal reaction. However, the teenager had placed too much hope in the relationship, expecting the girl to meet all the needs that were not being met elsewhere. This girl had her own problems and could not support him. The nurse also determines what the adolescent usually does to cope with difficult experiences and what has been tried thus far. Another area to assess is support: what supports are usually available to the adolescent and which are available at present. In the case study the boy's best friend was not available, and his mother significantly minimized the loss of his father because she was relieved that her husband was gone.

An important step in crisis intervention is a careful *suicide or homicide assessment.* The nurse must determine if the teenager has suicidal or homicidal ideas, intentions, and a plan. If so, it must be assessed whether the teen has the means to carry out the plan, how detailed the plan is, and whether the method is lethal. Factors that increase the likelihood of suicide are losses or failures, illness, use of alcohol and drugs, being an adolescent, being male, having a history of attempts, and experiencing hallucinations.

After the data are gathered, the next step is *to analyze all the information* and *to provide a cognitive explanation* of what is happening to the adolescent. In the case study the adolescent did not realize he was so vulnerable from previous losses and was relieved to know that he was in a crisis, suffering from depression, and that counseling could help. Another factor influencing his situation was that he was demonstrating signs of codependence, a result of growing up in a chemically dependent family about which he understood little. His mother, however, did understand, and she was surprised and relieved to know that her son's behavior was a result of several events and would respond to counseling.

The next step is *to make an appropriate referral* if the crisis worker does not provide treatment, or *to determine and implement a plan* to change the perception of the event, to provide or arrange situational support, and to develop coping skills. The nurse *terminates appropriately* and *follows up* to see that the plan was implemented.

CRISIS INTERVENTION IN CHEMICAL DEPENDENCY

There is a slightly different approach used to intervene when the adolescent or family is experiencing denial, usually in chemical dependence or substance abuse situations. Johnson (1986) and chemical dependence professionals call this type of crisis treatment strategy an *intervention.* As with traditional crisis intervention, the intervention is used by trained personnel. An intervention is not used with intoxicated, potentially violent, or mentally ill persons. There are eight steps in an *intervention* (Johnson, 1986). They are the following:

1. Make a list of meaningful persons who surround the chemically dependent person.
2. Form the intervention team.
3. Make written lists of specific incidents related to the drug or alcohol use that legitimize concern.
4. Find out about and make arrangements for treatment.
5. Name a chairperson.
6. Determine the order of confrontations.
   a. The first round is the list of incidents.
   b. The second round is the statement of limits.
7. Rehearse the intervention.
8. Follow through.

Nurses use crisis intervention in a number of settings. Psychiatric nurses may be employed as crisis therapists in a mental health center or other crisis counseling center, as staff nurses in inpatient units designed for crisis intervention only, or as staff nurses in inpatient settings where the hospital telephone serves as a hot line after business hours and particularly after 11 pm. School nurses regularly provide this service, especially if the nurse is functioning as the crisis and/or substance abuse coordinator for the school or school system. Emergency room and critical care nurses are in a position to refer or make arrangements for treatment for the adolescent who has attempted a suicide, experienced an accidental overdose, or suffered injuries related to misconduct or abuse.

Crisis Intervention in the Schools

High school and junior high or middle school students have so many problems that many school systems have established a student assistance program with a paid full-time coordinator to administer the program. The programs were originally designed for substance abusers, but they now also include such students as children of chemically dependent parents. The coordinator is assisted by volunteer school personnel and faculty who are trained in crisis intervention in the schools. School nurses are generally involved in the intervention teams.

Teenagers come to the attention of a teacher, counselor, nurse, or administrator through a number of ways. A student may be caught using chemicals at school, fighting, or causing other disturbances; he may self-report to a concerned faculty member or coach; or another student may talk to a faculty member about a friend's suicidal talk or abuse at home. Students rarely express concern about drug and alcohol use unless they are with peer counselors. If teachers are trained to notice symptoms of substance abuse, parental abuse, or depression, they may initiate intervention through the crisis team. The schools usually have policies and procedures for dealing with student crises. The school nurse, crisis coordinator, and administration should keep a list of known, reputable agencies or professionals who are skilled in assessing and treating adolescents and their families.

Pregnancy, sexually transmitted diseases, and eating disorders are likely to first come to the attention of the school nurse. The nurse uses crisis intervention techniques to assist the teenager to get medical help and talk to the family.

Many schools currently have support groups or programs for children of chemically dependent parents and for abused children. Intervention for at-risk teenagers is sometimes considered prevention, but because of the more advanced skills needed to provide this service, working with at-risk teenagers is included here. The purpose of these support groups is to provide adolescents with information about what is happening to them *(teaching)* and to assist them *to develop improved coping skills* and *to build self-esteem.*

When a student completes a suicide, the surviving students and teachers become very upset. Some students become suicidal and may imitate the suicide attempt. It is not uncommon to have several adolescent suicides within a few months to a year. As soon as possible, a specialist in dealing with suicide and its survivors should come to the school and hold meetings with students and staff. This person and additional counselors should be available to individual students for counseling and referral. This process is sometimes called *postvention* (Berkowitz, 1985).

Crisis Centers

Community mental health centers usually have a crisis service or department that is staffed 16 to 24 hours per day. The services may consist of same-day and walk-in appointments, individual or family counseling up to six appointments, and a telephone hot line staffed by trained volunteers. The crisis therapists also screen clients and refer them for hospitalization and emergency social services. Some crisis centers have overnight boarding or brief admissions. A psychiatrist may be on call. Other centers not only provide crisis intervention for the police department, but also accompany police officers to the scene of domestic violence or hostage situations. Nurses with bachelor's or master's degrees are employed as crisis counselors, as are persons from many other mental health disciplines.

Suicide Prevention Centers

Metropolitan areas usually have a suicide prevention service that may be separate from the crisis service in the same agency or may be handled by a separate agency. This program is geared specifically to preventing suicides, providing postvention service and training for volunteers, and educating the community. Suicide prevention centers provide hot lines, counseling, and referrals to other agencies for further treatment.

Emergency Rooms

The hospital emergency room receives patients who have attempted suicide and are in need of medical treatment for injury or overdose. The emergency department also sees patients who are suicidal but have not made an attempt, as well as people who are unmanageable because of mental illness or substance abuse. The physician or family may bring the suicidal or distressed person for assessment and referral, particularly if the hospital has a psychiatric service. Hospitals often employ a social worker or nurse clinical specialist to perform these assessments. Sometimes staff nurses from the psychiatric unit do assessments in the emergency room, but this precludes their caring for inpatients. Staff nurses should be very thoroughly trained for this role because the potential for legal liability is high. If the emergency department does not have these resources, emergency room nurses should make every effort to arrange for inpatient or outpatient care for suicidal or otherwise distressed teenagers. Emergency room nurses can be trained to do a lethality assessment, and policies and procedures may be developed to ensure the safety and treatment of suicidal, mentally ill, or substance-abusing adolescents needing treatment if there are no other options.

Toughlove

Toughlove (1980) is a self-help program developed by Phyllis and David York for parents whose teenagers are out of control. Teenagers who do not cooperate with their parents and teachers at all are usually substance abusing; the program is geared toward these children. The families are in frequent crisis and are taught through this program to use crisis to initiate change. The Toughlove program can be very helpful for families who have exhausted all options with a teenager who is completely uncooperative. Treatment is the preferred approach, but Toughlove is helpful when the family cannot get the child into treatment or for ultimately getting the adolescent to treatment. The program offers parents the following strategies:

1. Assessing whether the parents/family is in crisis
2. Taking a stand, which includes determining the "bottom lines," setting a structure, and permitting the teenager to experience consequences
3. Finding support in a Toughlove support group

The parent(s) choose a support team who will help with making decisions about limit setting, contracts for returning home, and arranging treatment. The purpose of the support team is to provide less emotional support for setting limits, which may be very hard for parents to do, especially if it means letting a child stay in jail or detention or having the court declare the child incorrigible or delinquent. The *Toughlove* book (York, 1989) makes it very clear about what kinds of behavior require Toughlove approaches. However, sometimes parents inappropriately apply these strategies to children who should not have them, to relieve themselves of parental responsibility or to justify punitive parenting.

Toughlove International provides programming for adolescents called *Toughlove for Kids* (York, 1987). The "kids" groups are run by professionals. The program includes a curriculum for a 39-week school course (York and others, 1986). The curriculum can be used as a positive approach to inschool suspensions or Saturday schools. Nurses should become familiar with the Toughlove groups in their clients' communities before referring to them.

There are many opportunities for crisis intervention with teenagers and their families. A list of resources for crisis intervention and at-risk adolescents is given in the box on p. 269. Nurses can be helpful through crisis intervention, therapeutic relationships, and referral because of their proximity to adolescents in so many situations.

Crisis Intervention Guide

1. Rapidly establish therapeutic relationship (through active listening and emphasizing)
2. Elicit and encourage expression of painful feelings
3. Discuss precipitating event (within past week)
4. Determine hazardous event (usually in past few months)
5. Assess balancing factors:
     perception of the event
       realistic or distorted
     coping skills
     situational supports
6. Assess suicide/homicide potential
     any significant relationships available for support
     suicidal ideas
     suicidal intent
     suicide plan:
       means to carry out available
       lethality of method
       well thought out plan
     presence of risk factors
       losses/failures
       illness
       use of drugs and alcohol
       adolescence, aging
       male
       hallucinations
       history of previous attempt(s)
7. Analyze the above
8. Plan and implement treatment plan (based on 4-6 weeks intervention, include anticipatory guidance)
9. Termination
10. Follow-up

Suicide Prevention/Intervention (Suicide call or attempt in your presence)

1. Establish rapport immediately
2. Reduce immediate danger — give simple commands
3. Obtain no-suicide contract
4. Place adolescent with someone else
5. Consider hospitalization if there is no one available for client
6. Continue with crisis intervention if immediate danger resolved
7. Follow-up

REFERENCES AND SUGGESTED READINGS

Aguilera DC (1990) Crisis intervention: theory and methodology, ed 6, St Louis, Mosby–Year Book, Inc.

Berkowitz IH (1985) The role of schools in child, adolescent and youth suicide prevention. In Peck ML, Faberow NL, and Litman RE, editors: Youth suicide, New York, Springer Publishing Co, Inc.

Caplan G (1951) A public health approach to child psychiatry, Mental Health 35:235.

Caplan G (1961) An approach to community mental health, New York, Grune & Stratton, Inc.

Cauce AM, Comer JP, and Schwartz D (1987) Long-term efforts of a systems-oriented school prevention program, American Journal of Orthopsychiatry 57:127-131.

Conley JF and Kendall J (1989) A school-based primary prevention group for children and alterations in health status, Journal of Child and Adolescent Psychiatric Nursing 2(3):123-128.

Cowen EL, Gesten EL, and Weissenberg RP (1980) An integrated network of preventively oriented school-based mental health approaches. In Price RH and Politser PE, editors: Evaluation and action in the social environment, New York, Academic Press.

Dixon SL (1987) Working with people in crisis, Columbus, Ohio, Merrill Publishing Co.

Edelson GA and Williams JC (1985) Child psychiatry consultation to a public high school: a developmental perspective, Journal of Child and Adolescent Psychology 2(2):105-109.

Johnson V (1986) Intervention: how to help someone who doesn't want help, Minneapolis, Johnson Books.

Kriechman A (1985) A school-based program of mental health services, Hospital and Community Psychiatry 36:876-878.

Lindemann E (1944) Symptomatology and management of acute grief, American Journal of Psychiatry 101:144.

Weissberg RP, Gesten EL, Rapkin BD, Cowen EL, Davidson E, Flores de AR, and McKim BJ (1981) Evaluation of a social problem-solving training program for suburban and inner city third-grade children, Journal of Consulting and Clinical Psychology 49:251-261.

York P and York D (1987) Toughlove: a self-help manual for kids, Doylestown, Penn, Toughlove International.

York P and York D (1989) Toughlove: a self-help manual for parents troubled by teenage behavior, Doylestown, Penn, Toughlove International.

York P, York D, and Dillemuth F (1986) The Toughlove kids program (curriculum) Doylestown, Penn, Toughlove Press.

Chapter 11

Strategies for the Therapeutic Milieu

The therapeutic adolescent milieu is the focus and responsibility of the nursing staff. The milieu described here, integrated with adequate assessment, traditional therapies, and appropriate pharmacological treatment, results in a significant improvement in adolescents and their families, low recidivism and high levels of staff morale and pride. The therapeutic milieu for adolescents is a complex, challenging arena for psychiatric nursing treatment. A great deal of information, practice and staff collaboration is needed to implement it successfully. This chapter, as well as Chapters 8 and 14, provide a base for this dynamic process.

Several ANA Standards of Child and Adolescent Psychiatric and Mental Health Nursing Practice (1985) apply to the therapeutic milieu:

STANDARD III: *Diagnosis*

THE NURSE, IN EXPRESSING CONCLUSIONS SUPPORTED BY RE-CORDED ASSESSMENT DATA AND CURRENT SPECIFIC PREMISES, USES NURSING DIAGNOSES AND/OR STANDARD CLASSIFICATIONS OF MENTAL DISORDERS FOR CHILDHOOD AND ADOLESCENCE.

STANDARD V-A INTERVENTION: *Therapeutic Environment*

THE NURSE PROVIDES, STRUCTURES, AND MAINTAINS A THERAPEU-TIC ENVIRONMENT IN COLLABORATION WITH THE ADOLESCENT, THE FAMILY, AND OTHER HEALTH CARE PROVIDERS.

STANDARD V-B INTERVENTION: *Activities of Daily Living*

THE NURSE USES THE ACTIVITIES OF DAILY LIVING IN A GOAL-DIRECTED WAY TO FOSTER THE PHYSICAL AND MENTAL WELL-BEING OF THE ADOLESCENT AND FAMILY.

STANDARD V-C INTERVENTION: *Psychotherapeutic Interventions*

THE NURSE USES PSYCHOTHERAPEUTIC INTERVENTION TO ASSIST ADOLESCENTS AND FAMILIES TO DEVELOP, IMPROVE, OR REGAIN THEIR ADAPTIVE FUNCTIONING, TO PROMOTE HEALTH, PREVENT ILLNESS, AND FACILITATE REHABILITATION.

Although there is some published discussion of the therapeutic milieu, little information exists on the specific activity of nursing personnel in the milieu. The information, milieu structures, and strategies presented in this chapter are based heavily on concepts from behavior and cognitive therapy and social skills training as well as basic principles of psychiatric nursing. Many variations of the milieu can be developed by use of additional therapeutical premises or by grouping adolescents by age or diagnosis. The description of the therapeutic milieu for adolescents is focused on interventions used by nurses in a milieu. The strategies may be easily modified for residential treatment and partial hospitalization or day treatment programs.

The notion of therapeutic environment began before World War II with the use of attitude therapy at the Meninger Clinic (Folsom, 1969). Attitude therapy was a prescription of staff attitude and behavior toward five types of patients in the hospital. This was developed at the request of direct care staff who were concerned about using the same approach with different types of patients. The notions of the therapeutic milieu (Bettleheim and Sylvester, 1948) and therapeutic community (Jones, 1953) were introduced shortly after World War II. With these models the focus of control for management of the unit shifted from the hospital hierarchy and staff to the patient group. With the introduction of psychotropic medication in the 1960s and shortened lengths of stay in the 1970s and 1980s, the original of therapeutic community has been modified to include the concepts of social learning theory. The assumption with the social learning model is that the patient has not learned adequate coping skills because of an "inadequate or unsafe interpersonal and physical environment" (Kunes-Connell, 1987). According to Jones (1968), the therapeutic environment is beneficial for the following reasons:

1. It fosters open communication between the individual and the environment.
2. It creates an environment in which persons can fully examine thoughts, feelings, and behaviors.
3. It properly sets limits on inappropriate behavior while supporting the individual in attempts to test new patterns of behavior.
4. It provides appropriate role models for behavior.

Skinner (1979) summarizes seven basic principles or assumptions underlying a therapeutic milieu:

1. The health in each individual is recognized and encouraged to grow.
2. Every interaction is an opportunity for growth.
3. The patient owns his own environment (participates in community government and activities).
4. Each patient owns his own behavior.

5. Peer pressure is a useful and powerful tool.
6. Inappropriate behaviors are dealt with as they occur.
7. Restrictions and punishment are to be avoided; (for adolescents, restrictions and consequences are logical and age appropriate).

A definition of the therapeutic milieu and a succinct summary of milieu therapy is provided by Kunes-Connell (1987):

> A therapeutic environment is a positive atmosphere in which the client has an opportunity to develop appropriate responses to individuals and situations that he encounters. Milieu therapy is a treatment mode in which personnel deliberately plan and structure the client's interpersonal and physical environment in an attempt to modify maladaptive behavioral responses while promoting more positive insights and responses. To effectively modify a client's maladaptive behavior, personnel must be comfortable in limit setting a client's inappropriate responses. To effectively promote insight, self-responsibility, and positive responses, the staff must function as role models and teachers of psychosocial skills. The treatment strategies of limit setting and teaching of psychosocial skills hold equal status in the therapeutic milieu and must be performed simultaneously.

Adolescents requiring inpatient care have not had—or have lost—the structure necessary in their family lives for gradual assumption of responsibility, increasing independence, and normal progression through developmental stages. This structure is applied in the milieu. The adolescent and the family can begin to rework the stages of growth and development. The focus of intervention in milieu therapy is the behaviors of the adolescent in the inpatient or day treatment environment. The adolescents are guided by a variety of strategies to replace nonproductive behaviors with more productive behaviors. The strategies are planned and developed according to the adolescent's length of stay, ability to understand, and behavior.

Peplau and others state that the therapeutic milieu has structured and unstructured elements. The structured elements include rules, policies, procedures, program schedule, privileges systems, and limit setting policies. The unstructured elements refer to "the complex system of interactions among patients, staff, other hospital personnel, friends and family members . . . ." (Peplau, 1982). Some nursing activities have been unstructured because either nurses were not taught specific strategies or none were available for psychotherapeutic interventions for limit setting, anger and aggression management, and skill development through goal setting. Thus structured milieu interventions should include skill development. Multidisciplinary collaboration is listed as a structured element because of its importance and frequency. The unstructured elements include the personal attributes of one-to-one and group informal interactions, self-esteem building, and role modeling. Teaching can be structured or unstructured. See the box on p. 276 for a list of the nursing interventions in the therapeutic milieu.

Structured Elements of the Therapeutic Adolescent Milieu

PROGRAM OF ACTIVITIES

The program of planned activities includes opportunities for quiet introspection, group therapeutic activities, group socialization activities, recreation and exercise,

Adolescent Psychiatric Nursing Strategies

Therapeutic milieu strategies

Unstructured elements

Caring	Role modeling
Staff attributes	Teaching
One-to-one and group informal interactions	Self-esteem building

Structured elements

Program of activities	Privileges
Therapeutic relationships	Goal setting and achievement: skill development
Staffing	
Surveillance	School
Rules	Teaching
Limit setting, anger, and aggression management	Multidisciplinary collaboration

Advanced practice strategies (clinical specialists)

Individual therapy
Group therapy
Family therapy
Multifamily group therapy

personal hygiene activities, family interactions, and school. The program also includes individual, group, family, and multifamily group therapy. The program is designed so that staff members have time to communicate between activities; adequate rest and sleep, opportunities for personal hygiene, and sufficient breaks for nutritional snacks and juices for the adolescents are also scheduled. Tables 11-1 and 11-2 give examples of a balanced schedule and a program of activities designed for two teams of eight adolescents. The boxes and table on pp. 281-287 may be useful for tracking and monitoring activities.

STAFFING

Nursing staffing is geared to a 1:4 or 1:3 ratio of staff to adolescents. The ratio is for direct care only. Trying to carry out unit clerk or charge duties is not possible with patient care responsibilities in an adolescent inpatient unit. One registered nurse and one child care worker, or two registered nurses assigned to the same eight adolescents is adequate for the program that is described here. If there are unusually aggressive, self-mutilating, or brain-injured adolescents present, an additional staff member may be needed. The staffing pattern used should be based on the assumption that emotionally disordered adolescents need a critical mass of adult support to keep acuity ratings from rising. Lack of staff results in anxiety and acting out by patients. Nursing personnel participate in, facilitate, or lead all activities to provide continuity and adequate supervision.

Text continues on p. 288.

Table 11-1   Adolescent Inpatient Schedule

Time	Monday	Tuesday	Wednesday	Thursday	Friday	Saturday	Sunday
7:00–7:45 AM	Wake up and shower	Wake up and shower	Wake up and shower	Wake up and shower	Wake up and shower	Wake up and shower	Wake up and shower
8:00–8:30 AM	Goals group	Goals group	Goals group	Goals group	Goals group	Goals group	Goals group
8:30–9:00 AM	Breakfast	Breakfast	Breakfast	Breakfast	Breakfast	Breakfast	Breakfast
9:00–10:15 AM	School	School	School	School	School	Family communication	Passes 11:00 AM–7:00 PM visiting
10:15–11:00 AM	(dining room)	(dining room)	(dining room)	(dining room)	(dining room)	10:00–11:00 AM (gym)	
11:00 AM–12:15 PM	Rec room	Group	Rec room	Group	Rec room	CD family group visiting	
12:15–12:45 PM	Lunch	Lunch Levels	Lunch	Lunch	Lunch	Lunch	Lunch
1:00–2:00 PM	Group (group room)	Crafts (kitchen)	Group (group room)	Crafts (kitchen)	Group (group room)	Planned activity and therapeutic home visits 11:00 AM–7:00 PM	Planned activities and therapeutic home visits 11:00 AM–7:00 PM
2:00–3:00 PM	Goal work	Chaplain group	CD group	Goal work CD group	Goal work	Goal work	Goal work
3:00–4:00 PM	Creative exp. I (group room)	Goal work	Creative exp. I (group room)	Goal work	CD group	Goal work	Goal work
4:00–5:00 PM	Motion therapy	Motion therapy	Motion therapy	Community meeting	Motion therapy	Motion therapy	Motion therapy

*Depends on access to Rec room.

Continued.

Table 11-1   Adolescent Inpatient Schedule—cont'd

	Dinner	Dinner	Dinner	Dinner	Dinner	Dinner	Dinner
5:00-5:30 PM							
5:30-6:30 PM *†*	Visiting	Visiting	Multifamily 6:00-7:00 PM	Visiting	Visiting	Visiting hours	Visiting hours
6:30-7:30 PM	Planned activity	Planned activity	Visiting	Planned activity	Planned activity	Planned activity	Planned activity
7:30-8:30 PM	AA meeting		Goal work	AA meeting	NA meeting		
8:30-9:00 PM	Snack	Snack	Snack	Snack	Snack	Snack	Snack
9:00-10:00 PM	Goals wrap up	Goals wrap up	Goals wrap up	Goals wrap up	Goals wrap up	Goals wrap up	Goals wrap up
10:00-10:15 PM	Lights out	Lights out	Lights out	Lights out	Lights out	Lights out	Lights out

*Depends on access to the Rec room.
†Depends on access to the YMCA.

Table 11-2   Adolescent Inpatient Schedule for Two Teams

Time	Monday		Tuesday		Wednesday	
7:00-7:45 AM	Wake up and shower		Wake up and shower		Wake up and shower	
8:00-8:30 AM	Goals group		Goals group		Goals group	
8:30-9:00 AM	Breakfast		Breakfast		Breakfast	
9:00-10:15 AM	School I (dining room)	Creative exp. II (kitchen)	School I (dining room)	Chaplain	School I (dining room)	Creative exp. II (kitchen)
10:15-11:00 AM		Goal work		Crafts II (kitchen)		Goal work
11:00 AM–12:15 PM	Rec room		Group I	Goal work	Rec room	
12:15-12:45 PM	Lunch		Lunch Levels		Lunch	
1:00-2:00 PM	Group I (group room)	School II (dining room)	Crafts I (kitchen)	School II (dining room)	Group I (group room)	School II (dining room)
2:00-3:00 PM	Goal work		Chaplain		Goal work	
3:00-4:00 PM	Creative exp. I (group room)	Group II (day room)	Goal work	Group II (day room)	Creative exp. I (group room)	Group II (day room)
4:00-5:00 PM	Motion therapy		Motion therapy		Motion therapy	
5:00-5:30 PM	Dinner		Dinner		Dinner	
5:30-6:30 PM	Visiting		Visiting		Multifamily 6:00-7:00 PM	
6:30-7:30 PM	Planned activity		Planned activity		Visiting	
7:30-8:30 PM					Goal work	
8:30-9:00 PM	Snack		Snack		Snack	
9:00-10:00 PM	Goals Wrap Up		Goals Wrap Up		Goals Wrap Up	
10:00-10:15 PM	Lights out		Lights out		Lights out	

Continued.

Table 11-2 Adolescent Inpatient Schedule for Two Teams—cont'd

Thursday		Friday		Saturday	Sunday
Wake up and shower		Wake up and shower		Wake up and shower	Wake up and shower
Goals group		Goals group		Goals group	Goals group
Breakfast		Breakfast		Breakfast	Breakfast
School I (dining room)	Crafts II (kitchen)	School I (dining room)	Creative exp. II (kitchen)	Family communication 10:00-11:00 AM (gym)	Passes 11:00 AM–7:00 PM
	Group II		Goal work		
Group I	Goal work	Rec room		Passes 11:00 AM–7:00 PM	
Lunch		Lunch			Passes 11:00 AM–7:00 PM
Crafts I (kitchen)	School II (dining room)	Group I (group room)	School II (dining room)		
Goal work		Goal work			
Goal work		Creative exp. I (group room)	Group II (day room)		
Community Meeting		Motion therapy			
Dinner		Dinner			
Visiting		Visiting		Visiting hours	Visiting hours
Planned activity		Planned activity		Planned activity	Planned activity
Snack		Snack		Snack	Snack
Goals Wrap Up		Goals Wrap Up		Goals Wrap Up	Goals Wrap Up
Lights out		Lights out		Lights out	Lights out

Adolescent Mental Health Unit Daily Point Sheet

NAME _____   **LEVEL 1:**   0-173 points (Monday)
DATE _____   0-137 points (Thursday)
LEVEL_____   **LEVEL 2:**   174-204 points (Monday)
POINTS   138-161 points (Thursday)
TO DATE _____

ACTIVITIES/RESPONSIBILITIES		POINTS EARNED STAFF INITIAL
Wakes up at 6:30 AM, out of bed, and vital signs taken		
Attends and participates in morning exercise group		
Showered and dressed in clean, appropriate clothing		
Completes morning chores on time (bed made, room neat)		
Attends and cleans up after self following breakfast		
GOALS GROUP	1. Is on time	
	2. Participates	
	3. Follows limits	
ACADEMIC INSTRUCTIONS	1. Is on time	
	2. Brings materials	
	3. Works without disturbing others	
	4. Remains quiet, in seat	
	5. Works on task	
	6. Completes assignments	
	7. Cleans up after self	
	8. Follows limits	
Attends and cleans up after self following lunch		
GROUP THERAPY	1. Is on time	
	2. Follows limits	
	3. Participates	
	4. Brings up issues with assistance	
	5. Brings up issues on own initiative	
	6. Gives feedback	
	7. Accepts feedback	
	8. Provides support	
OCCUPA- TIONAL THERAPY	1. Is on time	
	2. Follows limits	
	3. Participates	
	4. Brings up issues with assistance	
	5. Brings up issues on own initiative	
	6. Gives feedback	
	7. Accepts feedback	
	8. Provides support	
FREE TIME	1. Is constructive	
	2. Follows limits	
	1st SHIFT SUB-TOTAL	

From Middletown Regional Hospital, Adolescent Mental Health Program, Middletown, Ohio.

Continued.

Adolescent Mental Health Unit Daily Point Sheet — cont'd

NAME _____

DATE _____

LEVEL _____

POINTS

TO DATE _____

LEVEL 3: 205-225 points (Monday)

162-182 points (Thursday)

LEVEL 4: 226 points and up (Monday)

183 points and up (Thursday)

ACTIVITIES/RESPONSIBILITIES		POINTS EARNED STAFF INITIAL
GOALS WORK QUIET TIME	1. Is in room	
	2. Works on assignment	
	3. Is quiet, not disruptive	
SPECIAL TOPICS GROUP AND/OR GOALS WRAP UP GROUP	1. Is on time	
	2. Follows limits	
	3. Participates	
	4. Sets goal with assistance	
	5. Sets goal for self	
	6. Assists others with goal	
	7. Reviews goal achievement with group	
	8. Goal work complete	
	9. Brings up issues with assistance	
	10. Brings up issues on own initiative	
	11. Gives feedback	
	12. Accepts feedback	
	13. Provides support	
RECRE- ATIONAL THERAPY	1. Is on time	
	2. Follows limits	
	3. Participates	
	4. Interacts appropriately	
	5. Identifies a leisure activity or resource	
Participates in community clean-up activity		
FREE TIME	1. Is constructive	
	2. Follows limits	
RELAX- ATION GROUP	1. Is on time	
	2. Is quiet, not disruptive	
	3. Participates	
In room at appropriate time		
Lights out; is in bed at the appropriate time		
********BONUS POINTS********		
2nd SHIFT SUBTOTAL		
1st SHIFT SUBTOTAL		
− DEDUCTIONS		
TOTAL FOR THE DAY		

Deduction of Points as a Result of Inappropriate Behavior
One Point Deducted for Each Activity Checked and Initialed

ACTIVITY/BEHAVIOR	STAFF INITIAL
Refusal to participate in any structured activity	
Leaving a structured activity before completion of task without consent	
Use of inappropriate language (i.e., cursing, yelling, etc.)	
Refusal to respond to staff request to stop inappropriate behavior	
Disruptive behavior, or threatening behavior	
Abusing visiting privileges	
Abusing telephone privileges	
	TOTAL DEDUCTIONS	

SPECIAL CARE LEVEL: Time placed on: _____

Due to expire: _____

PLEASE NOTE: When placed on Special Care, it is to run for a period of **24 hours**, and you must successfully complete all Special Care requirements. If this is not accomplished, the 24-hour period may be extended.

BONUS POINTS: A *maximum* of three Bonus Points may be earned in any one day. Bonus Points are awarded for work that is deemed above that which is required for that particular group.

TELEPHONE

CALLS	TO WHOM	TIME OF DAY	STAFF INITIAL

Calls allowed

Level 1 = 1   1. _____

Level 2 = 2   2. _____

Level 3 = 3   3. _____

Level 4 = 4   4. _____

Levels 1 and 2: Calls are 5 minutes in length

Levels 3 and 4: Calls are 10 minutes in length

PLEASE NOTE: Incoming calls are allowed from family members only. With all other calls, a message will be taken and given to the person.

Middletown Regional Hospital, Adolescent Mental Health Program, Middletown, Ohio.

Gatehouse Levels System

Level	Participation	Sobriety	Responsibility	Individualized goals	Privileges
	Attends all program activities on the grounds	Complies with observed urines	Performs activities of daily living	Fill in own goals 1.	May receive calls from approved family members only at nurses' station; five minutes per call
Two (2) week entry period Status level	Listens actively Is respectful in groups Lets others finish Cooperates with psychological and educational Cooperates with complete physical examination-testing	Cooperates with substance abuse assessment Verbalizes in groups and one-on-ones substance abuse history and what brought you into treatment Displays appropriate behavior in AA/NA meetings onground Completes AA/NA and NA unit assignments	Signs in and out with magnet Knows rule book Does not communicate with other units Complies with any special diets Completes chores as assigned Has no exclusive or special relationships	2. 3.	

From Reichbach J and Spire-Porco K (1989) Levels system with a dual diagnosis adolescent population. Presented at National Advocates for Child Psychiatric Nursing, White Plains, NY. Courtesy of Four Winds Hospital, Katonah, NY.

Continued.

Gatehouse Levels System — cont'd

Level	Participation	Sobriety	Responsibility	Individualized goals	Privileges
LEVEL I	ALL ASPECTS OF PARTICIPATION OUTLINED ON ENTRY PERIOD + Accepts Confrontation Confronts others appropriately Accepts limits from staff members	Submits "life story" outline in written form Displays appropriate behavior in AA and NA meetings Completes AA and NA unit assignments	ALL ASPECTS OF RESPONSIBILITY OUTLINED ON ENTRY PERIOD + Sets up and follows through on one-on-ones	1. 2. 3.	Can vote in levels meeting Can initiate and receive calls Is eligible to go on off-grounds unit trip at staff discretion May attend off-grounds AA/NA meetings with staff approval May attend leisure education group May conduct unit tours for new admits May attend Alumni Picnic
LEVEL II	PREVIOUSLY OUTLINED + Identifies negative attention-seeking behaviors Identifies entitlement and "I want what I want when I want it" attitude	STEP I (AA) Preparation Acknowledges problems with addiction Tells "life story" Displays appropriate behavior in AA and NA meetings	PREVIOUSLY OUTLINED + Reports peer rule-breaking behavior Gets to individual and family therapy sessions on time	1. 2. 3.	1½ hour dinner pass May request 1 hour of personal time Is allowed on smoking couch unescorted May go to session unescorted May attend on-grounds hospital-wide activities such as dances and coffee house May attend alumni dance

Continued.

Gatehouse Levels System — cont'd

Level	Participation	Sobriety	Responsibility	Individualized goals	Privileges
LEVEL III	PREVIOUSLY OUTLINED + Owns up to part in any conflict Freely discusses self in groups and one-on-ones	Family cleans out room before first pass home Speaks at AA and NA meetings Works on getting a temporary sponsor	PREVIOUSLY OUTLINED + Gets to scheduled appointments (internist, hair cut) on time	1. 2. 3.	6-hour weekend pass May attend hospital-wide trips Eligible for election to community office May walk unescorted to scheduled appointments such as hair cuts and internist
LEVEL IV	PREVIOUSLY OUTLINED + Supports and helps others in groups Shows sensitivity to others' feelings	Sets up and cleans up at AA and NA meetings Attends home AA and NA meetings while out on pass Has a temporary sponsor	PREVIOUSLY OUTLINED + Provides leadership for peers through example	1. 2. 3.	12-hour weekend pass 3-hour weekend pass with sponsor May apply for on-grounds job May walk unescorted to and from job May have late curfew

Continued.

Gatehouse Levels System—cont'd

Level	Participation	Sobriety	Responsibility	Individualized goals	Privileges
LEVEL V	PREVI-OUSLY OUT-LINED + Recognizes signifi-cance of loss of supports	Sets up and cleans up at AA and NA meetings Establishes an out-side sup-port net-work Uses spon-sor	Engages lower-level peers in treat-ment Acts as pre-sponsor Runs meet-ings on weekends	1. 2. 3.	Overnight week-end pass 5-hour week-end pass with sponsor May see approved friend(s) while on pass
LEVEL VI	PREVI-OUSLY OUT-LINED + Says good-byes	Sets up and cleans up AA and NA meetings Establishes outside support network Uses spon-sor	PREVI-OUSLY OUT-LINED + Encourages peers to provide leader-ship to lower-level peers	1. 2. 3.	Overnight weekend pass 7-hour week-end pass with spon-sor May take walks up to 30 min-utes unes-corted with 2 or 3 same-sex patients; calls in every 15 mins. May see ap-proved friends while on pass

MULTIDISCIPLINARY COLLABORATION

Collaboration among nursing staff and among the various disciplines working with the adolescent in the therapeutic milieu is essential for consistency in interventions. Time must be scheduled for writing and updating the treatment plan and for communicating about the adolescents' behavior, goals and progress before group sessions and individual and family therapy. Milieu staff members also need time to meet and discuss communication problems, conflicts, scheduling problems, and milieu issues (Skinner, 1979). These times should be scheduled on an ongoing basis with compensation for time spent in these activities. Flexible staffing patterns help to reduce overtime.

RULES

The rules for the adolescent unit must be simply stated, available in a prominent place such as the bulletin board, and enforced in a consistent manner. The rules pertain to very basic issues that are found in school and the community at large. For instance, assaults, public displays of affection, illicit drug use, obscene language, and damaging property are not permitted. If such behaviors occur, the adolescent will experience the consequences. Adolescents need to know the rules and the consequences of disobeying them. Because disturbed adolescents often break rules as part of acting out, the unit has a written procedure for limit setting that is followed by all staff. All staff members, including therapists, psychiatrists, housekeepers, and volunteers, must know the rules and use the agreed-on process. Housekeeping staff and volunteers should be trained to report rule breaking to the nursing staff for processing. The box on p. 289 lists typical rules for adolescent units.

SURVEILLANCE

Constant *surveillance* is needed on an adolescent unit. Disturbed adolescents' poor impulse control and exaggerated propensity for testing limits can lead to potentially dangerous situations. One staff member should be with or know the whereabouts of each adolescent on a team of eight *at all times.* Checks or rounds every 15 minutes are not adequate for surveillance of adolescents. Documentation of the child's behavior every 15 minutes is done for adolescents at risk for suicide and running away, and for those in restraint and seclusion, according to state and agency policy. A staff/client ratio of 1:4 permits therapeutic interaction; one staff member can provide only observation to eight adolescents. Surveillance includes not only knowing where adolescents are physically but also observing for early signs of agitation, withdrawal and sadness, side effects of medication, self-induced vomiting, deliberate or inadvertent damage to hospital or patients' property, sexual acting out, and rule violations.

LIMIT SETTING, ANGER, AND AGGRESSION MANAGEMENT

Clear, consistent limit setting is a foundation of the adolescent therapeutic milieu. Adolescents in inpatient settings often have difficulty with impulse control and may act out by breaking rules and becoming aggressive. Many adolescents have not had clear, consistent limit setting in their families. Adolescents who have been abused become aggressive when their rage over this issue rises to the surface. The inability

---

Adolescent Rules

1. No hitting
2. No verbal abuse or name calling
3. Rooms must be straightened up and beds made before school starts
4. No slamming doors; no hitting walls or ceilings
5. Shoes must be worn for any activity or when off the unit; no revealing clothes such as short shorts or halter tops allowed
6. Music at a reasonable level; radios will be collected at 10:00 PM; no tapes allowed with privilege of Level 2 and above
*7. Smoking only during free time and in designated areas—dayroom and activity room in evening
   Two cigarettes every break (there are 6 breaks)
     8:15—8:30 AM
     10:00—10:10 AM
     12:45—1:00 PM
     3:30—3:45 PM
     5:15—5:30 PM
     8:45—9:00 PM
   Lose privilege of cigarettes if patients share with someone who is not allowed or smoke in a nondesignated area
8. No horseplay
9. No matches, lighters, or sharp objects; glass bottles and sharp objects such as scissors, razors, and blades will be kept locked in nursing station
10. No cameras
11. No food in rooms
12. No members of opposite sex allowed in rooms

   *A no-smoking policy is preferred and is the trend for adolescent programs.

---

of staff to manage acting out behaviors results in premature discharges, running away, injuries to patients and staff, high staff turnover, and chaos in the unit. The unit should have *no more than one* newly admitted very aggressive child on each team. After 1 or 2 weeks of treating the first child, the team can add a second highly aggressive child. If staff has no control over admissions, a 1:2 staff/patient ratio, or even a 1:1 ratio will be needed to work effectively with several very aggressive adolescents.

The staff must approach the process of limit setting with several basic premises: adolescents need limits to test as a part of normal growth and development, the focus of control should shift from external sources to the child's own resources as quickly as possible with each episode, and each attempt to exceed limits of acceptable behavior is a learning experience tied into the adolescent's individual goals relating to anger or impulse control.

A preventive or early intervention strategy used for anger control is the anger color chart. Each adolescent makes a color chart that depicts four or five mood stages (calmest to angriest) in colors that the adolescent chooses, using the adolescent's own labels to describe the stages. Next to each color, the adolescent writes down the behaviors that occur, the respective feelings, and what actions or techniques the child can use to become calm. The adolescent uses color visualization to determine where his feelings are located on the chart, then the adolescent visually moves down the colors to the calmest one. (Figure 11-1 is an anger chart, reproduced here in black and white). Other early anger management strategies that are taught during the first phase of milieu treatment are deep breathing and relaxation techniques. These tools can be used when identification of feelings becomes too overwhelming or painful; they are invaluable in assisting adolescents to express anger appropriately.

The *limit setting* process (see box on pp. 291-292) incorporates principles of reality therapy (Wubbolding, 1988; Jones and Jones, 1981). The process is designed to bring the adolescent's unacceptable behavior to his attention, remind him of the rule or expectation, assist him to name what he is feeling, help him to say what he really wants or needs, then allow him to choose an appropriate way to get the need met.

Out of control	Hit people Hyperventilate Punch walls Run away Throw things	Destroy property
Mad	Mad at others Cuss Yell Tune people out totally Urge people (egg them on) to fight	Set up other people Feel defiant Power struggle in effect
Frustrated	Lose eye contact Begin to tune people out Go off by self Turn radio up loud Breathe faster	Voice gets louder Use alcohol/drugs Set up power struggle
Anxious	Bite nails Tap foot Tap pencil/chew on pencil Twist hair Pace	Doodle on paper Write on self/clothing Have sweaty palms Feel shaky
Calm	Feel mellow Get relaxed Feel happy Talk to friends Listen to radio	

Figure 11-1 Anger chart.

Interactions with the adolescent are firm, respectful, age appropriate, patient, and problem solving in tone. Encouragement to cooperate and support are given. The more out of control the child is, the more directive the staff must be.

Time out is a strategy frequently used on adolescent units. Time out is a 5- to 15-minute period that an adolescent spends in a designated space away from the distractions of his room and the unit and where he is then assisted through the steps of finding a better way to get his needs met. Time out is not seclusion. It is a working, problem-solving technique used on an as-needed basis, prescribed regularly to impulsive adolescents, or chosen by the adolescent who is overstimulated or losing control. Time out is always used in conjunction with other strategies, including limit setting, contingency management contracting and levels systems, response-cost

---

Limit Setting/Behavior Processing
and
Time Out Procedure*

Pre-steps

1. Get the adolescent's attention to allow him/her to stop the unacceptable behavior without interevention.
2. Identify to the adolescent the feeling you perceive him to be experiencing (mad, sad, or scared).
3. Assist the adolescent to name the feeling he is having.
4. Remind the adolescent of the rule.
5. Ask the adolescent what he needs.
6. Ask the adolescent for a more appropriate means of getting the need met.
7. If the adolescent cannot come up with a suggestion, staff may assist in identifying an alternative solution to the problem. Start with identifying natural consequences.
8. If unable to do this, remind the adolescent of the consequences for disruptive behavior (time out, loss of activity or level privileges, trust, and self-esteem).

Time out

9. If the adolescent still refuses to alter direction of behavior, staff may verbally direct the adolescent to his room or the time out room until calm (giving the adolescent space away from the distractions of the unit to make a better decision).
10. Use the patient's room if at all possible; use the time out room if the adolescent is unable to maintain himself in his room or if prescribed by treatment plan or patient request. If the behavior continues to escalate, call for extra help. An RN must be present.
11. If the adolescent refuses time out, the staff will physically escort him to the time out room.
12. Time out is usually 5 to 15 minutes. Monitor every 5 minutes or as necessary, repeating steps 2 through 8.
13. If the adolescent is unable to remain in the time out room on his own, staff will stand in doorway to monitor and provide external controls.

*Staff should feel comfortable calling for extra support at any point in the procedure. At least 5 people should be available for transport and restraint.

Continued.

Limit Setting/Behavior Processing
and
Time Out Procedure — cont'd

14. If his behavior still escalates, staff may manually restrain the adolescent through approved techniques of aggressive patient management. Staff will focus on the adolescent calming himself. Remediation follows escalation.

Seclusion

15. If the adolescent's behavior continues to escalate and appears harmful to himself or others, RN may call a physician for a seclusion order. If an emergency situation exists, an RN may obtain this order within 1 hour after the procedure.
16. Seclude the patient, first removing the belt, shoes, and any sharp objects.
17. Begin special observation documentation. Monitor every 15 minutes or as necessary.
18. Establish criteria for removal from seclusion.
19. If the adolescent continues to escalate, an RN may call a physician for a medication order to assist the patient in calming himself.

Restraints

20. If the adolescent still poses a threat to himself or others, staff may exercise use of restraints.
21. Restraints should be applied, using hospital-approved techniques, so that the adolescent is not dangerous to others but reasonably comfortable. Female patients may have their feet restrained together instead of with the four-point application.
22. Establish criteria for removal.
23. Begin special observation documentation. Monitor at least every 15 minutes. Provide fluids, toilet, and range of motion (ROM) every 2 hours.
24. When the adolescent is calm, remediate and get him involved in the program as soon as possible.
25. Explain what consequences for rule violations will be applied and when.

---

techniques (such as losing points or privileges for certain behaviors), skill training for anger management, and counselling for underlying issues. See Chapter 8 for a description of these processes.

Time out is easy to comprehend but is a complicated procedure in practice. Parents, teachers, and child care staff in institutions need training and supervision to use the technique properly. It is necessary to train three shifts of staff to implement a procedure that takes only 15 minutes. It is not unusual to find time out being abused by staff members who are angered by an abusive and aggressive adolescent. Time out is over-used when it is extended to other behaviors, when positive reinforcement is neglected, and when it is extended beyond reasonable limits (Varley, 1984). Entering the seclusion room to assess the adolescent and provide care requires careful planning by the staff. Kendrick and Wilbu (1986) provides the following plan:

1. The nurse in charge gives a brief description of the patient (name, age, behavior, and level of control).

2. The nurse in charge outlines the purpose of entering the seclusion room.
3. The nurse in charge assigns staff members to specific responsibilities, including spokesperson, and one staff member to each limb of patient. Female patients will have their feet held together.
4. The nurse in charge reduces noise and activity level near seclusion room and gathers supplies.
5. The spokesperson tells the patient that staff is coming and to sit in the center of the room.
6. Staff members enter, with those assigned to the arms first, then those assigned to the legs.
7. The staff members, especially the spokesperson, should kneel on one knee or squat to be at eye level with the adolescent.
8. Provide care for patient and/or process with patient expectations and readiness for removal.
9. Assess for safety factors and the patient's level of agitation.
10. Leave the room in reverse order of entry.

When an adolescent does not respond to verbal interaction or the time out process, refuses time out, or is attempting to hurt himself or others, manual restraint is used. A *baskethold* is the preferred technique for most adolescents and can be used relatively easily by most staff members. The "basket" is a supporting, huglike hold that permits the staff member to continue interacting with the child or to bring the child gently to the floor until assistance arrives. The adolescent is manually restrained until he feels calm, usually no more than 15 minutes. Then remediation occurs. *Remediation* is processing with the adolescent what happened and how to prevent such behavior in the future, and letting the adolescent know that he is still cared about. Remediation reduces the humiliation of losing control and redirects the event into a learning opportunity. Remediation includes reintegrating the adolescent into the peer group.

Seclusion is used when the child's aggressive behavior continues to escalate after 15 to 30 minutes of manual restraint. The adolescent is placed in a seclusion room with the door locked to provide a safe place to become calmer. Frequent observation and interaction by the staff ensures the safety of the adolescent, lets the adolescent know he is not abandoned, and provides opportunities for remediation to begin.

The nursing staff team member assigned to the adolescent works with the child whenever possible; however, the staff member who initially confronts the adolescent should follow the process through if possible. The registered nurse should be aware of all time out procedures and must be present to authorize and supervise any manual restraint and seclusion. If the adolescent is kicking, screaming, or fighting, the staff must hold the adolescent to deal with him or her. The adolescent is restrained manually while being dealt with.

Seclusion is rarely used on units that are staffed properly, have a structured program, and use the limit setting process. Mechanical restraints are used rarely in the care of adolescents. Neither seclusion nor manual or mechanical restraints (leather restraints, restraint boats, or wraps) should be used unless less restrictive measures fail. These procedures are used only when the adolescent is in imminent danger to himself or others. Because these procedures deprive patients of basic civil liberties, much consideration must be given to their use, documentation of the use, standards of care, and actual care given to the adolescent receiving these procedures. Each incident should be reviewed concurrently or retrospectively as a part of the quality assurance program in the facility. It is critical that staff analyze the use of potentially punitive measures (Frietas and Pieranunzi, 1990). The Joint Commission on Accreditation of Healthcare Organizations (JCAHO) and the Health Care Financing Agency through Medicare require special reviews of these procedures. In fact, the American Academy of Child and Adolescent Psychiatry Peer Review guidelines (Stevenson and Duprat, 1989) state that the use of restraints four or more times in 24 hours and the use of seclusion or restraints more than five times in any 30 consecutive days is an automatic "reviewable occurrence." That is, each incident is a quality review problem and must be reviewed by a qualified child and adolescent psychiatrist.

As needed medication (PRN) for behavior control is also rare in adolescent psychiatry, except for extreme situations. Sedation prevents processing events and problem solving (Pond, 1988). It may be used for psychotic adolescents, but is used very early in the limit setting process. See Chapters 13 and 14 for interventions with psychotic adolescents and pharmacology for adolescents.

PRIVILEGE SYSTEM

Adolescent units have levels of privileges that the adolescents earn by keeping the rules, achieving their goals, and working in therapy sessions. The staff keeps track of progress during each level period. Staff members decide on the adolescents' advancement based on information recorded on levels input sheets regarding goal achievement, rule keeping, and working in therapy. This is deliberately somewhat subjective because parents make subjective decisions to permit more freedom based on adolescents' increasing responsibility. Tokens or points are often used but are not as desirable because most families do not follow through at home with point systems. Staff members also record the use of privileges on a tracking sheet so that adolescents cannot manipulate to gain extra privileges. Levels advancement occurs in meetings with the adolescents, where reasons for the advancement or retention are explained. Staff members on day and evening shifts rotate the responsibility of the meeting so that one shift or one particular staff member is not perceived to be the sole decision maker in this important process. The boxes on pp. 295-299 provide examples of several levels systems, level tracking sheets, and a level input sheet.

GOAL SETTING AND ACHIEVEMENT

Setting a goal every morning and determining every evening whether the goal was met provide the focus for each day for the adolescent and the staff. The goal setting is done in a "goals group." The group of staff and peers provides ideas. Adolescents who have been in the program for a while provide excellent peer role modeling for newer patients. The goals can be written on 3 × 5 cards so the children may keep them available. The goal may be transcribed onto the treatment plan each day. The adolescent records the goal and the activities performed to accomplish it in a notebook. An adolescent with severe learning disabilities can be assisted by a staff member or a peer to record the goal and related activities, or a typewriter or tape recorder may be used.

Text continued on p. 300.

Levels System

Responsibilities	Privileges

Level I

Accomplishes daily goals	Mail (sent and received)
Performs personal hygiene (teeth brushed, bathed, and clothes clean)	Planned recreation activities
Cleans room (bed made, clothes picked up, and dirty linen and trash put in proper place)	Immediate family visiting
Keeps schedule with assistance	Checking out of board games

Level II

Identifies positive behaviors	Two phone calls daily
Attends groups regularly	Radio during free time in room until 10 PM
Accomplishes daily goals	Supervised group walks
Cooperates with staff requests	Off-grounds recreation privileges (with parents' consent)
Controls aggressive behavior	Supervised trip to gift shop or cafeteria
Follows adolescent program rules	Weight training

Level III

Actively participates in groups	Bedtime at 11 PM on Friday and Saturday
Identifies feelings/thoughts/behaviors	Grounds pass of 15 minutes once per day (specify areas) with parental consent
Communicates in "I" statements	Visits from two friends
Accepts responsibility for accomplishments and mistakes	Radio with headset out of room during free time
Follows adolescent rules	Computer with supervision

Level IV

Shows evidence of being self-directed	Grounds pass of 30 minutes
Gives support and accepts support	Unlimited radio (may keep)
Initiates ideas for improvement	Four phone calls
Uses assertive communication	Parent-brought food
Follows adolescent rules	Bedtime at 12 PM on Friday and Saturday

From Good Samaritan Hospital and Health Center, Mental Health Inpatient Unit, Adolescent Track, Dayton, Ohio.

Adolescent Levels System

Level I

No telephone calls
Send and receive mail
Board games and cards
Planned activities
Group walks
No radios
Bedtime at 10 PM

Level II

One telephone call/level (10 minutes)
Radio until 10 PM
Bedtime at 11 PM on Friday and 10 PM Saturday
Vending machine (supervised)
Ping pong with supervision daily (limit 15 minutes) 3:30-4:30
Fifteen minutes of one-to-one with staff during activity

Level III

Two telephone calls/level (10 minutes)
Pool table with supervision limit daily (30 minutes) 3:30-4:30
Stereo room 15 minutes (volume limit−2)
Input in selection of weekend movies
Radio until 10 PM
Bedtime at 11 PM on Friday, 10 PM on Saturday
Use visitor lounge for visit (if open)
Parents may bring food to keep in office

Level IV

Three telephone calls/level 30 minutes for 1-3 calls
Stereo room 30 minutes daily (unsupervised)
Vending machine (unsupervised)
Walk family or peers to door
Skip breakfast on weekend
Keep radio all the time
Bedtime at 11 PM on Friday and Saturday

Level V

Identify special privileges from designated list

Continued.

Adolescent Levels System — cont'd

Level V*

Three telephone calls/level
Vending machine (unsupervised)
Walk family/peers to front door
Stereo room 30 min. daily
  (unsupervised)
Skip breakfast on weekend
Keep radio at all times

Gift shop (unsupervised)
Parents may take out to dinner one time for
  1 hour
One friend may visit for 1 hour
Stay up until 12 PM on Friday and
  Saturday

*Staff may identify special privileges from designated list.

Level Tracking Sheet

Level I

	Date		Date	
Responsibilities Accomplishes daily goal	Yes	No	Yes	No
Personal hygiene (brush teeth, bathe, and clean clothes)				
Clean room (make bed, pick up clothes, and put dirty linen and trash in proper place)				
Keeps schedule with assistance				
Privileges Mail sent and received				
Planned recreation activities				
Immediate family visiting				
Minister/counselor				
Checking out of board games				
Restrictions No phone calls				
No radios				
Bedtime 10 PM				

From Good Samaritan Hospital and Health Center, Mental Health Inpatient Unit, Adolescent Track, Dayton, Ohio.

Level Tracking Sheet				
Level III				
	Date		Date	
Responsibilities Accomplishes daily goal	Yes	No	Yes	No
Actively participates in groups				
Identifies feelings/thoughts/ behaviors				
Communicates in "I" statements				
Accepts responsibility for accomplishments and mistakes				
Follows rules				
Privileges Bedtime at 11 PM on Fridays and Saturdays				
Grounds pass 15 minutes once per day (specify areas) with parental consent				
Visits from two friends				
Radio with headset out of room during free time				
Computer with supervision				
Restrictions Natural consequences				

Level Input Sheet

Name _____   Level _____
Total # of goals achieved _____
Date last raised _____

Behavior improvements
Date

Behavior problems
Date

Guidelines to raise to next level
Date

Goals that can be accomplished in 1 day are set. An adolescent who has a severe attention deficit disorder, a borderline IQ, or severe impulse or aggression problems may have goals that can be met as often as every hour. The goals are action oriented. The child must interact with others, role play, verbalize understanding, make lists, write feelings in a letter, or perform other activities. These learning activities engage the adolescent in increasing self-awareness and internalizing new interpersonal and social skills. The staff uses the therapeutic techniques described in Chapter 8 to coach goal setting and achievement.

Goal setting and skill development (Table 11-3) follow a four-phase sequence:
1. Basic skills development and problem definition
2. Self-awareness development: identifying feelings and behaviors, linking feelings and behaviors, and identifying beginning alternative behaviors
3. Changing behavior: expressing feelings, wants, and needs; getting wants and needs met appropriately; managing anger and aggression; and developing insight into the child's own and others' behavior
4. Integrating and terminating: maintaining gains at home and school, preparing for difficult situations, preparing for placements, identifying and arranging support, and saying good-bye

The four phases can be achieved in about 4 weeks in acute inpatient settings; they can be expanded to as many weeks as appropriate for various settings. The phases are accomplished according to the adolescent's and family's ability to progress through them and the time available for treatment.

During the first phase (basic skills and problem definition) the adolescent identifies those areas that are causing problems and those that contributed to admission to the treatment program. Adolescents also learn two basic communication skills: "I" statements (see the box on p. 302) and active listening. The anger chart is drawn toward the end of the first week to help the adolescent begin to identify and manage anger. An example of a first week goal is: "I will use an "I" statement with a peer, a staff member, and my parents today." The adolescent is also taught deep breathing and relaxation. During the second phase, adolescents identify feelings they are experiencing, specific problem behaviors they engage in, and situations that are difficult for them. Adolescents usually need a great deal of assistance in identifying feelings. To begin with, feelings are categorized into *mad, sad, glad,* and *scared.* "Mad" is the easiest feeling to identify, and the anger chart helps the child to notice the state of his body, match his thoughts with the physical response, then name the response or feeling. The "My Special Feelings" box on p. 302 is a learning material related to feelings.

Problem behaviors and situations are viewed as social deficits or deficits in other skills. When the adolescent identifies feelings and receives validation of them from staff, he is able to begin to identify problem areas. For instance, an adolescent may determine that he curses if he feels angry when teased by his peers. He can then learn to deal with teasing in a new way. The Structured Learning approach is excellent for teaching social skills to adolescents. Every adolescent unit should have a copy of *Skillstreaming the Adolescent* by Goldstein and others (1980). See Chapter 8 for an extensive discussion of skill development and goal setting and a list of materials and programs to use in this process. Assertiveness training activities should be included

Table 11-3   Goal Setting and Skill Development Progression

Outcomes	Activities
Phase one: basic skills and problem definition	
Basic skills	
"I" statements	"I" statements practice
Listening	Active listening
Basic anger management	Relaxation techniques
	Anger management (anger chart)
Identifying problems	Identifying angry feeling
	List problems (get information from parents, siblings, peers, and other staff about this)
	Write in journal what happened I "trashed" my room, etc.
	Skillstreaming group VI skills
Phase two: self-awareness	
Identifying feelings: mad, sad, glad, or scared	Complete feeling sheet and discuss with primary nurse
Identifying behaviors needing change (also ones that work)	Identify situations side that precipitate feeling
Linking behaviors and feelings	Responses to situations in *Skillstreaming* Group III skills
Identifying beginning alternative behaviors	*Skillstreaming* group IV and V
	Using "I" statements
	Giving and receiving feedback
Phase three: changing behavior	
Expressing feelings and wants	*Skillstreaming* Group I, II, IV, and V skills
Getting wants, needs met appropriately	Complex goals requiring interaction with peers, family, staff
Managing anger and aggression	Goals to break resistance and practice managing difficult situations
Developing insight into own and others'/family's behavior	Goals developed with family and group therapist at this point
	Role plays/sculptures
Phase four: integrating and terminating	
Maintaining gains at home and school	Various *Skillstreaming* exercises
Preparing for difficult situations at home, school	Role playing
	Any of the *Skillstreaming* skills or choices
Preparing for placements	Exercise
Identifying and arranging supports	
Saying good-bye	Good-bye activities

"I" Statements

"I" statements are used to accept responsibility for your own feelings and to give a clear message as to how you feel, why, and what you want or need.

I feel (mad, sad, scared, glad)_____

Because _____

And I want/need _____

There are hundreds of "feelings" words, but to simplify things, concentrate on the basic four: mad, sad, scared, and glad.

Example:

Wrong:

"What's the matter with you?! Can't you tell time?! You're grounded!!"

Right:

"I feel angry because you're late, and I want you to go to your room until we talk later."

My Special Feelings

I am happy when _____   I am really good at _____

I get angry when _____   I get excited when _____

I hope that _____   I feel safe when _____

I am good at _____   I need _____

I am afraid of _____   I am thankful for _____

I am ashamed of _____   I am lonely when _____

I feel sorry for _____   I am proud of _____

for all adolescents in the second phase (self-awareness). During this period the adolescent is learning new behaviors from various formal groups and informal sources in the program.

If resistance prevents therapeutic progress, an adolescent with sufficient ability to abstract can be taught the various psychological defense mechanisms. See the box on p. 304 for an adolescent level description of defense mechanisms.

Identifying defense mechanisms usually helps the adolescent to recognize blocks to progress and then develop some goals to work through the blocks. If resistance persists, various techniques can be used to reduce it. These are described in detail in Chapter 14.

During the third phase (changing behavior), the adolescent is pressured with confrontation and support to practice new skills in situations similar to real-life circumstances. Typically, during this week the child is developing insight, which is often painful, and the work of family therapy is very intense. The goals set each day usually relate to skills and strategies the child will practice or try in stressful family, peer, group, or classroom situations. The amount of pressure applied is determined during treatment planning sessions. The child's ego strength, intelligence, family progress, and probable posthospital placement are taken into consideration. Collaboration between milieu, individual, group, and family therapists is critical during this period.

The fourth phase (integrating and terminating) is the period of integration and preparation for discharge. The adolescent may attend school or spend additional time at home with family members to ease transition. Teachers, outpatient therapists, and probation officers attend the discharge conference with the family and staff. Situations that are anticipated as difficult are role played. Good-byes are said, and termination is completed. Discharge preparation provides many goals to be achieved.

For 4 weeks, daily goal setting in the inpatient setting or longer in other settings is related specifically to the adolescent's problems. This results in improved impulse control and problem-solving ability; appropriate expression of feelings, needs, and wants; and most important, elevation of self-esteem.

FAMILY PROGRAMS

Parents or other guardians are an integral part of the therapeutic milieu. Many adolescent units severely limit parent visiting. If families are not available for the nursing staff to teach, role model, and provide emotional support, the adolescent and family will have less opportunities to learn and practice improved communication. (For a list of communication topics, see the box on p. 305). In acute settings the formal family program consists of a family assessment and social history, two family therapy sessions, a didactic series of information, a multifamily therapy group, and a discharge summary meeting with other important after-care personnel. In residential or day treatment, the sessions are spread out over longer amounts of time. In addition to the structured program, the nursing staff members assist families to develop and practice new skills for parenting, managing a difficult teenager, and developing social support with other families in the milieu. The nurse also collaborates closely with the family therapist in developing goals for the adolescent in relation to family treatment goals. See Chapters 12 and 14 for more information on family interventions.

Learning About Defense Mechanisms

1. Withdrawal or avoidance — turning the attention away from a troublesome problem (daydreaming in a pleasant world where problems either do not exist or are easily solved)
2. Repression — ridding the conscious mind of unpleasant or painful thoughts or memories (blotting out an unpleasant experience, such as death of a close friend)
3. Rationalization — making excuses for events because the real reasons are too hard to face (telling yourself that not getting something you really wanted was for the best)
4. Compensation — trying to make up for personal lacks or shortcomings, real or imaginary, by developing other goals or abilities; most often used to overcome feelings of inferiority (developing a strongly extroverted, outgoing personality to make up for lack of beauty)
5. Projection — overcoming inferiority or guilt by blaming other people or objects (blaming the baseball bat when you strike out)
6. Displacement (transfer) — transferring emotions such as anger or love from one object or person to another (smashing a chair or banging your fist against a wall in the middle of an argument instead of attacking the other person)
7. Sublimation — channeling socially unacceptable drives into acceptable behavior (becoming a boxer, football player, or wrestler to provide an outlet for your urge to be tough or masculine)
8. Idealization — believing people or situations to have qualities of excellence or perfection they may not possess to make them fit your own "ideal" (seeing your boyfriend or girlfriend as perfect)
9. Conversion — turning an unconscious emotional conflict into a physical illness (getting an upset stomach the day of final exams)
10. Regression — retreating to earlier forms of behavior or to past situations and experiences to avoid what is difficult in the present (regression must not be confused with conscious enjoyment of memories; a regressing person unconsciously wants to relive successful experiences from the past because he or she is unhappy with the present) (an adult playing hopscotch with children to avoid having to make friends with adults)
11. Identification — imitating another person or putting yourself in another person's place (imitating the walk, talk, or manner of a movie or television star)
12. Reaction formation — developing an attitude opposite to your true feelings, often replacing one extreme with the other (having the urge to drink, and overcoming it by becoming a crusader against drinking)

THE THERAPEUTIC CLASSROOM

Since school is a major part of every adolescent's life, the inpatient adolescent attends school daily. The purpose of the therapeutic classroom is to assess the adolescent's school adjustment and achievement, to determine appropriate posthospital educational placement, to maintain the child's academic progress while in the hospital, and to assist the adolescent to cope in the classroom setting. The teacher should be certified in learning and behavior disorders and mental retardation for grades 7

Adolescent Family Program Communication Group Topics

I. **Family stress**

    A. Causes of stress and symptoms
    B. Rating of stress level (life change scale)
       Stress is the product of changes and adjusting to changes (divorce)
    C. Types of symptoms that are caused by stress (overload symptoms scale)
    D. Ways to reduce stress (relaxation)

II. **Effective parenting**

    A. Ineffective methods of parenting
       1. Permissive
       2. Autocratic
    B. STEP program philosophy for effective parenting (*STEP-Teen Parent Handbook*
       may be borrowed from the unit)
    C. Characteristics of equality between family members
    D. Goals of adolescent misbehavior (attention, power)
    E. Effective parenting methods (consistency, communication)
    F. Organizing family meetings
    G. Role playing

III. **Nonverbal communication**

    A. Illustration
    B. Definition
    C. Importance
    D. Types of nonverbal cues
    E. Improving skills

IV. **Family communication styles**

    A. Placater
    B. Blamer
    C. Computer
    D. Distracter
    E. Leveling (effective)
    F. Role playing

---

through 12. Serving as the coordinator between the program and the child's home school, the teacher completes discharge planning with the school. The classroom is a part of the milieu; the child may have daily goals related to school, the same limit-setting process is used, and the teacher is heavily involved in assessment and treatment planning. A nursing staff member assists the teacher in the classroom, and the teacher is given a report on the child's progress and daily goal before class.

Unstructured Aspects of the Therapeutic Milieu

STAFF ATTRIBUTES

The most important element of the unstructured milieu is the individual staff members. A mix of personalities, experiences, ethnic groups, and sexes helps recreate the adolescent's normal environment and prevents homogeneity. Although diversity in the staff group is essential, several common characteristics must be present. For instance, all staff members must have the capacity to love and empathize with teenagers and their families. They also must be able to let go of their attachment when the child leaves. The manager or supervisor of the program realizes that this capacity to love is vital to the unit but is also a potential cause of burnout. Thus a key role of the supervisor is to treat staff members with love and respect. The manager must recognize their strengths, give them room and encouragement to grow, process difficult terminations and feelings about a child's pain, and help them find meaning for suffering. This managerial support is a combination of clinical supervision and management strategies for clinical staff.

Another required characteristic of staff members is the belief that *everyone has the capacity to grow and change.* This attribute gives families and adolescents hope. Staff members must also have the ability to set limits. Underlying the capacity to love, a hopeful attitude, and the *ability to set limits* is a high level of self-esteem. Working in a program such as one of those described in this book enhances and nurtures these qualities in staff, as well as in patients. The caring, nurturing and hopeful attitude permeate all interactions with adolescents in the milieu. The behavioral and cognitive approaches so important for disturbed adolescents will not be effective if they are not implemented with caring and support.

ONE-TO-ONE INTERACTIONS

One-to-one interactions are an important part of the milieu. Each adolescent's treatment plan directs the tone, focus, and frequency of these interactions with staff members. Conversation with the adolescent includes processing events as they arise, working on goal achievement, limit setting, friendly small talk, and some humorous "joking around." The tone of interaction is similar to the attitude therapy approach (Folsom, 1969). For instance, for an adolescent who is suicidal and hopeless, a kind, active, friendly approach is used; for an adolescent who is angry and paranoid, a passive, friendly approach without touching is used, at least initially. The focus may be on expressing feeling, solving problems, or any area that is the focus of treatment that day or week of the program. The frequency of interpersonal contact is dictated by the severity of the child's disturbance, the need for increased surveillance for the child's or others' safety, and whether dependence or independence is being encouraged. All verbal and nonverbal communication from staff members to the adolescent is designed to enhance self-esteem. The staff members convey that they like and care for the adolescent but do not accept inappropriate behavior. If a staff member becomes angry or upset with an adolescent's behavior, the staff member uses "I" statements to let the adolescent know the behavior was upsetting. The appropriate time for this is usually during remediation or as soon after the incident as possible. If a staff member handles a situation poorly or causes a misunderstanding, an apology should be offered.

ROLE MODELING

Role modeling is another important factor in a therapeutic milieu. Direct care staff members serve as positive male and female role models for the adolescents and their parents. The staff's positive attitude, good communication and limit setting skills, good manners, good health habits and grooming, teamwork, and positive reinforcement of progress demonstrate good mental health and positive interpersonal interaction.

TEACHING

Teaching specific content occurs in structured and unstructured ways in the program. Parent education groups are structured sessions with didactic and experiential approaches. The content includes communication, parenting, and stress. Nurses teach adolescents and parents about psychotropic and other medications. Sexuality and contraception can be taught in classes or individually, and pregnant teenagers receive prenatal teaching. On-the-spot teaching of parenting skills occurs regularly. Frequent, continuous orientation to the program; information about what, where, and when activities are occurring; and explanations and demonstrations of the various skills needed are all forms of teaching.

The therapeutic milieu for adolescents is a complex, challenging arena for psychiatric nursing treatment. A great deal of information, practice and staff collaboration is needed to implement it successfully. This chapter, as well as Chapters 8 and 14, provide a base for this dynamic process.

REFERENCES AND SUGGESTED READINGS

Bettleheim B and Sylvester E (1948) The therapeutic milieu, American Journal of Orthopsychiatry 18:191.

Coleman JC (1987) Working with troubled adolescents: a handbook, London, Academic Press Inc, Ltd.

Folsom JC (1969) Attitude therapy as a communication device, Transactions, spring:18-26.

Freitas L and Pieranunzi V (1990) Ethical issues in the behavioral treatment of children and adolescents, Journal of Child and Adolescent Psychiatric Nursing 3(1):3-8.

Goldstein A, Sprafkin R, Gershaw NJ, and Klein P (1980) Skillstreaming the adolescent, Champaign, Ill, Research Press.

Jones M (1953) The Therapeutic Community, New York, Basic Books, Inc, Publishers.

Jones M (1968) Beyond the therapeutic community, New Haven, Conn, Yale University Press.

Jones V and Jones L (1981) Responsible classroom discipline, Boston, Allyn & Bacon, Inc.

Kendrick DW and Wilbu G (1986) Seclusion: organizing safe and effective care, Journal of Psychosocial Nursing 24(11):26-28.

Kunes-Connell M (1987) Therapeutic environment and the therapeutic community. In Norris J, Kunes-Connell M, Stockard S, Ehrhart PM, and Newton GR, editors: Mental health–psychiatric nursing: a continuum of care, New York, John Wiley & Sons.

Peplau H (1982) Some ideas about nursing in the psychiatric milieu. Presented at Boulder Psychiatric Institute, Boulder, Colo.

Pond VE (1988) The angry adolescent: treatment versus containment practices, Journal of Psychosocial Nursing 26(12):15-17.

Reichbach J and Spire-Porco K (1989) Levels system with a dual diagnosis adolescent population. Presented at National Advocates for Child Psychiatric Nursing, White Plains, N.Y.

Skinner K (1979) The therapeutic milieu: making it work, Journal of Psychiatric Nursing and Mental Health Services, August 17:38-44.

Stevenson K and Duprat MM (1989) Child-adolescent psychiatric illness: guidelines for treatment resources, quality assurance, peer review and reimbursement, Washington, DC, American Academy of Child and Adolescent Psychiatry.

Varley WH (1984) Behavior modification approaches to the aggressive adolescent. In Keith CR, editor: The aggressive adolescent, New York, Macmillan Press.

Wolf M (1977) A review of literature of milieu therapy, Journal of Psychiatric Nursing and Mental Health Services 15:26-32.

Wubbolding RE (1988) Using reality therapy, New York, Harper & Row Publishers, Inc.

Chapter 12

Psychotherapy and Expressive Therapies

Patricia Clunn
Christina R. Hogarth

STANDARD V-D

THE CHILD AND ADOLESCENT PSYCHIATRIC MENTAL HEALTH SPE-
CIALIST USES ADVANCED CLINICAL EXPERTISE TO FUNCTION AS A
PSYCHOTHERAPIST FOR THE CHILD OR ADOLESCENT AND FAMILY
AND ACCEPTS PROFESSIONAL ACCOUNTABILITY FOR NURSING
PRACTICE.

Psychiatric nurse clinical specialists are prepared to work with clients according
to specific age-groups (adult, child, adolescent, geriatric), using individual, family,
and group interventions by completing a master's program in psychiatric mental
health nursing. National certification by the ANA as a clinical specialist (CS) in
mental health nursing requires postmaster's degree clinical psychotherapeutic
practice supervised by a member of the core mental health disciplines and successful
completion of the standardized ANA certification examination. Certification (C) as
a nurse generalist requires supervised postbaccalaureate clinical practice and
successful completion of the standardized ANA certification examination, in
addition to other criteria. Thus certification serves as a measure of quality assurance
for nurses who provide psychotherapy in their practice.

Although clinical nurse specialists are prepared to provide individual, family, and
group psychotherapies, other nurses working in family-centered or inpatient
psychiatric agencies find it necessary to acquire these skills, and many staff nurses
provide these interventions under the supervision of master's- or doctoral-prepared
nurses or clinicians from core mental health disciplines (Hamyion, 1983). These staff
nurses have unique opportunities to help disturbed adolescents in in-patient settings.
Hospitalization makes them more available than those seen in mental health clinics
or private office visits. Staff nurses need an understanding of the principles and
purposes of the various therapies, so that they can augment these therapies, and
collaborate with the clinical specialist or interdisciplinary team member therapists.

The core mental health disciplines prepare clinicians to provide psychotherapy to adolescents individually, with their families, and in groups. Regardless of the clinician's specialty discipline, the techniques of psychotherapy are based on the same theories and require the professional accountability of all practitioners who provide therapy. Nursing psychotherapy is distinguished from that of other mental health disciplines on the basis of its concepts, history, and practice (Flaskerud, 1984). It is especially suited to provide culturally relevant nursing therapy, integrating physical and mental health concepts and involving and managing the family, milieu, and other social systems.

It is important to be aware that not all practitioners in the field of psychiatry have the training needed to qualify them as therapists. For example, not all psychiatrists have completed the additional educational requirements and clinical work required for board certification in psychoanalysis, nor have all psychiatrists completed the additional training required to conduct family and group psychotherapy. Most clinical psychologists are trained in individual and group therapies but not in family therapies. Psychiatric social workers generally are trained in individual, group, and family therapies.

School—with strong academic and social influences on the adolescent—is a major part of the adolescent's world. Special educators, school counselors, and school nurses are often prepared to provide mental health services. Because most adolescents spend a major part of their day in school settings, these professionals often are the first to identify an adolescent's mental health problem and are available for psychotherapeutic interventions (Miller, 1974). Counselors and special educators with preparation at the master's-degree level often provide individual, group, and family therapy, as well as including psychoeducative therapies that are a significant aspect of the adolescent's overall therapeutic program.

The provision of other therapeutic modalities, such as occupational, music, art, recreational, and dance therapies, is the domain of clinicians, another group of adolescent mental health workers, and most of these experts have completed advanced education and training programs in these special areas. Most adolescents prefer action—that is motor activities and physical expression—to verbal communication, and these "expressive" interventions can be therapeutic in and of themselves. They often are used to help the adolescent client gradually become available for the "talk" therapies.

Theoretical Approaches to Adolescent Psychotherapy

This chapter provides an overview of the theory, rationale, techniques, and evaluation procedures of some of the most frequently employed psychotherapies in the treatment of adolescents. Although the theoretical basis of treatment is similar to that of adult therapy, adolescent treatment presents unique challenges. Adolescents are neither grown-up children nor miniature adults, and their treatment cannot be viewed as scaled-down adult therapy. Adolescent psychotherapists need an expanded knowledge base of the human condition and a specific perspective concerning what constitutes therapy or counseling, terms used interchangeably in much of the literature. Factors such as stages of adolescent development, environments, and reasons for entering therapies influence the approach to therapy. Because developmental considerations are critical in the therapeutic interactions with adolescents, most experts claim that therapists experienced in working with younger children adjust their psychotherapeutic approaches more easily to working with adolescents than do therapists whose previous experience has been with adult clients.

In the United States at present there are a variety of schools of thought on adolescent psychopathology, each with specific, related interventions. No one philosophy predominates, and there is considerable diversity with competing paradigms, fragmentation, and rivalry among theorists and the treatment methods they espouse. There are remarkable geographical differences in the dominant theories and therapies used with adolescents, a result of the concentrations of different clinical "schools of thought" at various medical, nurse education, and training centers in the country (Lazare, 1979).

The major contemporary psychotherapeutic models for adolescent treatment discussed in this chapter are behavioral-cognitive, psychoanalytic, interpersonal, social, systemic (family systems), and group therapies. Other influential systems include the existential school and various forms of psychotherapy that have emerged from the humanistic school, such as gestalt therapies and transactional analysis. Many of the procedures and techniques have in common the goal of helping the adolescent to develop a sense of mastery, combat social isolation, restore the person's feelings of group relatedness, and aid in personal rediscovery (or discovery) of the meaning of life. The models differ in their philosophical explanations of the root of the adolescent's problems: early childhood, recent past, and present. Furthermore, in therapy with adolescents, important elements are the youngster's age and the tasks of adolescents, as well as the role of parents and significant others. All of these elements are viewed differently by the various schools of therapy. However, the aim of all forms of psychotherapy and intervention strategies is to help adolescents feel better in relation to both their inner and outer worlds.

BEHAVIORAL THEORY AND THERAPY

The behavioral approach is one of the most popular psychotherapeutic interventions currently in use, and its major proponents in the United States are Wolpe, Eysenck, and Beck. Behavioral theory and research are rooted in learning theory concepts and behavioral analysis of symptoms (Klerman and Millon, 1986). This approach was initially developed in laboratories for experimental psychological research. Most behavioral techniques and methods have been proved effective in such laboratories before they are applied to clinical situations.

Behavioral theories attribute abnormal or deviant behavior to learning, environmental influences, and the response of others to behavior. Deviant and dysfunctional behavior patterns caused by anxiety and neurosis are viewed as being controlled by a number of stimuli conditions, which may be completely unknown to the person exhibiting the behaviors. These stimuli, which are externally (environmentally) or internally (cognitively) controlled, provide the basis for the two major types of interventions: operant and cognitive behavior modification.

The task of the behavioral therapist is to determine the environmental factors that are associated with these undesirable behaviors. Behavioral therapists use behavior modification, behavior therapy, and cognitive behavior therapies. Although these terms are used interchangeably, nurses need be aware of the distinct focus of each. Most of the major theorists and behavioral therapies first appeared during the 1950s and provided the philosophical base of most individual behavior therapy and behavior modification techniques that are used today.

Individual behavioral approaches with adolescents with behavior problems are based on the various theories and therapies supporting individual behavioral changes. *Group behavioral therapies with adolescents* have a wide variety of applications in this age-group. There are four major types of group behavioral therapies (Brown and Prout, 1989):

- Operant group therapy, which views the social environment of the group as a microlaboratory, with appropriate behavior increased and inappropriate behavior decreased through the use of operant techniques and principles.
- Modeling and behavior rehearsal, which applies social learning theory models to a group. Observational learning assumes that the person learns simply by observing behavior and its consequences; thus adolescents learn from group peers. Behavior rehearsal consists of role playing and the trying on certain behaviors by group members, whose performance is then critiqued and discussed by group peers.
- Cognitive behavioral training in social skills, noted by adolescents as one of the important areas of concern. Most extensively and widely developed training, these group protocols usually include relaxation procedures and dealing with real-life stressful situations.
- Social skills training, which focuses on teaching prosocial skills and cognitive behavior training (Gresham and Ledmanek, 1983).
- Group procedures for reducing anxiety.

Adolescents' difficulties with peer relations are understood in context of the development of cognitive controls. The concept of cognitive control explains the way individuals coordinate information from the external environment with the affects, fantasies, and motives from their internal environment to remain in control of the information. Cognitive controls mediate between the influences of personality and motivation on one hand and cognition on the other, and they evolve into an enduring aspect of the individual's cognitive functioning and adaptive style. Thus cognitive control therapy, initially used with adolescents with attention deficit disorders, has shown to be useful for aggression and impulsiveness.

Peer therapy is used for better-adjusted adolescents to affect change in their social system. Peer interaction can provide opportunities for learning to control aggression, improving perspective-taking abilities, and engaging in intimate relations (Raskin, Lamhand, and Martsolf, 1990). When adolescents are withdrawn and isolated, they benefit more from interactions with younger peers whose social development is similar to theirs. The school setting is a natural environment for these types of behavioral interventions (Siepker and Kandaras, 1985).

When planning behavioral therapies designed to improve adolescent social interactions, therapists need to make an initial distinction between internalized and externalized peer disorders. For example, a physically abused adolescent who is aggressive with peers may do best in individual behavioral therapy (Gilbert, 1988), whereas a neglected youth who is withdrawn with peers might benefit from peer group therapy. The goal is to provide and facilitate the development of more adaptive ways of dealing with expression and regulation. For appropriate planning the clinician needs to understand the adolescent's developmental level in relation to expression of affect (Stanisz, 1990).

Behavioral theories are based on the principle that behavior is changed by the administration or withholding of rewards. In purely behavioral terms a desired behavior is encouraged with concrete rewards such as food, stickers (gold stars), and other similar immediate reinforcers. Principles of behavior therapy are used in privilege systems in adolescent inpatient units, as well as in a few specialized situations in adolescent psychiatry. Sometimes a desensitization program is used for phobias. In youngsters with borderline or low intelligence, head injuries, or severe attention deficit disorders, an hourly program of reinforcers is used to elicit positive behaviors and self-control. Behavior therapy typically is not used as a treatment philosophy for individual therapy. Generally, behavior programs are used to change habits, such as smoking and overeating, and they provide an adjunct to insight-oriented therapy.

COGNITIVE THEORY AND THERAPY

The basic premise of cognitive theory is that values and beliefs govern people's behavior and responses to situations. These beliefs can be rational, irrational, or distorted (Beck A, 1979; Ellis and Grieger, 1978). Feelings can be appropriate or inappropriate to the situation because of beliefs about the event. Cognitive therapy techniques assist the adolescent to develop realistic or rational beliefs, which results in appropriate feelings. Reality therapy (Wubbolding, 1988) includes the concept of understanding, identifying, and satisfying needs and wants. Cognitive therapists use a variety of active, directive techniques to reframe irrational beliefs and to help the adolescent identify and use new ways of thinking and behaving. The principles of reality therapy are widely used in schools, law enforcement agencies, group homes, and residential treatment centers. Reality therapy is recommended for adolescent inpatient programs, especially for limit setting and behavior processing (Brown and Prout, 1989).

HUMANISTIC AND EXISTENTIAL THEORIES AND THERAPY

Humanistic theorists believe that each person is the best source of self-information. The self is viewed holistically—physically, emotionally, socially, and spiritually. Individuals are viewed as accountable to themselves for growth and achieving their human potential, or self-actualization. The humanist is concerned with the experience of self in the moment (although this moment may be connected to the past). Existential issues such as the meaning of pain, suffering, loneliness, and joy are explored to transcend painful experiences.

Humanistic and existential therapists believe in an active, positive regard and empathy (Carkhoff and Truax, 1967). The humanistic therapist assists the adolescent to become aware of thoughts, feelings, and behaviors as they occur in the here and now. Gestalt therapy (Perls, 1970) is based on an active, experiential process in which the therapist directs the adolescent through creative encounters with various aspects of the self or "unfinished business" in the person's life. Self-awareness is a significant focus of Gestalt therapy, and changes in behavior are developed in the therapy session itself (Zinker, 1977).

PSYCHOANALYTICAL THEORY AND PSYCHOANALYSIS

Freudian psychoanalytical concepts that led to psychoanalysis as therapy have been modified to include ego psychology and self-psychology. The therapeutic emphasis is on intensive, insight-oriented, dynamic psychotherapy and psychoanalysis. Major proponents in the United States include Erikson, Mahler, Kohut, and Kernberg (Millon and Klerman, 1988).

Sigmund Freud, the founder of psychoanalysis and psychoanalytical psychotherapy, described psychoanalysis as the procedure by which mental processes are investigated and neurotic disorders are treated, as well as a body of information that describes human behavior (Weisz and Benoit, 1989). Psychoanalysis, which has a deterministic, biological foundation, is based on the premise that behavior is largely beyond the realm of conscious awareness. Anxiety and repression are key concepts. Initially, psychoanalytical theory focused on tension reduction and instinctive drives that are modified during the psychosexual developmental process.

The fundamental issue in psychic development is learning to tolerate anxiety related to the psychosexual developmental phase and to develop defenses in an adaptive fashion. In the psychoanalytical treatment process with adolescents, defenses are analyzed to uncover conflicts arising from sexual and aggressive drives. The two key phenomena in psychoanalysis are transference and resistance. Freud believed clients with severe forms of psychological disturbances—those with psychoses—could not benefit from psychoanalysis.

Adolescent psychoanalytical therapy is adapted from classical Freudian psychoanalysis and psychodynamic understanding of human development. Psychoanalysis has broadened its scope and now includes psychoanalytical psychotherapy and other forms of therapy. These therapies are based on psychodynamic principles and unconscious processes. They focus on defense mechanisms and intrapsychic conflict, which are attributed to an imbalance among the id, the ego, and the superego. The techniques of psychoanalysis and other major types of psychoanalytical psychotherapy used with adolescents differ from those used with adults (see box on p. 317).

Contemporary adolescent psychoanalysts, such as Laufer (1981), stress that adolescent psychopathology must be understood developmentally as a breakdown in the formation of a final sexual organization. The major developmental tasks of critical concern are separation-individuation from the family, promotion of significant peer relationships, development of positive self-esteem and sexual identity, and control of sexual drives and adaptation to sexual norms.

Psychoanalytical psychotherapy focuses on creating a dependency relationship in which the adolescent is dependent on the therapist inasmuch as the central assumption is that the neurotic conflict will emerge in the relationship and be worked through in the transference context. The therapist must provide a comfortable environment that offers the adolescent relief from the outside world, which the young adolescent may view as hostile, critical, and unacceptable. The analyst is both friend

Psychoanalytical Psychotherapies

Psychoanalysis

Goal is to reorganize character structure and to diminish defenses. Use of free association; focus on interpretations, resistances, and transferences. Use of the couch. Therapy sessions of about 50 minutes four to five times a week for 2 to 5 or more years. Requires adolescents who have relatively mature personalities, positive life situations, and are motivated for long-term, stable, therapeutic alliance.

Insight therapy

Goal is resolution of selected conflicts, removal of limited pathological defenses. Free association and transference deemphasized; emphasis discussions of current interpersonal events. Insight refers to adolescent's emotional and intellectual understanding of dynamics through "corrective emotional experiences." Psychotropic drugs also may be used. Meetings usually last for ½ to 1 hour, one to three times a week, for a few sessions or for several years. Requires adolescent with fairly adequate ego strength, such as an older adolescent with some infantile conflicts that influence current reactions to situations.

Relationship therapy

Goal is growth of relatively immature personality through relationship with therapist that offsets prior inadequate and poor significant relationships. Includes group, family methods; uses other therapists and agencies. Meets one to two times per week; may last a month to several years. Requires adolescents with capacity for growth. Relationship therapies performed by many psychiatric social workers, nurses, and psychologists.

Supportive therapy

Places more emphasis on support then do other analytical interventions to restore adolescent to prior status during a period of crisis, emotional turmoil, or decompensation. Provide reduction of anxiety and fear and helps adolescent tolerate unchangeable situations. Therapist actively intervenes, advises, selects, and directs discussions. Psychotropic drugs are used, as are occupational therapies, hospitalization, and family contact. Sessions are brief, but may include lifelong contacts, as occurs with psychotic adolescents. Nonpsychiatrist physicians and other mental health workers may provide supportive therapies.

Brief psychotherapy

Distinguished by a limitation in number of therapy sessions, agreed upon in advance of therapy with the adolescent or defined by its focus on one specific symptom or problem. Developed as an alternative to long-term therapies cited previously. Focus on current problem, avoids transference issue, character problems, regression, dependency. Often used with adolescents needing guidance, help with developmental progression, or specific task mastery. Best for well-functioning adolescents. Requires careful psychoanalytical diagnosis. May be limited to six 1-hour sessions. Used to facilitate emotional development (Gray, 1978), with goal of keeping anxiety to a minimum. Performed by a variety of mental health professionals.

Modified from Stuart GW and Sundeen SJ, (1991) Principles and practices of psychiatric nursing, St. Louis, Mosby–Year Book, Inc.

and role model and must be firm, understanding, and objective. There is considerable difficulty in creating a positive transference because adolescents often mistrust adult values and attempt to assert their own independence. Thus this tenuous psychoanalytical relationship with the adolescent has been labeled a "fragile alliance" (Meeks, 1971). Bryt (1966), another well-known adolescent psychoanalyst, suggests modifications of psychoanalytical treatment goals with adolescents to include the following:
- Development of a consistent sense of self
- Ability to use foresight and have fun
- Desire to be with others and capacity to be alone
- Understanding that other people are neither all to one's liking nor are they all unlikable
- Gain in confidence in the ability to make choices, with the understanding that some options are worse and some better

INTERPERSONAL THEORY

The migration of many European psychoanalysts to the United States before World War II initiated the "Americanization" of European psychoanalytical theories, which evolved into the major theoretical "schools" that continue today. American scientists included psychocultural components, which distinguished American psychiatric theories from the purer, classic European theories.

Sullivan's interpersonal theory (1953), developed by an American for the American culture, exemplified these changes. The focus of this theory is on relationships between and among people and emphasizes society's role as the creator of personality. Sullivan's theory reflects its integration of anthropological concepts, such as those concerning verbal and nonverbal communication, participant observation, the use of themes, theme analysis, and the assumption that one's cultural perspective is at least partially shaped by the language of that culture. Sullivan's therapeutic methods, in contrast to classical psychoanalysis, were applicable to inpatients, including adolescents diagnosed with severe psychoses such as schizophrenia, and provided nursing staffs with many interventions and nursing management techniques.

INVESTIGATIVE NURSE PSYCHOTHERAPY

Hildegard Peplau (1952, 1964), a leader in psychiatric nursing therapy was strongly influenced by Sullivan's interpersonal theory and creatively developed concepts and approaches for nursing therapy. She also drew on the theories of Maslow and Symonds which in turn were influenced by Freud, Fromm, and Pavlov (Marriner-Torney, 1989), to develop a method of psychiatric nursing therapy that continues today (Lego, 1982).

Peplau's theory provided a self-directed nurse practice model for therapeutic interventions and psychotherapy with seriously disturbed, psychotic clients at a time when most psychiatric nurses worked with clients hospitalized in large state institutions. Her theory revolutionized psychiatric nursing in the early 1950s, providing a nursing framework and technique of interpersonal nursing interventions, a major contribution to scientific base of nursing. Most of the literature on nurse-client relationships since the publication of Peplau's text in 1952 is based on her theoretical concepts (Lego, 1980). As Peplau's interpersonal concepts were applied to other clinical areas of nursing, her theory brought about a "second-order" change in the discipline of nursing (Sills, 1978).

Most nurses are introduced to Peplau's theory of nurse-client interpersonal relationships during their basic psychiatric education in programs in which inpatient settings are used for clinical experiences. Before the development of special units, adolescents were assigned to adult units of patients for student learning. Most faculty members who teach in clinical training programs base their client selection on what Schofield (1974) called adolescents diagnosed with schizophrenia with the YAVIS syndrome, the tendency to treat *y*oung, *a*ttractive, *v*erbal, *i*ntelligent, and *s*uccessful persons. As a result of this bias against work with older clients (Beck, 1979), most nurses have their first supervised psychiatric nurse-client relationship with adolescents.

For more than 40 years Peplau was instrumental in developing, expanding, and teaching mental health nursing as a science and in researching and writing about the role of psychiatric nursing. She influenced the development and focus of master's degree programs in psychiatric nursing and the role of the clinical specialist as nurse psychotherapist. Peplau and other early psychiatric nursing leaders set standards for master's degree programs for clinical nurse specialists so that these students acquired the same competence in theory and practice required of the other core mental health professionals.

Peplau's investigative psychotherapy continues to be taught as a basic framework in many master's degree programs that prepare clinical specialists and continues to influence the psychotherapeutic framework currently used by practicing nurse psychotherapists (Sills, 1978).

Peplau's psychodynamic theory-based nursing model emphasized the client's psychobiological experiences and concepts such as needs, frustration, conflict, anxiety, and learning. Experimental learning is the process that underlies the investigative approach to psychotherapy (Peplau, in Field, 1979).

Peplau's theory applied with adolescent patients stresses Sullivan's theory of the developmental period of adolescence. It divides adolescence into several stages: preadolescent, early adolescent, and late adolescent. Many of the competencies that emerge during the adolescent period in the normal developmental process are important for successful psychotherapy and are summarized in the following material.

One concept important to Peplau's interpersonal theory is the chum relationship in adolescence. Through this intense friendship with another adolescent of the same sex, adolescents develop the basis for intimacy and love in both same- and opposite-sex relationships (Field, 1979). The adolescent's self-worth is validated in the chum normal relationship, and the adolescent learns to respond to and care for another. In therapeutic work with adolescents, nurses use consensual validation and enchance communication techniques to help the adolescent with reality.

Another concept of special value to the nurse psychotherapist who uses Peplau-based therapy with adolescents is the concept of the self system. Sullivan (1963) defined the self system as consisting of the "good me," "bad me," and the uncanny, unreal experiences of the "not me." The concept of self may be modified at numerous steps along the person's developmental path; it progresses from association with parents and siblings to teachers and peers and, during adulthood, to employers, coworkers, and mates. However, the fundamental components of the self system are established early in life and reflect the influence of the messages significant others on the forming personality. The sequential steps of this concept of the self are as follows:

1. Appraisals of the person by significant others occur.
2. These appraisals are heard and incorporated by the growing child because they are repeated over and over by the significant other.
3. The child or individual acquires the actions that implement the appraisals.
4. The person begins to sort his or her own behaviors into the "yes me," "no me," and "not me" categories.
5. The person sets up situations to maintain the encouraged or repeated appraisals in order to hear them again and again. If this reinforcement does not occur, anxiety will ensue, no matter how irrational it may be.

Field (1982) gives the example of a client who told the nurse therapist that she (the client) was mean, ugly, and nasty. The therapist disagreed and told the client she was not ugly, indeed, that she was very attractive. After the session the client cut her face with broken glass. This incident illustrates that after years of reinforcement of a negative self-image, an individual is gravely threatened when that self-image is contradicted. Thus therapists are cautioned to listen rather than attempt to provide reassurance that the therapist's observations differ from the client's perceptions. Gradually, with work, adolescent clients can alter a negative self-image and become increasingly able to sort out facts and truths about themselves and begin to perceive anew those experiences that led to the need for therapeutic assistance. Peplau's therapy is especially useful when long-term therapy is indicated.

The three major aspects of long-term nursing psychotherapy are diagnosis, prognosis, and treatment. This psychotherapy is in contrast to short-term therapy approaches and crisis interventions, which are used to provide brief therapy to assist an otherwise well-functioning person during a difficult time. Long-term nurse psychotherapy provides the immediate supervision and treatment the adolescent needs in an extreme state of dysfunction. Adolescents with problems that involve distinctly psychotic behavior rather than neurotic maladjustments require long-term therapy.

As in all forms of psychotherapy, the initial step is the formulation of the adolescent's diagnosis according to classic concepts and use of DSM-III-R categories. As the therapeutic relationship proceeds, however, more dynamic interpretations of the adolescent's behavior emerge, and these are not limited by categorization. It is essential that the nurse therapist ascertain if the adolescent is being treated with psychopharmacological agents, because with these medications highly disturbed adolescents may be more amenable to talk therapy. If psychotropic drugs are not being used, the therapeutic styles and goals of psychotherapy need to be adjusted.

Indications for long-term therapy include the adolescent's history of psychotic breaks with reality since early childhood, bizarre behaviors over extended periods of time, and violent or extreme acting-out episodes. A long history of severe disturbances makes it reasonable to expect that because it took many years for the severe disturbance to develop, the process of helping the adolescent will be lengthy. Etiological factors may consist of a combination of biochemical imbalances and environmental and interpersonal assaults on the personality (Field, 1982).

With profoundly disturbed or psychotic adolescents, talk therapy may be deferred or provided concurrently with other therapeutic techniques, such as art and music therapy and vocational and group experiences, which often help the person become more available for talk therapy (Field, 1982). Free and others (1986) present an interesting case example, illustrated with the artwork of an adolescent hospitalized for psychoses whose treatment included the integration of art and music into psychotherapy. The parallels in the adolescent's progress with the different therapists illustrates the development, expansion, and resolution of the chum relationship discussed earlier.

Establishing rapport is the crux of nursing therapy. The initial bonding between the adolescent and therapist is essential for the interpersonal process to succeed. Often adolescents think it is a disgrace for them to be in therapy or hospitalized, that it denigrates their value as human beings. They think that they ought to be able to solve their own problems, a feeling especially intense in adolescents who are experiencing profound drives toward mastery and independence. Thus it is important that adolescents feel that one person, the therapist, understands what they are thinking and feeling and that this understanding is conveyed through an accepting and caring attitude. This approach provides an environment in which the adolescent can begin to feel comfortable about expressing feelings and thoughts. The therapist represents reality to the adolescent. Because getting in touch with reality is difficult, the initial stages of therapy often are fraught with testing and tribulations. The therapist provides a model for the adolescent; some adolescents idolize their therapist whereas others hate them, and the nurse needs to learn how to comfortably handle both transference extremes. No matter how adolescents act, feel, or speak, they need to know the therapist is there to help.

It is most therapeutically effective if the adolescent can describe and discuss a single event in detail so that the therapist can imagine being in the same situation. The recall of specific scenes provide useful material for exploration. No detail in these recountals is unimportant, because connections and patterns emerge that can be analyzed. Five or ten sessions often are required before the adolescent with severe disorders usually feels comfortable enough to describe specific events and interactions; it is important to avoid rushing. Initially, encouraging adolescents to talk about neutral events in their lives, as well as pleasant experiences, enhances trust. As these exchanges continue over a period of time, the therapist facilitates the emergence of themes by eliciting a recountal of the adolescent's feelings at certain times. The identification of themes assists the therapist in directing the exploration of more complex and often misperceived experiences.

Anxiety, which usually is the most visible manifestation of discomfort of severely disturbed persons, is shown by squirming, fingernail biting, hand twisting, and body scratching, especially when they are describing a difficult situation. On the other hand, when adolescents say that talking about certain things makes them feel less miserable and anxious and physical manifestations of distress decrease, the adolescent is beginning to express feelings that previously were repressed and distorted. These are signs of therapeutic progress.

To ascertain the person's habitual "relief behaviors," therapists often ask adolescents what they usually do when they feel really anxious and upset. As causes of anxiety are identified and related to other people or situations in the adolescent's life, the anxiety itself will diminish and the clients will begin to feel more comfortable. Thus the adolescent has developed competence in facing problems that previously were ignored and felt to be too painful to acknowledge consciously.

There are few criteria to evaluate the adolescent's progress in working toward improvement or recovery. In the dynamic engagement between two persons—in this case the therapist and the adolescent—the therapist's intuitive sense often proves to be more telling than formal standards (Fields, 1982) (See box on p. 323).

In addition to theme analysis the nurse therapist uses language and teaches language to the adolescent. Teaching also occurs through the use of analogies. The therapeutic process deals with problems such as auditory and visual hallucinations, delusional ideas, silence, withdrawal, and dependency. Termination of therapy entails the gradual weaning of adolescents from their attachment to the therapist, and it requires dealing with positive and negative transference.

Peplau's theoretical framework has been tested and expanded during the last four decades, and numerous case studies describing the applications of Peplau's theory to nursing psychotherapy can be found in the literature (Thompson, 1986).

Group Psychotherapy

Group psychotherapy is the treatment of emotional disorders to effect change by means of group processes. Adolescents are particularly suited to group therapy because of their need for intense peer relationships.

TYPES OF GROUPS

There are many types of groups, including self-help groups, support groups, therapeutic groups, and psychotherapy groups. Self-help groups include Alcoholics Anonymous, Weight Watchers, and many others that have no professional leader. Support groups for persons with various illnesses or problems are sometimes led by a professional and are designed to develop coping mechanisms. Therapeutic groups have specialized themes, and the leader, often a nurse, uses a combination of didactic and experiential exercises to provide information and develop skills. Group psychotherapy is insight oriented and led by a therapist with at least a master's degree. A fully qualified group therapist has had formal training in group dynamics, personality development, and emotional disorders. In addition, the therapist has participated in group therapy and has completed supervised leadership of group therapy.

Yalom (1985) states that there are 11 therapeutic factors in therapeutic groups, especially group psychotherapy. These factors are listed and defined in Table 12-1. Groups can be psychoanalytical, cognitive, or humanistic-existential in their approach.

Meaningful Indications of Improvement or Movement Toward the Resolution of Conflicts

The adolescent's appearance may change. May dress with more or less care; facial expression may become more strained or more relaxed. It is anticipated that when difficult truths are being faced, tension will increase. However, as troublesome events and feelings move toward resolution, relaxation of tension will follow in expression and bodily movements.

A change will occur in relation to anxiety. The adolescent who was speaking rapidly may begin to express self in more calm and reflective ways. The adolescent's pattern of twisting things may change. The therapist should be alert for changes in appearance, speech, and body posture.

Aspects relating to the sessions themselves will change. The adolescent who has been late or reluctant to come to the interviews may appear early and say to the therapist, "You're two minutes late."

The adolescent may become possessive of the therapist and the location in which the sessions take place. If another adolescent intrudes, the first adolescent may say, "Get out of here, this is my time." Some of the reasons for possessiveness are that deep confidences are now being shared and very private feelings are being shown and discussed. On numerous occasions this may be the first time that the adolescent has been able to ventilate and confront feelings and thoughts that have been buried for years. No wonder the need for privacy and confidence are very strong!

The adolescent will begin to recognize the therapist as a person by remembering his or her name, by making comments about the therapist's dress, way of speaking, or general demeanor. The adolescent may begin to emulate the therapist's speech, bodily movements, and actions.

As the therapeutic session nears completion, the adolescent may say, "I know my time is up, but there is one more thing I want to say before we stop." Or the adolescent may say, "Since we started five minutes late, can we continue for another five minutes?"

The adolescent may evidence an acute awareness of what therapy is about. Compared with the earlier interview comment, "What do you want me to talk about?" the adolescent now says, "Last time, when we stopped, I was talking about my high school experience. I want to continue with that," which is evidence that the adolescent is beginning to perceive the relatedness between events of the past and present feelings.

The adolescent will begin to edit errors of speech, think carefully, and weigh words before speaking. The ability to focus on specific events and persons increases steadily, a marked distinction to diffuse thinking that may have been present at the beginning of therapy.

Evidence of genuine internalized insights will occur. When the therapist hears the adolescent say, "I know now why I did that," or "I know now why I felt that way," one can be assured that real progress is being made.

Table 12-1   Yalom's Therapeutic Factors

Factor	Definition
Imparting information	Receiving didactic information and advice
Instillation of hope	Increasing hopefulness of group members
Universality	Realizing that others experience same thoughts, feelings, and problems
Altruism	Sharing part of oneself to help another
Corrective reenactment of primary family group	Alter learning experience previously obtained in families
Development of social interaction techniques	Increasing awareness of social interactions and developing social skills
Imitative behaviors	Increasing skills by imitating behaviors of others in group
Interpersonal learning	Engaging in wider range of interpersonal exchanges, thereby increasing each member's understanding of responsibility and complexity of interpersonal relationships and decreasing each member's interpersonal distortions
Existential factors	Helping members deal with meaning of their own existence
Catharsis	Expressing feelings previously unexpressed
Group cohesion	Feeling attraction for group and other members

Modified from Yalom ID (1985) The theory and practice of group psychotherapy, ed 3, New York, Basic Books Inc., Publishers.

PRACTICE OF GROUP THERAPY

Performing group therapy requires monitoring the verbal and nonverbal communication among group members for content and process. Content is the actual meaning of the words. Process means the underlying themes with which the group is grappling and the personal interactions among group members. Based on the needs of the group, the group leader chooses themes and facilitates the discussion of the process that occurs. The group therapist works in the "here and now" (Yalom, 1985). Keeping the conversation focused on the present process helps adolescents understand their relationships with group members, assists them to develop insight into the history of that behavior, and gives them the opportunity to try new ways of interacting in the group. Transference that develops among group members and between group members and the leader is observed by the leader and dealt with according to the group's phase and purposes. The therapist also must be aware of countertransference among group members. The leader builds a group culture and group norms that permit and encourage self-disclosure to the group members rather than to the therapist. As the group matures, the members assume responsibility for maintaining norms, processing the dynamics, and staying "here and now."

Communication techniques used in group therapy are similar to those of individual therapy. However, the therapist monitors the communication process of the group as a whole as well as that among various members. Corey (1985) lists 22 communication skills used in group therapy:

Active listening. Paying total attention to the speaker's verbal and nonverbal communication

Restating. Putting a member's comment into different words to clarify the meaning

Clarifying. Responding to unclear or confusing messages by focusing on underlying meanings and helping someone sort out confusing thoughts or feelings

Summarizing. Pulling together important elements of a group interaction

Questioning. Asking open-ended questions (questions that open up alternatives and new areas of self-investigation), such as "What are you experiencing?" "How are you dealing with . . .?"

Interpreting. Offering tentative hypotheses concerning certain patterns of behavior. Interpreting requires considerable skill, and timing is critical.

Confronting. Pointing out behaviors or discrepancies between verbal and nonverbal messages in a tactful way

Reflecting feelings. Responding to the emotional content of what was said

Supporting. Providing encouragement and reinforcement, particularly when group members are self-disclosing, explaining painful feelings, or taking risks

Empathizing. Sensitively grasping the subjective experience of the adolescent

Initiating. Getting the group restarted or introducing a meaningful theme after a period of work

Goal setting. Helping members set goals

Evaluating. Determining what the process is for the group and for individual members, especially at the end of the session

Giving feedback. Providing specific, descriptive information about a member's behavior

Suggesting. Suggesting alternative ideas or courses of action that enhance an individual's movement toward independence

Protecting. Safeguarding members from unnecessary psychological risk

Self-disclosure. Revealing information about oneself to encourage self-disclosure of members (used very selectively)

Role modeling. Demonstrating honesty, openness, assertiveness, and empathy

Dealing with silence. Silence must be assessed, with leader intervention geared toward dealing with the reasons for the silence

Blocking. Interrupting counterproductive behaviors in a group

Facilitating. Opening up clear and direct communication and helping members assume increasing responsibility for the direction of the group, including (1) focusing on resistances and explaining them, (2) encouraging members to openly express feelings and expectations, (3) teaching members to focus on themselves and their feelings, (4) teaching members to talk directly and plainly to each other, (5) creating a safe climate, (6) providing support, (7) fostering member-to-member interaction, (8) encouraging open expression of conflict, (9) helping members integrate what they are learning in their everyday lives, and (10) helping members achieve closure on unfinished business by the end of the session

Terminating. Wrapping up work for the session or the entire group as well as individual work within a session

PHASES OF GROUP THERAPY

The traditional outpatient psychotherapy group consists of 8 to 10 adolescents who meet regularly over an extended period, during which the group moves through several phases of growth. Yalom (1985) describes three stages of group development. The initial stage includes orientation, hesitant participation, search for meaning, and dependency. During this stage the members are adjusting to each other and the group setting, and there is considerable dependence on the therapist. Disclosures are tentative because little trust has developed and members are defining group therapy and their roles in it. The second stage includes conflict, dominance, and rebellion. This period is rather stormy; group members are vying for power, which includes attacking the group leader. This comes from the inevitable disappointment that follows idealizing the leader during the initial stages. The third stage is group cohesiveness. This is the working phase, characterized by the development of intimacy among the members.

INPATIENT GROUP PSYCHOTHERAPY

Because inpatients are often not in treatment for the length of time required for traditional group therapy, significant modifications must occur. Yalom (1983) recommends a process-oriented approach wherein the group facilitator is more active and directive. Inpatients are, of course, more disturbed, stressed, and anxious than are outpatients, and the therapist may have to manage difficult behavior and situations in the group. By nature, adolescents need more structure than do adults. A nurse should cofacilitate the psychotherapy group so as to assist with behavior management and provide continuity of care regarding group activity and its implications for the milieu. In an adolescent program that lasts about 4 weeks, the group can become cohesive, and considerable work can be accomplished. Inpatient group psychotherapy has been determined to be desirable and effective for inpatients (Yalom, 1983) and for adolescents (Gardner, 1988).

THERAPEUTIC DIDACTIC GROUPS

Psychiatric nurses can provide information to groups of adolescents and their families through lectures or videotapes, followed by a discussion or practice activity and discussion. This method is used in a variety of settings. Some of the many topics that are suitable for such groups are assertiveness, anger management, social skills, physical and psychological development, family dynamics, depression, chemical dependence, codependence, values clarification, sexuality, psychoeducation for schizophrenia, bipolar illness, attention deficit disorder, and medications. It is imperative that staff nurses have time built into their daily schedules to prepare adequately for group work. Nurses may resist involvement in group practice because they have neither adequate preparation time nor supervision and assistance. The box on p. 327 provides a model for planning didactic groups.

Family Therapy

Family therapy is the use of interpersonal and communication techniques to affect change in the family system. A family therapist has the minimum of a master's degree,

---

Therapeutic Didactic Group

Structure of content for session of 1 to 1½ hours
1. Topic
2. Definition of topic: definition is literature based (for example, anger, assertiveness)
3. Discussion or activity to determine how definition fits members
4. Instruction in one or two new strategies for managing problem/topic (strategies are literature based): lecture, video, demonstration
5. Practice: role play (best method), activity sheets, games
6. Discussion and wrap up
7. Homework (optional): goal work; should be congruent with treatment plan

---

with formal and experiential training in the practice of family therapy. Usually postgraduate training is necessary to achieve expertise. Advanced training institutes in major cities, which often are based on a particular theory and methods, provide various certifications.

In adolescent outpatient treatment, family therapy may be the treatment of choice or an adjunct treatment, or occasionally it may not be used at all. In inpatient treatment, family therapy is an extremely important aspect of care. The adolescent in inpatient treatment typically has considerable family dysfunction and is dependent on the family for support, sustenance, and limit setting. Allowing the family problems to go untreated is a disservice to the adolescent.

PRACTICE OF FAMILY THERAPY

Family therapists are very active and directive. They often are required to have a larger-than-life approach to intervene in families who have had several generations to develop their systems of communication, roles, rules, and ways of relating to persons and groups outside the family boundary. The family therapist is respectful, uses humor, and operates on the belief that families behave as they do because they are in pain or have not been exposed to other options. A family therapist uses a "no-fault" approach to family problems. Virginia Satir (1983) describes a number of roles family therapists play and techniques they use (see box on p. 328).

Other therapeutic techniques available to the nurse, family therapist, and the family are homework assignments, paradoxical injunction, and sculpting. Homework assignments might require family members to engage in one recreational activity together during the following week, to eat one third of their meals together, or to verbally reinforce each family member once each day. Paradoxical injunctions are instructions to perform the opposite of what is intended, also called "the therapeutic bind" (Lantz, 1978). Sculpting is a technique wherein the family physically enacts an experience without words, then "freezes." The sculpture expresses the feeling tone without word games and is a powerful device for assisting families to understand their relationships. The therapist instructs the family members to individually arrange the sculpture as they would like it to be, thereby initiating change with action (Papp, 1976).

Roles and Techniques of the Family Therapist

1. The therapist creates a setting in which people can, perhaps for the first time, take the risk of looking clearly and objectively at themselves and their actions. The therapist does this by being confident and giving the family confidence.
2. The therapist is not afraid; she asks questions without frightening the family members; she gets a family history and gets the facts.
3. The therapist shows adolescents how they look to others.
4. When the therapist asks for and gives information, she does so in a matter-of-fact, nonjudgmental, light, congruent way.
5. The therapist builds self-esteem.
6. The therapist decreases threat by setting the rules of interaction: no interrupting, acting out, or speaking for anyone else.
7. The therapist decreases threat by structuring the family sessions so that they have an end, by not taking sides, and by reporting any subgroup work back to the family group.
8. The therapist decreases threat by reducing the need for defenses. She reduces fear by dealing with anger as hurt, by showing that pain and other forbidden topics are all right to look at, and by burlesquing basic fears.
9. The therapist decreases threat by handling loaded material with care, moving from least threatening to more threatening, relating feelings to facts, using idiomatic language (such as "hit the roof,") and moderate profanity, and avoiding psychiatric jargon. The therapist traces hostile behavior and feelings to the underlying issue.
10. The therapist restores individual accountability for thoughts, feelings, and behaviors to the individual family members; reminds them that each person is in charge of himself or herself; checks out pronouns (such as "they"), and forbids tattling.
11. The therapist helps the adolescent to see how past models influence expectations and behavior.
12. The therapist delineates roles and functions by clarifying and by direct teaching.
13. The therapist completes gaps in communication and interprets messages; this includes separating the relationship part of a message from its content, pointing out discrepancies in communication, and spelling out nonverbal communication and double-bind messages.

Modified from Satir V (1983) Conjoint family therapy, ed 3, Palo Alto, Calif, Science & Behavior Books.

ROLE OF THE STAFF NURSE IN INPATIENT FAMILY THERAPY

The role of the staff nurse in inpatient family therapy is to complement the work of the family members in the milieu. The nurse clarifies communication, teaches the parents limit setting and parenting techniques, and assists the adolescent with preparing for family sessions. The nurse may role play a family scenario in a group or a one-to-one session to give the adolescent practice in making "I" statements, not interrupting, or bringing up painful issues in the family session. The nurse and family therapist collaborate in enhancing family treatment. The nurse also may cofacilitate the family sessions.

MULTIFAMILY GROUP THERAPY

Multifamily group therapy ranges from providing support and information, to actual group therapy with a group of families, to the practice of family therapy with individual families in the presence of other families, followed by group processing of their work. Multiple family groups in the inpatient setting provide a natural support network that continues to exist after discharge, reassures families that they are not alone in their difficulties (universality), and provides hope when they see other families growing and changing. Furthermore, a multifamily group provides assessment data and understanding of family functioning for staff members who do not see the family in treatment sessions.

Expressive Therapies

OCCUPATIONAL THERAPY*

In inpatient psychiatric settings, occupational therapy programs are valuable components in treatment programs for adults, adolescents, and children.

In a broad sense, occupational therapy uses activity to promote healing. Individuals who pioneered the profession believed a person's health was influenced by "the use of muscles and mind together in games, exercise and handicraft, as well as work" (Wade, 1964). Work, exercise, and play have long been recognized for their healing qualities.

Toward the end of the nineteenth century, work became a therapeutic change agent in the United States in the field of mental health. In a 1982 presentation, psychiatrist Adolf Meyer stated that "the proper use of time in some helpful and gratifying activity appeared to be a fundamental issue in the treatment of the neuropsychiatric patient." Meyer believed that a person's life must be balanced in the areas of work, play, rest, and sleep. He said, "We have come to realize more than ever that while some mental disorders are due to toxic conditions, others are due to conflicts in normal activities, and a cultivation of fruitful interests is the sanest and only efficient point of attack." Meyer believed treatment of the mentally ill should blend work and pleasure and should include recreation and productivity. He also believed that patients needed to have a realization of reality and a sense of actuality, which could be achieved through opportunities to do, to plan, and to create.

Meyer's beliefs had a major impact on the philosophy and history of occupational therapy as a profession. As the profession has evolved, an accepted definition of occupational therapy developed. According to the American Occupational Therapy Association, it can be defined as follows (Hopkins and Smith, 1972):

the art and science of directing man's participation in selected tasks to restore, reinforce and enhance performance, facilitate learning of those skills and functions essential for adaptation and productivity, diminish or correct pathology, and to promote and maintain health. Its fundamental concern is the capacity, throughout the life span, to perform with satisfaction to self and others those tasks and roles essential to productive living and to the mastery of the self and the environment.

---

* This section contributed by Barbara MacPherson, ORTL.

Most occupational therapists practice in hospitals, rehabilitation centers, schools, and community centers. Therapists are trained in mental health and in physical disabilities. Their education focuses on the study of the biological and behavioral sciences, pathological conditions, and occupational therapy techniques. A registered occupational therapist must obtain a bachelor's degree from an accredited occupational therapy program, must complete a minimum of 6 months of full-time fieldwork experience, and must pass the American Occupational Therapy Association's certification examination. Many states also require licensure. Because of the demand for occupational therapists, certified occupational therapy assistant programs were created. After completion of an accredited 2-year assistant program, 3 months of full-time fieldwork is required. The individual also must pass a certification examination and must obtain a license in those states that require licensure.

In a psychiatric setting, focus of therapy is on assisting in the diagnostic process and improving the individual's ability to function in society within the limits of the disability. The adolescent may be assessed in a variety of situations, including an individual session for gathering information and a task-oriented session in which the therapist can observe and assess an individual's functional skills (work habits, concentration, ability to follow directions). Adolescents generally are seen in discussion group settings to assess communication skills.

Treatment may include individual or group sessions, as appropriate for the adolescent. Sessions incorporate activity to promote an increased sense of self-worth, to improve performance in skills (problem solving, communication, activities of daily living), and to express feelings.

Occupational therapy often is seen as a nonthreatening therapy. Activities serve as a bridge for communication, especially for adolescents with issues of trust; thus this therapy is especially effective with children and adolescents. Because the emphasis is on "doing," occupational therapy may be more comfortable for the adolescent than are traditional verbal therapies particularly for children and adolescents hospitalized in mental health and substance abuse programs who have learning disabilities or mild to severe cognitive impairment. Some examples of occupational therapy groups are listed in Table 12-2.

ART THERAPY

Art therapists hold master's degrees and receive training in personality development, psychopathology, counseling, and eliciting artistic expression. They are of course artistically talented and creative. In addition to completing course work, art therapists are supervised in practicums at various settings. They usually are certified or licensed.

Through the use of client drawings and paintings, the art therapist assesses and treats issues and pathology. Art therapy is especially valuable for adolescents (and adults) who have difficulty expressing themselves verbally. The therapist assists them to reveal thoughts and feelings and to release anger, anxiety, and aggression through drawings.

RECREATION THERAPY

Recreation therapists may be trained in a college program for recreation therapy, or an occupational therapist may obtain additional training in this area; all recreation

Table 12-2   Occupational Therapy Groups

Group	Purpose
Task-oriented group using crafts/art media	Aid in gaining diagnostic information, observation, and work to enhance functional skills and interaction skills
Life skills groups (self-esteem, values clarification, communication, anger management, self-concept, problem solving)	Provide outlet for feelings through activity and discussion, opportunities to explore new skills, practice skills, and gain training for life skills
Activities of daily living groups (cooking groups, money management)	Teach skills in activities of daily living
Recreational groups	Provide outlets for emotions, energy, and tension; stimulate spontaneity; and allow for play and interaction

therapists are certified. For adolescents, recreation therapy includes a program of physical exercise and games that releases energy and develops physical and social skills. The recreational therapist also provides information about the availability of appropriate leisure activities, which is particularly important for antisocial adolescents and those with problems of substance abuse.

DANCE AND MUSIC THERAPY

Dance and music are used as recreational and therapeutic activities. Some recreational therapists also have training in dance therapy. However, dance and music therapists are relatively scarce at present; their preparation requires a master's degree in these specialized areas.

Trends in Psychotherapy

NEUROBIOLOGY

Historically, biological therapy is the oldest form of therapy; rooted in the nineteenth century schools of biology and medicine, it emphasizes psychopharmacology.

Advances in the neurosciences and biological psychiatry have provided the impetus for a number of mental health psychotherapists (Gottshalk, 1990) from the various disciplines to emphasize the need to adapt psychotherapies to these newer approaches. McKeon (1990) emphasizes that the new technologies offer psychiatric mental health nurses the opportunity to promote change and redirect energy and excitement to newer models in caring for the seriously mentally ill. These include development of expanded forms of assessment and new techniques of psychotherapy.

Gottshalk (1990), a psychologist, suggests that many mental health professionals have overlooked the fact that there is a specific biological basis for many of the traditional forms of psychotherapy. For example, psychological theories based on memory and learning as processes result in transient or permanent changes in brain chemistry. Also, psychological stress precipitates localized cerebral and systemic biochemical changes, and voluntary recall of an emotion-tinged memory activates concomitant localized glucose metabolism and peripheral autonomic nervous system processes. Research in psychotherapy has demonstrated that the communication process can normalize such changes to the extent of the human organism's capability. These findings provide potential areas of expansion in psychotherapy. Pothier (1988) has also stressed the need for nurses to emphasize the holistic perspective that has prevailed in nursing and to explore the biophysiological responses related to and supporting nursing therapies.

CROSS-CULTURAL COUNSELING AND PSYCHOTHERAPY

During the past few decades most mental health clinicians have added to their practices an increasing number of clients from cultures different from their own, requiring considerable changes in traditional psychotherapeutic methods (Dahl, 1989). The changes coincide with a growing emphasis on the clinician's ethical responsibility to attend to the consumer's cultural perspective and health care expectations. Psychocultural concepts are now viewed as an integral part of all psychiatric practice, confirmed by the proliferation of position statements by professional organizations that emphasize the clinician's ethical responsibility to know the adolescent's cultural values before delivering mental health services.

Psychiatric nurses historically have emphasized cultural concepts in their psychotherapeutic interventions; however, many of these concepts need reevaluation and updating in light of new theories and therapies. Several cultural frameworks have been developed that have been used to develop nursing curricula, as education changes practice. For example, Leninger's transcultural nursing theory (Boyle and Andrews, 1989) is currently used in a number of basic nursing education programs. National practice standards and publications, such as those for child and adolescent psychiatric nursing, also emphasize psychocultural concepts in practice for clinicians (ANA, 1985).

Each culture has specific expectations for their young; thus cultural traditions often cause intergenerational conflicts that affect the younger person's physical, social, emotional, and affective development. Clinicians who work with adolescents and their families are confronted with special psychocultural challenges, including the family's child-rearing patterns, the family's and adolescent's world view, and the adolescent's individual traits. These components need be considered within the cultural context of the adolescent's presenting psychiatric problem and psychotherapeutic interventions.

Current practice models avoid ethnocentric evaluations of group practices and beliefs that do not take into perspective the reality of that cultural group. This shift was accomplished largely by the efforts of cross-cultural clinicians and researchers with minority backgrounds, who encouraged discarding the deficient model. Current models in the area of minority research emphasize positive features of cultural variation and the cultural context of development. These changing perspectives and clinical applications are reflected in the current literature in contrast with the earlier focus on theory. For example, Sue and others (1982) include examples of the clinical cases, and Comas-Diaz and Griffith (1988) provide case applications of cross-cultural counseling within the context of the biopsychosocial model.

CULTURAL-SPECIFIC DISORDERS

Culturogenic stress. There are different perspectives concerning culture stress or shock, which is defined as an abrupt, disorganizing reaction as a result of exposure to a new culture. Culture or "reality" shock is a term familiar to most nurses through the work of nurse-anthropologist Kramer, whose research related the concept of cultural shock to recently graduated nurses who experienced "bicultural" difficulties when they entered the hospital work setting. Having absorbed the idealistic values promoted in preparatory programs, they were confronted by a conflicting reality in the workplace (Kramer and Schmalenberg, 1978).

Culture shock occurs when a person who has adhered rigidly to old, familiar ways has to adjust to a new environment. With migration, for example, comes many additional traumas. Not only are old cultural values in conflict with values in a new culture or setting; changes often include changing roles and loss of sources of support. Many young adolescent clients experience reality shock when they advance to high school or move to a different type of community, for example, from rural to urban.

In some instances, cultural values protect people from culturogenic shock. It has been observed that different cultural groups exposed to similar stress display different responses as a result of these value protections. For example, in cultures that value extended family relationships, there is less stress in child rearing when several family members help new parents; thus the extended family system serves a protective function. Adolescent pregnancy, for example, is less traumatic for girls from these cultures.

Posttraumatic stress disorder is an example of a DSM-III-R diagnosis that is culturally influenced, depending on how the adolescent's specific culture deals with and expresses stress. Initially this diagnosis was limited to military personnel and to refugees following migration, especially those who have resettled after major traumas, such as being physically beaten or raped or witnessing the killing of relatives and loved ones in concentration camps during war. This diagnosis has been expanded to include adults and adolescents who have been victims of rape, incest, severe accidents, and incidents involving the death of others (Lyons, 1989).

Clinicians who work with families from various cultures need to be highly sensitive to the fact that the family's cultural values can place adolescents at an even higher risk for emotional conflict. Thus the nurse's language in presenting and discussing the mental health problem and/or diagnosis should be based on a clear understanding of the parents' world view and their cultural values and beliefs about mental disorders. The assessment interview should convey interest and foster a safe atmosphere in which ethnocultural identity conflicts can be disclosed, inasmuch as these areas can significantly affect the therapeutic situation. Jacobsen (1988) has developed a series of stages and suggested questions to manage the ethnocultural assessment (see boxes on pp. 334-335), which has been adjusted to the adolescent client.

Presenting behaviors and complaints commonly reported and observed in adolescents that are encountered in cross-cultural treatment settings include anger, tantrums, irritability, depression, sadness, loneliness, anxiety, psychomotor and verbal hyperactivity or retardation, school adjustment problems, social withdrawal, and somatic complaints.

Ethnocultural Assessment

Stage I

Obtain information about the adolescent and adolescent's family ethnocultural heritage. For example, culture of origin for both maternal and paternal lines of the family and delineation of ethnic heritage. Parents place of geographical origin is insufficient to understand complex multicultural-multiethnic backgrounds. A single, readily identifiable attribute of a person, such as name or language spoken, is not useful and implies an assortment of stereotyped cultural characteristics.

Stage II

Circumstances leading to the family's ethnocultural problem. How does the young person understand the events leading to the transitions from the culture of origin? If culture of origin is in state of sociopolitical transition that led to the move, what are the family's thoughts and feelings about these events? Although relocation may have been recent or generations in the past, the person's historical account is needed to understand perspectives on the "family myth." Recounting this history can be cathartic and can set the stage for the therapeutic alliance. For example, Hispanic adolescents whose grandparents came to the United States to avoid the Castro regime may hold their grandparents' myth of returning to Cuba, whereas those whose parents go back and forth between the United States and the islands for temporary, seasonal employment, as do Puerto Ricans, have different cultural concepts.

Stage III

On the basis of the adolescent's and the parent's intellectual and emotional perceptions of the development of the family's niche in the host society since translocation: (1) Have family members stayed together or are they dispersed? (2) What has the family's relationship been with other members of its original ethnoculture? (3) Is the family better or worse off than before translocation? (4) Has the adolescent internalized the family's sagas? This data provide a background for the adolescent's entrée to the world at large and are predictors of the adolescent's future success or failure in terms of the larger public's perception. This stage is critical to developing a contextual framework within which to place adolescent's subjective experiences.

Modified from Jacobsen FM (1988) Ethnocultural assesment. In Comas-Diaz L and Griffith EEH, editors, Clinical guidelines in cross-cultural mental health, New York, John Wiley & Sons, Inc.

Continued.

Formulating a cross-cultural diagnosis begins with defining normality and abnormality in members of other cultures and establishing the child-rearing practices and expectations of adolescents held by that culture. The clinician needs to be aware of the following factors (Helman, 1984):

1. The extent to which cultural factors affect some of the diagnostic categories and techniques of Western psychiatry
2. The role of the youth's culture in helping her or him to understand and communicate her or his psychological distress
3. How the behavior is viewed by parents and other members of their cultural group, and whether the abnormal behavior is viewed as beneficial to the group or not

---

Ethnocultural Assessment — cont'd

Stage IV

The adolescent's view of his or her cultural adjustment as an individual, distinct from the family. Need to ask the adolescent's feelings regarding sense of ethnocultural integration, which may be quite different from that of other family members, particularly older generations. Is the adolescent striving to become more American, disavowing the norms and customs of the ethnocultural background? Is the adolescent striving assertively to resist acculturation? Perception of one's ethnocultural identity may be key for coping skills of many people. For example, elderly, first-generation immigrants may resist acculturation, rejecting "loose" American attitudes about parental respect. Disapproval helps older generations ensure continuity of family support to which they were entitled in their cultural of origin. Thus they ward off terrifying loss of social support that may accompany younger family members' acculturation to mainstream American dominant culture.

Stage V

It is important to recognize that young people of other ethnic groups may have no prior knowledge of the process of psychotherapy and thus may need considerable explanation and reassurance.

---

4. Whether the specific cluster of symptoms, signs and behavioral changes shown by the adolescent are interpreted by the family and their community as evidenced of a culture-bound psychological disorder

Guidelines for engaging adolescents and their families of other cultures in therapy. Allen (1988) suggests the following considerations are important when engaging adolescents and their parents of other cultures in culturally sensitive psychotherapy.

1. Avoid assuming the adolescent and parents are absolutely likely or unlikely to have any particular life problem, personality disorder, illness, mode of presentation, or attitude to therapy; that is, do not stereotype. For example, despite the frequent nature of somatic characteristics, do not automatically expect them to be present.
2. Assess the adolescent and family's understanding of psychiatry and psychotherapy, as well as to what extent he or she was adequately prepared by the referring agent. Try to understand the model the family is using as well as the degrees of contribution of cultural conditioning and intrapsychic defenses.
3. Given the fact that the adolescent is a unique composite of biological, psychological, social, spiritual and political attributes, all these need careful assessment. Once a proper clinical assessment is made, it is possible to begin validating needs conveyed by the youth and family's understanding, and help them make the link between nonpsychological and psychological models, if possible. The use of diagrams, day-to-day examples and experiential demonstrations are useful.
4. As well as doing a conventional history and mental status assessment, try to assess the cultural influences, socialization patterns, and culturally determined adaptive traits that have operated at the client's particular point on the color-class spectrum.
5. Approach cultural issues cautiously but advisedly while assessing the cultural awareness,

openness, flexibility, general defensiveness and other ego strengths of the family. Share interest in and knowledge of the culture or subculture and seek to learn from them.

6. Avoid being judgmental and show respect for the strengths of the cultural background. Also, avoid being condescending, overenthusiastic, phony and prescribing.

7. Use a degree of formality, depending on the cultural relatedness of the family. Given many culture's concern about respect, it is best to start with a warm but friendly attitude.

8. If the family has a strong religious world view, suggesting a member of the clergy is appropriate. Be prepared to elicit tactfully information about the use and views relating to nontraditional healers. Be prepared to collaborate with these nontraditional healers, and to rely on cultural brokers as necessary. Encourage parents to become as involved as possible in parent-student school activities, such as the PTA, and other areas of the adolescent's formal educational experiences.

9. People of other cultures often have their own dialects that are valid language forms used to express their rich cultural heritage and deep emotions. Learn as much as possible about the client's ethnic group and culture, especially the group's preferences. The ability to help clients develop pride in their native language and culture is enhanced if the clinician can speak the same language. Become familiar with the specific culture's available literature in the area of mental health, such as the book by Constantino and others, *Cuento Therapy: Folktales As a Culturally Sensitive Psychotherapy for Hispanic Children* (listed in references).

10. To provide for parents and adolescents not "losing face" with one another, arrange for separate interview opportunities so that father, mother, and adolescent can ventilate grievances, explore values and roles and help discover means of conflict resolution between and across generations. Refrain from using the adolescent as an interpreter in family sessions.

11. When dealing with psychotic clients, look for the meaning and form in terms of factors such as cultural confusion, stresses, coping mechanisms and secondary gains.

12. If working with migrants and relocated families wishing to return to the original residence, avoid suggesting returning as a solution to adjustment problems.

Culturally sensitive interventions

Fragmented ethnocultural identification. Ethnocultural identity is an important component of one's total identity.

In the United States, ethnocultural transitions probably occur more frequently than in other countries, due, in part, to the relatively large influx of immigrants and because Americans have a propensity to move more frequently than do people in other countries.

Adler (1975) has identified a five-stage developmental process that is a useful therapeutic tool in which the adolescent and the family progress through class-cultural transitions and culture shock.

1. Initial contact with a second culture, where the client is insulated by his or her culture of origin

2. Disintegration, where awareness of being different results in depression and withdrawal

3. Reintegration, where the second culture is rejected through anger and rebellion.

4. Autonomy, where the client is able to negotiate different situations culturally, thus surviving new experiences

5. Independence, where ethnocultural, social and psychological differences are accepted and enjoyed. The client is able to exercise choice and responsibility, and to discern the cultural aspects of everyday interactions and circumstances age appropriately.

When ethnocultural assessment confirms that the adolescent's self-identification is fragmented, the therapist actively fosters the adolescent's identification with his or her ethnocultural origin by means of three major therapeutic functions (Comas-Diaz and Jacobsen, 1988):

1. Reflection, whereby the therapist mirrors the ethnocultural pieces of the fragmented self, and acknowledges the pervasive influence that ethnicity and culture have on the client's life. The therapist underscores aspects of the adolescent's life that reveal ethnocultural identity conflict: "It is difficult for you to see yourself as Cuban" or "You avoid people from your community because they remind you of being Cuban." These statements communicate awareness of the fragmented ethnocultural self.
2. Education, whereby the therapist guides the client through a reformation of ethnocultural identity, providing a "safe" environment where the adolescent can examine conflicted identity. By using direct approaches, the therapist helps the client examine inconsistencies between aspects of his or her own ethnic background, and between other ethnocultural values and those of the second culture.
3. Mediation, whereby the therapist helps the adolescent integrate his or her ethnocultural self into a consolidated sense of self. The therapist helps the client connect different aspects of the self to achieve a more integrated identity. Restoring a sense of identity may require resolving cultural conflicts within the family, between the family and community and/or between the adolescent and the wider context in which the adolescent and family function. During mediation, the therapist encourages the adolescent to verbalize existing identity conflicts; enunciations such as "It is confusing to you because at times you feel like a Cuban and at other times you feel like an American" helps clients to name the identity conflict and hence initiate the reintegration process.

The problem of adolescents requiring assistance in cultural reorientation occurs frequently in multicultural health care setting, and provides opportunities for primary prevention interventions. Usually this reorientation is a basic and universal clinical problem despite psychocultural variations. Cultural insights help shape psychotherapeutic interventions; goals can be integrated into traditional approaches such as psychodynamic, behavioral, and existential therapies. The box on p. 338 illustrates a process of cultural reorientation developed by Allen (1988) for use with the major traditional psychotherapeutic interventions. The outline provides a guide for clinicians beginning to develop cross-cultural counseling skills (adolescent psychiatric nurses) are useful in community agencies such as schools, where conducting individual, sibling, and "life change groups" is a productive intervention.

Culturally sensitive psychotherapies. The usefulness of psychotherapy based on psychoanalytical theory with adolescents who are socially and culturally removed from the Western concept of middle class has been a long-standing dispute. Dahl (1989) claims that while psychoanalysis is advisable, it requires significant changes in techniques to establish a therapeutic relationship that is meaningful for adolescents of other cultures. It is important to understand the specific culture's view of the origin of illness and how healing is effected. Dahl holds that role expectations and culture-specific communicative interactions are the central elements to be explored and considered, and that cultural empathy includes acceptance of the adolescent's cultural self-image. He stresses that the need to work within an accepted, established therapeutic paradigm is not eliminated because of an adolescent's cultural orientation.

Culturally Sensitive Adolescent Psychotherapy

1. Cultural self-assessment and insight information. Clinician helps the adolescent identify:
   A. Areas of psychocultural confusion
   B. The relationship between evident features of history, social disintegration and psychological disorder
   C. The adolescent's universalism and openness, for example, the extent to which his or her cultural cognition includes timeless values and represents an open (versus closed) system
2. Cultural reevaluation — review of cultural strengths. The clinician helps the adolescent discover and analyze:
   A. Positive survival strengths throughout one's national history and involving one's ethnic group
   B. Daily individual social manifestations of coherence-producing values
   C. Cultural traits, such as humor, old world–new world contrasts, cosmopolitanism, hospitality, articulateness (oral traditions), high achievement motivation (social mobility), strong interpersonal values (commonality)
   D. Common face-to-face indigenous support systems, for example, friendships, extended family-tenement yards, religion, friendly societies such as Scouts, church activities, and after-school sports
   E. Specific cultural folklore and arts
   F. Achievements of individuals and the region on the world scene
3. Cultural reevaluations — establishing criteria of adaptiveness of cultural values. The adolescent is assisted in evaluating the role of cultural values in:
   A. Promoting physical, psychological, and spiritual health
   B. Promoting human rights, self-esteem, dignity
   C. Promotion universalism and openness
   D. Promotion social integration
4. Cultural goal settings. The young person sets goals for achieving:
   A. Newly desired adaptive versus maladaptive cultural values and behaviors in terms of one's assessment and reevaluations
   B. Internality versus externality

Modified from Allen, EA (1988) West Indians. In Comas-Diaz L and Griffith EEH, editors, Clinical guidelines in cross-cultural mental health, New York, John Wiley & Sons, pp. 328-329.

Clinicians who work with clients of other cultures need adhere to the same traditional, professionally defensible or "tested and proved" paradigms of therapy. They must be guided by the principles of established therapies, no matter the approach: group, individual, play, behavior modification, or other method. Expectations of both parents and adolescents should be considered in goal setting for treatment and integrated into the clinicians' own professional theoretical frame of reference. Regardless of culture, clinicians need to evaluate the psychological strengths and adaptations of both youngster and family and to monitor indicators of developmental progress and signs of stress. Understanding the family's world view, combined with the clinician's identification with his or her own body of professional knowledge, experience, and accountability, is essential in the provision of safe care in all psychotherapeutic interventions.

Somatopsychic nurse therapy. Nursing psychotherapy is distinguished from psychotherapy as it is practiced in other mental health disciplines because of its conceptual base, history, and mode of practice (Flaskerud, 1984). It is especially suited for culturally relevant nursing therapy as it integrates physical and mental health concepts, and involves the family and social system.

One culturally relevant nursing therapy, somatopsychic therapy—developed by Flaskerud in 1987—was designed specifically for work with Vietnamese and Filipino clients in the United States. It has been successfully adapted and applied in clinical work with adolescents and families of other cultural groups, especially adolescents for whom somatization is a major symptom. The aim of this nursing psychotherapy is the provision of therapy congruent with the client's beliefs about health and illness, deemphasizing the stigma associated with mental illness and reintegrating the young person into the family and social group. The anticipated effects of the treatment are that the client's level of functioning will improve.

The following eight factors, specified in somatopsychic therapy (Flaskerud 1987), have been adapted to the psychiatric nursing of adolescents:

1. Therapists are master's-prepared clinical specialists in adolescent psychiatric nursing who share the adolescent's language and culture and are called nurse-counselors to avoid the stigma associated with mental disorders. They possess the physical and mental assessment skills and specific adolescent intervention knowledge and experience needed to function as therapists. Their education is congruent with the client's expectations of health professionals.

2. Assessment of the adolescent includes psychiatric, functional, developmental, and physical areas, with attention given to those areas in which somatic complaints are focused. This attention to somatic complaints legitimizes somatization as an appropriate, acceptable means of expressing distress.

3. Pharmacotherapy specific to the client's diagnosis is prescribed and instructions given by the nurse-counselor to the adolescent and the family.

4. Brief family-centered therapy is the treatment approach. The focus is on current problems, using situational or crisis-oriented family techniques. Families are told the treatment will last 3 months on the first visit, and the problem is discussed and treated as the family's problem, not the individual adolescent's.

5. Therapy is active, directive and includes giving direct advice and guidance. The nurse therapist is viewed by the family as the knowledgeable authority, and the family is given special roles and involved in the regimen, customary in many cultures.

6. Therapy includes encouraging the adolescent to conform with the family values, and the family to forgive the adolescent's transgressions and accept the adolescent back into the family. The family is reassured the problems are manageable and given specific directions on managing behavior problems. Work with other important social system, such as schools and teachers, helps the family develop a strong support network with others.

7. Referrals are made for social, economic, and legal problems that usually accompany psychological distress.

8. Families are asked about self-treatment measures and alternate kinds of food and home remedies, such as herbal teas and diet treatments, as cold and hot foods, and encouraged to follow these customs. Attention needs be given to possible contraindications of folk remedies with prescribed medications, and the clinician and family seek alternatives that meet both value systems. They are encouraged to continue consulting traditional healers and clergy and activities congruent with their cultural beliefs about healing.

Nonspecific cultural interventions. In child and adolescent psychotherapy, multimodal interventions have been traditional, inasmuch as child and adolescent psychotherapists consider the multiple lines of development and use several kinds of interventions simultaneously. The use of multiple interventions means that the concurrent strategies require distinctive monitoring. Thus, a hyperactive male adolescent who is experiencing relocation difficulties and whose family is of another culture could be treated with medication and with individual therapy to improve his low impulse control and enhance his ethnic identity. He would participate in a behavior group to improve interpersonal skills and would meet in parent and sibling sessions with the therapist providing him support in directing and airing parental ethnocentric adaptation conflicts and in assisting him to cope with the demands of his "two world views."

ECLECTIC INTEGRATIVE PSYCHOTHERAPY

Since 1975, research on the various forms of psychotherapy has shown most psychotherapies are equally effective (Luborsky and others, 1975, Smith and others, 1980). These findings have altered the traditional notions of the "one model" world view. Most clinicians use a variety of therapeutic methods and eclectic interventions (Omer and Alon, 1989).

The new eclectic world view in the culture of psychiatric treatment emphasizes many nonspecific factors. It has stimulated a search for integrative and eclectic principles that guide clinicians in whatever their choice, or choices, of interventions. Several efforts to define the principles of these strategy have appeared in the literature in response to suggestions that clinicians seek to identify strategies that serve as unifying concepts for various psychotherapies. Omer (1989) has begun to develop and test principles toward this end, and the list developed thus far includes adolescent intervention (see boxes on pp. 341-343).

Integrative Strategic Principles of Psychotherapy

Principle No. 1. Define a hierarchy of therapeutic goals. When movement toward a goal is blocked, move toward goals that come next in that hierarchy. Goal choices are most important because choice and definition organize strategic planning and execution. Hierarchy provides for greater therapeutic flexibility than does a single goal. Suggested "rules of thumb" for ordering of goals:

1. Define a central goal that is consistent with the adolescent's central complaint, in terms that the adolescent understands and accepts. Define a major goal that answers adolescent's request. For a family or another system, there may be discrepancies in help requested by different members. Clinician needs to define a goal acceptable to all members or ally with a member of the adolescent system with whom a common goal can be worked out.

2. A goal needs to be defined well enough so that it is clear when it has been attained or when it is being approached. Clinician should be able to say "we are about half the way to the goal." Goals such as "attainment of emotional maturity" are too hazy for modern criteria. A goal is easily understandable by adolescents if formulated in simple words, or words similar to theirs.

3. Modify behaviors that reinforce the central problem.

4. Work on behavioral and mental avoidances. Seek areas avoided by adolescents as avoidance, a major concern in all therapeutic methods; behaviorists stress avoidance of adverse stimuli; existentialists, of responsibility; psychodynamic therapists, of forbidden emotions; and interpersonal therapists stress avoidance of intimacy.

5. Ineffective repetitive solutions. Adolescent's attempted solutions often maintain the very problems they should solve. For example, the child is kept incompetent by the parents despite constant efforts. Intrapersonal and interpersonal solutions need to be sought to strengthen the adolescent's competence.

6. Rigid patterns, rules, myths. Irrational do's and dont's, strongly held myths, particularly proximal to the major problem. Psychodynamic therapists try to uncover the repressed origins of rigid behaviors, cognitive therapists show the adolescent their irrationality, and systemic therapists attempt to explore problem by paradox.

7. Unreflective dysfunctional (automatic and impulsive) behavior. If automatic and habitual, it is carried out without conscious participation; if impulsive, it is ruled by an apparently irresistible drive and is stronger than attempts to control. Insight-oriented therapists try to increase control by awareness; behaviorist to block the behaviors' situational triggers; existentialists to help adolescent to "own them"; systemic therapist to derail them through counter rituals.

Modified from Omer H and Alon N (1989) Principles of psychotherapeutic strategy, Psychotherapy vol 26, Fall 1989, pp. 282-289.

Continued.

Integrative Strategic Principles of Psychotherapy — cont'd

8. Pursue changes that best trigger other positive changes. Reverse of above, which aims to decrease problem-maintaining behaviors. This principle furthers the spread of problem-opposition. Therapists almost universally approve change: adolescent's interdependence, efficacy, assertiveness, assumption of responsibility, and creativity. "Good guys" of psychotherapy: avoidance, ineffective solutions, unreflective dysfunctional patterns, rigid rules; "bad guys": common denominators of all therapeutic problems.

9. Define goals to fit resources and constraints, that is, reality principle of psychotherapy. Violated when constraints of time and money are ignored, for example, adolescent in acute crisis given lengthy diagnostic test; clinics with high patient-personnel ratio specialize in depth therapies; and disregard of cultural background.

Principle No. 2. Perform small interventions to test the adolescent's reactions and to introduce a beginning change in the problem area. The principle of active diagnosis, assessing adolescent responsivity to the therapist, mini-intervention testing of adolescent's reaction (called a probe by Haley, 1977). Problem helps formulate strategy, and a diagnosis should include how adolescent reacts to being questioned, confronted, supported, directed. Probes meet this need; they are the scouts of psychotherapeutic endeavor.

Examples: Short-term psychodynamic therapist preforms a trail interview to check prospective adolescent's reactions to interpretations. A family therapist asks parents to set limits to their adolescent's behavior during the session to check the family's readiness to set down boundaries. A behavior therapist gives a writing task to an enuretic boy to assess his readiness to cooperate.

Principle No. 3. Avoid attacking points of maximum resistance unless certain of overcoming them. By avoiding major resistance areas, therapist turns instead to more accessible ones. When a dynamic psychotherapist circumvents a highly sensitive area in favor or an alternative exploration, or when processing a traumatic episode is opposed, the therapist focuses on matters of daily living.

1. If therapist feels sure major resistance can be overcome, attempt may be worthwhile, for example, direct attack, intense in vivo exposure for phobias and obsessions. Ordeal therapy commits adolescent to therapeutic task of such difficulty that giving up the symptom is preferable to withstanding the ordeal. Massive confrontation of a adolescent's avoidance of responsibility is seen in reality therapy.

2. The areas of maximum resistance and adolescent's central complaint seldom coincide. Addressing central complaint deepens therapeutic alliance, whereas resistance weakens it. High resistance can be function of particular approach chosen to address central issue, and once awakened, is often taken as showing adolescent's lack of motivation for change. Present principle encourages clinicians to change their strategy rather than blame the adolescent for the opposition. Occasionally a new approach will change entrenched resistance to cooperation.

Continued.

Integrative Strategic Principles and Psychotherapy — cont'd

Principle No. 4. Exploit timing (crises, life transitions, beginning of therapy), or create them by surprising moves. Most therapist agree that crises and life transitions provide propitious time for therapeutic intervention. Crises cause suffering that motivate adolescents for hard work; tend to suspend rules and routine that prevent change; highlight inadequacy of previous adjustment.

1. Paradoxical that when adolescent seems weakest, readiness for action is greatest. Practitioners from different orientations view the opportunity presented by crisis differently. For example, psychodynamic therapists see crisis as a time in which defenses are weak and unconscious processes accessible. Existentialist views crisis as boundary situations that confront people with their finiteness, challenge their freedom and responsibility, and create a sense of solidarity absent from daily living. Family therapists find crisis opportunities for structural changes. Crises are unique items that call for quick therapeutic decisions.
2. Life transitions unfreeze stable arrangement, for example, the therapist taking advantage of an anniversary date. People in stages of transition are prone to soul-searching and reassesment of relationships and priorities.
3. At the beginning of therapy adolescent is more ready for action, still flexible. However, premature movements can create unexpected moves that disorganize adolescent's rigid patterns. Example: Surprise intentionally pursued, as in Alexander and French's corrective emotional experience (1946). Therapists are instructed to act in ways that counter the adolescents' transferential experience. Surprises are what most positive critical incidents in psychotherapy are. Paradoxes and therapeutic rituals, as in Milan school of family therapy are useful, for example, when the family expects a paradox, therapist does not deliver one.

Principle No. 5. Concentrate on the therapeutic influence so as to achieve maximum impact at strategic points.

Principle No. 6. Mobilize allies or others that advance therapeutic goals.

Principle No. 7. Stabilize partial achievements.

Principle No. 8. When therapist or adolescent is paralyzed between competing therapeutic goals, follow a direction that may advance therapy either way.

Principle No. 9. Prepare a line of retreat that allows for continuing therapy after interventions that may fail:
1. The straightforward approach
2. Camouflaging failures
3. The tactical use of failures

Principle No. 10. When a whole strategy fails, change the therapeutic framework or redefine goals.

REFERENCES AND SUGGESTED READINGS

Alexander F and French TM (1946) Psychoanlytic therapy: principles and applications, New York, Ronald Press.

Altshuler KZ (1990) Whatever happened to intensive psychotherapy? American Journal of Psychiatry 147:428-433.

American Nurses' Association Council on Psychiatric and Mental Health Nursing (1985) Standards of child and adolescent psychiatric and mental health nursing practice, Kansas City, Mo, The Association.

American Psychiatric Association (1980) Diagnostic and statistical manual of mental disorders, ed 2, Washington, DC, The Association.

American Psychiatric Association (1987) Diagnostic and statistical manual of mental disorders III-R, ed 3, Washington, DC, The Association.

Arnstcin RL (1984) Young adulthood: stages of maturity. In Offer D and Sabshin M, editors, Normality and the life cycle, New York, Basic Books Inc, Publishers.

Bateson G, Jackson D, Haley J, and Weakland J (1968) Toward a theory of schizophrenia. In Jackson D, editor, Communication, family, and marriage, Palo Alto, Calif, Science & Behavior Books.

Beavers W (1977) Psychotherapy and growth: a family systems perspective, New York, Brunner/Mazel Inc.

Beck A (1979) Cognitive therapy of depression, New York, The Guilford Press.

Beck C (1979) Mental health and the aged, Advances in Nursing Science 1:79-87.

Beeber LS (1989) Enacting corrective interpersonal experiences with the depressed client: an intervention model, Archives of Psychiatric Nursing 3:211-217.

Blos P (1962) On adolescence: a psychoanalytic interpretation, New York, Free Press of Glencoe.

Bowen M (1978) Family therapy in clinical practice, New York, Jason Aronson, Inc.

Boyle JS and Andrews MM (1989) Transcultural concepts in nursing care, Glenview, Ill, Scott, Foresman/Little Brown College Division, Scott Foresman & Co.

Brown DT and Prout HT (1989) Behavioral approaches. In Brown DT and Prout HT, editors: Counseling and psychotherapy with children and adolescents, ed 2, Brandon, Vt, Clinical Psychology Publishing Company.

Brown DT and Prout HT, editors (1989) Counseling and psychotherapy with children and adolescents, ed 2, Brandon, Vt, Clinical Psychology Publishing Co.

Bryt A (1966) Modification of psychoanalysis in the treatment of adolescents. In Jules H, editor, Adolescence, dreams and training, vol 9, Science and psychoanalysis, New York, Grune & Stratton, Inc.

Carkhoff R and Truax C (1967) Toward effective counseling and psychotherapy, Chicago, Aldine Publishing Co.

Cole M (1981) The zone of proximal development: where culture and cognition create each other, Center for Human Information Processing, San Diego, Calif, University of California Press.

Comas-Diaz L and Griffith EEH, editors, (1988) Clinical guidelines in cross-cultural mental health, New York, John Wiley & Sons, Inc.

Committee on Ethnic Minority Human Resources Development (1985) Position paper: issues and concerns regarding the preparation of psychologists for service and research with ethnic minority populations, Washington, DC, American Psychological Association.

Constantino G, Malgady R, and Rogler LH (1985) Cuento therapy: folktales as a culturally sensitive psychotherapy for Hispanic children, Hispanic Research Center, New York, Fordham University.

Corey G (1985) Theory and practice of group counseling, ed 2, Monterey, Calif, Brooks/Cole Publishing Co.

Dahl C (1989) Some problems of cross-cultural psychotherapy with refugees seeking treatment, American Journal of Psychoanalysis 49:19-32.

Davidson JR (1989) Individual psychotherapy. In Johnson BS, editor, Psychiatric–mental health nursing adaptation and growth, Philadelphia, JB Lippincott Co.

Ellis A and Grieger R (1978) Handbook of rational emotive therapy, New York, Springer Publishing Co Inc.

Engle GL (1971) Sudden and rapid death during psychological stress: folklore or folk wisdom? Annals of Internal Medicine 74:771.

Erikson EH (1963) Childhood and society, ed 2, New York, WW Norton & Co Inc.

Favazza AR (1985) Anthropology and psychiatry. In Kaplan HI and Sadock BJ, editors, Comprehensive textbook of psychiatry/IV, volume 1, ed 4, Baltimore, Williams & Wilkins.

Field WE, editor (1979) The psychotherapy of Hildegard E. Peplau, New Braunfels, Tex, PSF Productions.

Field WE (1982) Long-term psychotherapy. I. Advances in psychiatric mental health nursing (Lesson 4, 1:26), Villanova, Penn, Pro Scientia, Inc.

Field WE (1982) Long-term psychotherapy. II. Advances in psychiatric mental health nursing (Lesson 5, 1:26), Villanova, Penn, Pro Scientia, Inc.

Flaskerud JH (1987) A proposed protocol for culturally relevant nursing psychotherapy, Clinical Nurse Specialist 1:150.

Flaskerud JH (1989) Transcultural concepts in mental health nursing. In Boyle JS and Andrews MM, Transcultural concepts in nursing care, Glenview, Ill, Scott Foresman/Little Brown College Division, Scott Foresman & Co.

Ford DH and Urban HB (1963) Systems of psychotherapy, New York, John Wiley & Sons, Inc.

Frank JD (1973) Persuasion and healing: a comparative study of psychotherapy, Baltimore, Md, The Johns Hopkins University Press.

Free K, Tuerk J, and Tinkleman J (1986) Expressions of transitional relatedness in art, music and verbal psychotherapies. The Arts in Psychotherapy 13G:197-213.

Freitas, Laud Pieranuwi VR (1990) Ethical issues in the behavioral assessment of children and adolescents, Journal of Child and Adolescent Psychiatric and Mental Health Nursing 3:3-8.

Freud A (1969) Adolescence as developmental disturbance. In Kaplan G and Lebovici S, editors, Adolescence: psychological perspectives, New York, Basic Books Inc, Publishers.

Freud A (1965) Normality and pathology in childhood, New York, International Universities Press.

Freud A (1937) The ego and mechanisms of defense, London, Hogarth Press.

Freud S (1953) Remembering, repeating and working through. The standard edition of the complete psychological works of Sigmund Freud, vol 132, London, Hogarth Press (originally published in 1914).

Fromm-Reichman F (1950) Principles of intensive psychotherapy, Chicago, University of Chicago Press.

Gardner RA (1988) Psychotherapy with adolescents, Cresskill, NJ, Creative Therapeutics.

Geknan C (1984) Culture, health and illness, Bristol, UK, John Wright & Sons.

Gilbert CM (1988) Sexual abuse and group therapy, Journal of Psychosocial Nursing and Mental Health Services 26:19.

Gresham FM and Lemanek KL (1983) Social skills: a review of the congitive-behavioral training procedures with children, Journal of Applied Developmental Psychology 4:239-261.

Grossman F and Freet B (1978) A cognitive approach to group therapy with hospitalzied adolescents. In Freeman A and Greenwood VB, editors: Cognitive therapy applications in psychiatric and medical settings, New York, Human Sciences Press.

Haley J (1977) Problem-solving therapy, San Francisco, Jossey-Bass.

Hamric AB (1983) The clinical specialist. Role and Development. In Hamric A and Spross J, editors: The clinical specialist in theory and practice, New York, Grune & Stratton, Inc.

Hautman MA (1979) Folk health and illness beliefs, Nurse Practitioner 4:23.

Helman C (1984) Culture, health and illness, Bristol, England, John Wright & Sons.

Henderson G and Primeaux M (1981) Transcultural health care, Reading, Mass, Addison-Wesley Publishing Co, Inc.

Hill L and Smith N (1985) Self-care nursing: promotion of health, Englewood Cliffs, NJ, Prentice-Hall Inc.

Hopkins H and Smith N (1972) Occupational therapy: its definition and functioning, American Journal of Occupational Therapy 26:204.

Hopkins H and Smith N (1988) Wiliard and Spackman's occupational therapy, Philadelphia, JB Lippincott Co.

Horowitz M, Maramar C, Krupnick J, Wilner N, Kaltreider N, and Wallerstein R (1984) Personality styles and brief psychotherapy, New York, Basic Books Inc, Publishers.

Jacobsen FM (1988) Ethnocultural assessment. In Comas-Diaz L and Griffith EEH, editors, Clinical guidelines in cross-cultural mental health, New York, John Wiley & Sons, Inc.

Janosik EH and Phipps LB (1982) Life cycle group work in nursing, Monterey, Calif, Wadsworth, Inc.

Karasu TB (1980) The ethics of psychotherapy, American Journal of Psychiatry 137:1502-1514.

Kiev A (1974) Magic, faith and healing, New York, The Free Press.

Kinzie JD (1978) Lessons from cross-cultural psychotherapy, American Journal of Psychotherapy 32:510.

Klein M (1932) The psycho-analysis of children, London, Hogarth Press.

Kleinmann A (1981) Patients and healers in the context of culture, Berkeley, University of California Press.

Kleinmann A (1982) Neurasthenia and depression: a study of somatization and culture in China, Cultural Medicine Psychiatry 6:117-190.

Klerman GL (1986) Historical perspectives on contemporary schools of psychopathology. In Millon T and Klerman GL, editors, Contemporary directions in psychopathology, New York, The Guilford Press.

Kluckholm C (1944) The influence of psychiatry on anthropology in America during the past one hundred years. In Hall JK, editor, One hundred years of American psychiatry, New York, Columbia University Press.

Lantz JE (1978) Family and marital therapy, New York, Appleton-Century-Crofts.

Laufer M (1980) On reconstruction in adolescent analysis. In Feinstein S, Giovacchini P, Looney J, Schwartxberg A, and Sorosky A, editors, Adolescent psychiatry, vol 8, Chicago, University of Chicago Press.

Lazare L (1979) Outpatient psychiatry, Baltimore, Williams & Wilkins.

Lebra W (1976) Culture-bound syndromes: ethnopsychiatry and alternate therapies, Honolulu, The University Press of Hawaii.

Lego S (1980) The one-to-one nurse-patient relationship, Perspectives in Psychiatric Care 18:67-87.

Leighton AH (1982) Relevant generic issues. In Gaw AG, editor, Cross-cultural psychiatry, Litton Mass, John Wright & Sons.

Leininger M (1978) Changing foci in American nursing education: primary and transcultural nursing care, Journal of Advanced Nursing 3:155-166.

Levy R (1982) The new language of psychiatry, Boston, Little, Brown & Co.

Lewin K (1935) A dynamic theory of personality: selected papers, New York, McGraw-Hill Book Co.

Liaschenko J (1989) Changing paradigms within psychiatry: implications for nursing research, Archives of Psychiatric Nursing 3:153-158.

Licht S (1948) Occupational therapy source book, Baltimore, Williams & Wilkins.

Lin KM and Finder E (1983) Neuroleptic dosage for Asians, American Journal of Psychiatry 140:490-491.

Luborsky L and Crits-Christoph P (1990) Understanding psychotherapy: the core conflictual relationship theme method, New York, Basic Books, Inc, Publishers.

Lyons JA (1989) Posttraumatic stress disorder in children and adolescents. A review of the literature. In Chess S, Thomas A, and Hertizig ME, editors: Annual progress in child psychiatry and child development, New York, Brunner/Mazel, Inc.

Mahler M (1971) A study of the separation-individuation process and its possible application to borderline phenomena in the psychoanalytic situations, Psychoanalytic Study of the Child 26:404.

Marriner-Torney A (1989) Nursing theorists and their work, cd 2, St Louis, The CV Mosby Co.

McClary CL, Zahrt L, Montgomery JH, Walker H, and Petry JR (1981) Wellness: the mode in the new paradigm, Health Values 19:8.

McGoldrick M, Pearce JK, and Giordano J (1982) Ethnicity and family therapy, New York, The Guilford Press.

McKay N (1981) Melanie Klein's metapsychology: phenomenological and mechanistic perspective, International Journal of Psychoanalysis 62:187.

McKeon KL (1990) Introduction: a future perspective on psychiatric mental health nursing, Archives of Psychiatric Nursing 4:19.

McNany GW (1990) Psychobiological indices of bipolar mood disorder: future trends in nursing care, Archives of Psychiatric Nursing 4:29.

Meeks JE (1971) The fragile alliance: an orientation to outpatient psychotherapy of the adolescent, Baltimore, Williams & Wilkins.

Merram F (1978) The group approach in nursing practice, ed 2, St Louis, The CV Mosby Co.

Meyer A (1982) The philosophy of occupational therapy, Archives of Occupational Therapy 1:1.

Miller D (1974) Adolescent psychology, psychopathology, psychotherapy, New York, Jason Aronson, Inc.

Miller D (1980) Family maladaptation reflected in drug abuse and delinquency. In Sugar M, Responding to adolescent needs, Jamaica, NY, Spectrum Publications.

Miller D (1983) The age between: adolescents and therapy, New York, Jason Aronson, Inc.

Miller D (1986) Attack on the self: adolescent behavioral disturbances and their treatment, Northvale, NJ, Jason Aronson, Inc.

Millon T and Klerman GL (1986) Contemporary directions in psychopathology, New York, The Guilford Press.

Minuchin S (1974) Families and family therapy, Cambridge, Mass, Harvard University Press.

Minuchin S (1982) Families and family therapy, Archives of Occupational Therapy 1:1.

Minuchin S and Fishman H (1988) Family therapy techniques, Cambridge, Mass, Harvard University Press.

Mishne JM (1986) Clinical work with adolescents, New York, The Free Press.

Monti PM, Abrams DB, Kadden RM, and Cooney NL (1989) Treating alcohol dependence: a coping skills training guide, New York, The Guilford Press.

Moos RH and Ruhst R (1982) The clinical use of social-ecological concepts: the case of an adolescent girl, American Journal of Orthopsychiatry 52:111-122.

Moritsugu J and Sue S (1983) Minority status as a stressor. In Felner R, Jason L, Moritsugu J, and Faber S, editors, Preventive psychology: theory, research and practice in community interventions, New York, Pergamon Press, Inc.

Orque MS and Block B (1988) Culture, ethnicity and nursing. In Potter P and Perry AG, editors, Fundamentals of nursing, ed 2, St Louis, The CV Mosby Co.

Orque MS, Block B, and Monrroy LS (1983) Ethnic nursing care, St Louis, The CV Mosby Co.

Papp P (1976) Family choreography. In Guerin PJ, editor, Family therapy, New York, Gardner Press Inc.

Paskar KR, Lamb J, and Martsofl DS (1990) The role of the psychiatric/mental health clinical specialist in an adolescent coping skills group, Journal of Child and Adolescent Psychiatric Mental Health Nursing 3:47-51.

Paul EL and White KM (1990) The development of intimate relationships in late adolescence, Adolescence 98:375.

Pedersen PB, Lonner WJ, and Draguns JG, editors (1981) Counseling across cultures, Honolulu, The University of Hawaii Press.

Pedersen PB and Marsella AJ (1982) The ethical crisis for cross-counseling and therapy, Professional Psychology 13:492-500.

Pedersen PB, Sartorius N, and Marsella AJ, editors (1984) Mental health services: the cross-cultural context, Beverly Hills, Calif, Sage Publications Inc.

Peplau HE (1952) Interpersonal relations in nursing, New York, GP Putnam's Sons.

Peplau HE (1964) Basic principles of patient counseling, ed 2, Philadelphia, Smith, Kline & French Laboratories.

Peplau AE (1975) Basic principles of patient counseling, New Braunfels, Tex, PSF Productions.

Perls F (1970) The Gestalt approach, Palo Alto, Calif, Science & Behavior Books.

Piaget J (1958) The growth of logical thinking from childhood to adolescence, New York, Basic Books Inc, Publishers.

Piaget J (1963) The origins of intelligence in children, New York, WW Norton & Co, Inc.

Pothier P (1988) Point/counterpoint, Archives of Psychiatric Nursing 2:259.

Prince R (1980) Variations in psychotherapeutic procedures. In Triandis HC and Draguns JG, editors, Handbook of cross-cultural psychology, vol 6, Psychopathology, Boston, Allyn & Bacon, Inc.

Prince R (1987) Alexithymia and verbal psychotherapies in cultural context, Transcultural Psychiatry Review 24:107-118.

Reed PG (1987) Spirituality and well-being in terminally ill hospitalized adults, Research in Nursing and Health 10:335-344.

Regier DAS and Burke JD (1985) Quantitative and experimental methods in psychiatry. In Kaplan HI and Sadock BJ, editors, Comprehensive textbook of psychiatry/IV, vol 1, ed 4, Baltimore, Williams & Wilkins.

Riegel RF and Meacham JA, editors (1976) The developing individual in a changing world, Chicago, Aldine.

Rowe J (1988) Attachment theory and milieu treatment of children, Journal of Child and Adolescent Psychiatric Mental Health Nursing 1:66-76.

Sarason IG and Sarason BR, editors (1985) Social support: theory, research and applications, Dordrecht, The Netherlands, Martinus Nijhoff.

Satir V (1983) Conjoint family therapy, ed 3, Palo Alto, Calif, Science & Behavior Books.

Satir V (1988) The new peoplemaking, Mountain View, Calif, Science & Behavior Books.

Schmalenburg C and Kramer M (1979) Coping with reality shock: voices of experience, Wakefield, Mass, Nursing Resources, Inc.

Schofield W (1974) Psychotherapy: purchase of friendship, Englewood Cliffs, NJ, Prentice-Hall, Inc.

Secrest L (1977) On the dearth of theory in cross-cultural psychology: there is madness in our method. In Poortinga YH, editor: Problems in cross-cultural psychology, Amsterdam, Sweets and Zeitlinger.

Shea SC (1988) Psychiatric interviewing: the art of understanding, Philadelphia, WB Saunders Co.

Siepker BB and Kandaras CS, editors (1985) Group therapy with children and adolescents. New York, Human Sciences Press.

Smith NL, Glass CN, and Miller TI (1980) The benefits of psychotherapy, Baltimore, Johns Hopkins University Press.

Smoyak S, editor (1975) The psychiatric nurse as family therapist, New York, John Wiley & Sons, Inc.

Spector RE (1979) Cultural diversity in health and illness, New York, Appleton-Century-Crofts.

Stanisz MM (1990) A support group for inpatient abused adolescents, Journal of Child and Adolescent Psychiatric and Mental Health Nursing 3:14-17.

Steiger N and Lipson J (1985) Self-care nursing: theory and practice, Bowie, Md, Brady Communications.

Still JV (1984) How to assess spiritual needs of children and their families, Journal of Christian Nursing 1(1):4-6.

Sue DW and Sue D (1977) Barrier to effective cross-cultural counseling, J Counseling Psychology 24:420.

Sue S, Ito J, and Bradshaw C (1982) Ethnic minority research: trends and directions. In Jones EE and Korchin SJ, editors, Minority mental health, New York, Praeger, Publishers.

Sullivan HS (1953) The interpersonal theory of psychiatry. In Perry HS and Grawel ML, editors, The collected works of Harry Stack Sullivan, New York, WW Norton & Co, Inc.

Sullivan HS (1962) Schizophrenia as a human process, New York, WW Norton & Co, Inc.

Szapocznik J, Foote FH, Perez-Vidal A, Hervis OE, and Kurtines W (1985) One person family therapy, Miami, University of Miami School of Medicine.

Szapocznik J, Kurtines W, and Fernandy T (1980) Bicultural involvement and adjustment of Hispanic American youth, International Journal of Intercultural Review 4:353-365.

Szapocznik J and Truss C (1978) Intergenerational sources of role conflict in Cuban mothers. In Montiel M, editor, Hispanic families, Washington DC, COSSMHO.

Taft R (1978) Statement on ethics, Adopted by the International Association for Cross-Cultural Psychology, July 29.

Tapp JL (1981) Studying personality development. In Heron A and Kroeger E, editors, Handbook of cross-cultural psychology, vol 6, Psyhopathology, Boston, Allyn & Bacon Inc.

Thompson L (1986) Peplau's theory: an application to short-term individual therapy, Journal of Psychosocial Nursing 24:26-31.

Tietjen AM (1989) The ecology of children's social support networks. In Belle D, editor, Children's social networks and social supports, New York, John Wiley & Sons Inc.

Tomm K (1984) One perspective on the Mikan's systems' approach, Journal of Marital and Family Therapy 10:113-125.

Torrey EF (1969) The case for the indigenous therapist, Archives of General Psychiatry 20:365-373.

Triandis H and Draguns J, editors (1980) Handbook of cross-cultural psychology, 6 vols, Boston, Allyn & Bacon Inc.

Tseng WS and McDermott JF (1981) Culture, mind and therapy: an introduction to cultural psychiatry, New York, Brunner/Mazel Inc.

Valente SM (1990) Clinical hypnosis with school-age children, Archives of Psychiatric Nursing 4:131-136.

Walsh F (1982) Conceptualizations of normal family functioning. In Walsh F, editor, Normal family processes, New York, The Guilford Press.

Ward C (1980) Spirit possession and mental health: a psychoanthropological perspective, Human Relations 33:49-163.

Watzlawick P, Beaven J, and Jackson D (1967) Pragmatics of human communication, New York, WW Norton & Co Inc.

Weidman H (1975) Concepts as strategies for change, Psychiatric Annals 5:116-518.

Weisz F and Benoit C (1989) Psychoanalytic approaches. In Brown ST and Prout HT, editors, Counseling and psychotherapy with children, ed 2, Brandon, Vt, Clinical Psychology Publishing Co.

Werner E (1979) Cross-cultural child development, New York, Brooks/Cole Publishing Co.

Westley FR (1982) Merger and separation: autistic symbolism in new religious movements, Journal of Psychoanalytic Anthropology 5:137-154.

White GM (1982) The role of cultural explanations in "somatization" and "psychological-ization," 16:1519-1530.

Whiting BB (1980) Culture and social behavior: a model for the development of social behavior, Ethos 8:95-102.

Whiting BB and Whiting JWM (1975) Children of six cultures: a psychocultural analysis, Cambridge, Mass, Harvard University Press.

Wilkinson CB and O'Connor WA (1982) Human ecology and mental illness, American Journal of Psychiatry 139:985-990.

Wilson EO (1975) Sociobiology: the new synthesis, Cambridge, Mass, Harvard University Press.

Winnicott DW (1977) The piggle, New York, International Universities Press.

Wubbolding RE (1988) Using reality therapy, New York, Harper & Row Publishers, Inc.

Yalom ID (1983) Inpatient group psychotherapy, New York, Basic Books Inc, Publishers.

Yalom ID (1985) The theory and practice of group psychotherapy, ed 3, New York, Basic Books Inc, Publishers.

Youniss J and Sjmollar J (1985) Adolescent relations with mothers, fathers and friends, Chicago, University of Chicago Press.

Ziegler VE and Briggs JT (1977) Tricyclic plasma levels: effects of age, race, sex and smoking, Journal of the American Medical Association 238:2167-2169.

Zinker J (1977) Creative process in Gestalt therapy, New York, Random House, Inc.

Chapter 13

Psychopharmacology

Norman L. Keltner

STANDARD V-F. *Intervention: Somatic Therapies*

THE NURSE USES KNOWLEDGE OF SOMATIC THERAPIES WITH THE CHILD OR ADOLESCENT AND FAMILY TO ENHANCE THERAPEUTIC INTERVENTIONS.

Adolescent psychopharmacology is one dimension of a comprehensive approach to the nursing care of adolescents with mental health disturbances. Although there are many approaches to treatment, none lends itself to scientific scrutiny and replication of effort more readily than does psychopharmacological intervention. It is by far the most research-based dimension of psychiatric nursing. This avenue of intervention holds much promise, but risks are associated. Beyond having the ability to work with adolescents and understanding the scientific foundation of drug therapy, the psychiatric nurse must be aware of the various strategies for effective administration of drugs: surveillance, teaching, collaboration, and advocacy (see box on p. 352). In addition, the nurse must be aware of the nursing implications for each drug administered, understand the side effects of these drugs, be aware of drug interactions, be on the alert for toxic reactions, and the nurse must also teach the parent. Only when these methods of psychopharmacology have been added to appropriate psychosocial interventions can the patient receive maximal benefit from psychiatric nursing care.

Psychopharmacologic Treatment of Attention Deficit Hyperactivity Disorder

Attention deficit hyperactivity disorder (ADHD) is the most common pediatric behavioral disorder. It has been estimated that up to 20% of all school-age children have it (LaGreca and Quay, 1984); but a more accurate estimate is 2% to 3%. Until recently it was thought that ADHD was outgrown at puberty because of the developmental changes that take place at that time. Cantwell (1985) found that ADHD symptoms persist into adolescence in 50% to 80% of the cases, indicating a greater incidence of this disorder in adolescents than previously thought. One third

---

Nursing Strategies for Effective Administration of Psychopharmacological Agents To Adolescents

Surveillance

1. The nurse must monitor for a response, side effects, and patient compliance.

Teaching

1. The nurse must teach the adolescent and family about the drug to be administered and obtain consent for drug therapy.
2. The nurse must teach other staff members about drugs.

Collaboration

1. The nurse must inform the physician of the patient's response to the drug.
2. The nurse should provide outpatient therapists, school nurses, or other school personnel with the rationale for a certain drug and information about the drug dosage, action, side effects, and response.
3. The nurse must arrange with the family the way prescriptions will be filled and monitored and should explain the need to communicate drug information to all caregivers of the adolescent.

Advocacy

1. The nurse must work to establish policies and procedures for appropriate administration and surveillance in all settings.

---

continue to show signs of ADHD into adulthood. Boys are three times more likely than girls to have ADHD, and six to nine times more boys than girls seek professional intervention (American Psychiatric Association, 1987). ADHD is related to other adolescent problems such as antisocial behavior, substance abuse, and poor school performance. Academically, adolescents with ADHD are about 2 years behind their peers (Munoz-Millan and Casteel, 1989).

Central nervous system (CNS) stimulants are the drugs most commonly used to treat children, but they are used less often in adolescents, particularly older adolescents. It is a commonly held opinion among many professionals working with ADHD that when the hyperactive individual reaches puberty, stimulants lose their effect. A number of authors question this belief (Safer and Krager, 1988; Clampit and Pirkle, 1983; Cantwell, 1977; Lerer and Lerer, 1977), noting their own and other clinical studies that indicate stimulants are as useful for adolescents as they are for younger children. Despite the facts that ADHD persists into adolescence and adulthood and that stimulants continue to be effective, some professionals prefer other psychotropic drugs.

ADHD is characterized by inattention, impulsiveness, and hyperactivity. Fidgeting and restlessness are more prominent in adolescents than is hyperactivity. All of these deficits cause a problem for the adolescent in school who is expected to sit still and listen.

CENTRAL NERVOUS SYSTEM STIMULANTS

Safer and Krager (1988) found that between 1975 and 1987 the percentage of public middle school students receiving medication for hyperactivity or inattention rose from 0.5% to 3.68%, and between 1983 and 1987 the percentage of public senior high school students rose from 0.21% to 0.40%. This research conservatively estimates that 750,000 youths (including 5.96% of all elementary public school children) received medication for hyperactivity in 1987 and predicts that one million will be receiving medication in the early 1990s. Of the school-age children taking stimulants, 25% are in special education classes (Safer and Krager, 1988).

The most commonly used drugs in the treatment of ADHD are the amphetamines, usually dextroamphetamine (Dexedrine) and methylphenidate (Ritalin). Of the two, methylphenidate is used more often — about 93% of the time (Safer and Krager, 1988). However, these drugs are frequently not used in adolescents, particularly older adolescents, partly because of the aforementioned belief that these drugs are not as effective after childhood and partly because of the potential for abuse by the patient, siblings, or peer group.

Nonetheless, cerebral stimulants used in conjunction with counseling are effective. Improvement for the ADHD patient means the ability to control behavior, to pay attention, and to learn. In short, these drugs give the adolescent an opportunity to succeed in school. The *stimulant* has a *calming* effect. This so-called paradoxical effect can be explained by the theory that low levels of these drugs stimulate inhibitory neurons in the central nervous system (CNS), thus producing an overall CNS "depression." Another view suggests that low doses of CNS stimulants, by stimulating the child's immature reticular activating system, enable the motor cortex to respond appropriately to external stimuli. Presumably these effects are caused by the CNS stimulant's ability to increase the levels of dopamine, norepinephrine, and serotonin. Although many drugs used in the treatment of childhood behavior disorders simply make the child more "manageable," CNS stimulants directly affect the problem behavior.

Dextroamphetamine (Dexedrine). According to Safer and Krager (1988), dextroamphetamine accounts for only 3% of the medication given for ADHD. Children 6 years old and over may be given 5 mg once or twice per day, with an increase of 5 mg per day at weekly intervals as needed. Spansules are available and may be given once daily in the mornings (to prevent insomnia). When the child enters adolescence, the dosage should be reevaluated. Tolerance in ADHD patients is rarely reported. The dosage for these patients should not exceed 40 mg of dextroamphetamine per day. Since abuse potential is high (although evidence that children themselves abuse is not convincing), amphetamines are schedule II drugs. The American Academy of Pediatrics recommends that dextroamphetamine dosage should be approximately half of the methylphenidate dosage.

Methylphenidate (Ritalin). In children older than the age of 6, 5 mg of methylphenidate before both breakfast and lunch is recommended. If needed, the daily dosage may be increased by 5- to 10-mg increments at weekly intervals. The optimum daily dosage is 0.3 mg/kg. Some research indicates that greater levels of methylphenidate (for example, 0.6 mg/kg) may be counterproductive (American Journal of Nursing, 1985). Although 0.3 mg/kg per day may not correct all social behavior concerns, it is an appropriate amount to increase learning ability. Children should receive no more than 1 mg/kg per day or a total of more than 60 mg per day regardless of weight. The sustained-release form (Ritalin-SR) may be substituted for divided dosages. Abuse potential exists with methylphenidate, so it is a schedule II drug.

Pemoline (Cylert). Pemoline differs chemically from the amphetamines and methylphenidate and is used exclusively for ADHD. It is well absorbed, has a long duration of action (12 hours), and is excreted partially unchanged (approximately 50%) in the urine. Although in the past it was assumed that a therapeutic effect took about 4 weeks to develop, recent work suggests that a therapeutic effect starts within 2 days.

Pemoline causes less cerebral stimulation than the other two CNS stimulants do. Side effects are similar to those of the amphetamines and methylphenidate. Dosage for children older than the age of 6 is 37.5 mg daily in the morning. Because pemoline has a long half-life, it can be given once per day. The daily dosage may be increased by 18.75 mg at weekly intervals up to a maximum of 112.5 mg per day. The usual maintenance dosage is 56.25 to 75 mg per day. Pemoline has low abuse potential and is a schedule IV drug (Table 13-1).

Nursing Implications

Side effects. Side effects of CNS stimulants include nervousness, tachycardia, insomnia, anorexia, stomach ache, symptoms of depression (sadness and crying), weight loss, and temporary growth retardation (both height and weight). Insomnia and anorexia are best handled by dosage timing; for instance, anorexia can be minimized by giving the drug with meals, and insomnia is reduced by giving the last dose at least 6 hours before bedtime. Methylphenidate has somewhat fewer sympathomimetic effects than do the amphetamines. Brown and Sexson (1989) reported a significant increase in diastolic blood pressure in adolescent boys receiving methylphenidate. Close monitoring of blood pressure is recommended. Sometimes a paradoxical worsening of ADHD can occur with methylphenidate. If this occurs, the drug should be withheld. Although much concern exists about the danger of these drugs, they are among the safest of the psychotropics in use.

Interactions. CNS stimulants used in the treatment of ADHD—for instance, dextroamphetamine and methylphenidate—are well absorbed from the gastrointestinal tract and distributed throughout the body. They begin to have an effect within 1 hour or less. Although methylphenidate is completely metabolized by the liver, dextroamphetamine is excreted unchanged in the urine. When the urine is acidified, amphetamines are excreted more quickly (the half-life decreases). Acidifying agents include ascorbic acid and fruit juices. On the other hand, if urine is alkalinized (for example, as with sodium bicarbonate), amphetamines are reabsorbed and have a prolonged effect because amphetamines are not metabolized in the liver (the half-life increases). Because stomach ache is a side effect of amphetamines, a parent might be tempted to give the child medication containing sodium bicarbonate. In practice, the parent or nurse should not give an over-the-counter (OTC) product for an upset stomach that would alkalinize the urine. To do so would intensify the effect of the amphetamine. OTC drugs for colds and hay fever also increase sympathomimetic

Table 13–1   Comparison of Central Nervous System Stimulants Used in Treating
ADHD

	Half-life (hrs)	Starting dosage	Maximum dosage (mg/day)
Dextroamphetamine	6-8	5 mg qd or bid	40
Methylphenidate	1-3	5 mg breakfast 5 mg lunch	60
Pemoline	8-12	37.5 mg in AM	112.5

effects and should be avoided. Other drug interactions with CNS stimulants are numerous. CNS stimulants increase the serum levels of antidepressants and decrease the effects of antihypertensives (therefore increasing blood pressure). When given with antipsychotic drugs or CNS depressants, the effects of the CNS stimulants are reduced. In fact, antipsychotic drugs can be used to treat overdoses of CNS stimulants. Monoamine oxidase (MAO) inhibitors, and sympathomimetics (including OTC preparations) can cause hypertension when given with CNS stimulants.

Toxicity. Amphetamine overdose may be fatal. If symptoms of overdose are observed (the patient is hyperalert and talkative and has tremors, exaggerated startle reflex, paranoia, hallucinations, confusion, and tachyarrhythmias), notify the physician and arrange for hospitalization. Urinary acidification speeds up elimination, activated charcoal slows absorption, and gastric lavage can rid the body of the unabsorbed drug. The nurse should monitor for vital signs and reduce environmental stimuli. Further information on protocols for an amphetamine overdose can be found in other texts.

Parent teaching. When adolescents and teenagers are members of families, the parents must take the ultimate responsibility for their compliance to dosage schedules. Because of their important role in psychopharmacology, parents deserve special consideration in teaching about all the drugs mentioned in this chapter. Parents need to be aware of the abuse potential of CNS stimulants and should keep them away from other siblings. Parents should be advised to assess for "cheeking" (when the pill is placed in side of mouth but not swallowed) and hoarding, which can result in the storing up of these drugs and thus potential overdose.

Parents must be taught to tolerate some hyperactivity and not automatically to seek an increase in dosage or increase it on their own. The optimum daily dosage for methylphenidate (0.3 mg/kg) does not always reduce the hyperactive behaviors to the degree parents would like, so the parents must be encouraged to live with some less-than-ideal behavior. Because of the appetite suppression and delayed growth caused by amphetamines, parents should be taught to weigh their child on a weekly basis. Long-term growth problems apparently do not occur; recent research indicates that methylphenidate does not noticeably impair growth during early adolescence (Vincent and others, 1990). Nevertheless, as with all psychotropics, a drug-free "holiday" is warranted to assess the continued need for the drug. Eventually adolescent patients must be taught to administer and monitor these drugs themselves to assume responsibility for their own care.

TRICYCLIC ANTIDEPRESSANTS

As already noted, CNS stimulants are the drugs most often used to treat ADHD; however, approximately 30% of children receiving these drugs do not improve. Other drugs have been tried with varying degrees of success. Tricyclic antidepressants (TCAs) have been used to treat of ADHD; they seem to have more side effects than do the CNS stimulants and, according to some clinicians, have short-lived results. On the other hand, TCAs have four potential advantages over stimulants: (1) they have a longer duration of action, (2) they may be given as a single dose, (3) plasma levels can be confirmed, and (4) they have little potential for abuse (Gastfriend and others, 1984).

Dosages for ADHD are lower than those for depression. Gastfriend and others (1984) found improvement in 11 of 12 adolescent patients using desipramine. Starting dosages were 10 to 25 mg per day; mean dosages after the fourth week of study were 1.57 mg/kg. Pliszka (1987) found that overall, TCAs were not as effective as CNS stimulants; however, they were effective for highly anxious ADHD patients. Bupropion (Wellbutrin), a new antidepressant, has also been prescribed in the treatment of ADHD with some success.

Nursing Implications

Side effects. Gastfriend and others (1984) reported these significant side effects associated with desipramine in an adolescent population with ADHD: drowsiness (50%), postural dizziness (25%), weight loss and decreased appetite (25%), headache (16%), insomnia (8%), and racing thoughts (8%). Other common side effects of TCAs include dry mouth, sedation, and cognitive problems.

Interactions. Three categories of interactions are associated with TCAs: those that cause CNS depression, those that cause cardiovascular and hypertensive effects, and those that result in additive anticholinergic effects. Although an adolescent is unlikely to come into contact with all the interactants that could cause these effects, many interactants are readily available and tempting in our drug-taking society.

CNS depressants such as alcohol, anticonvulsants, and benzodiazepines (for example, Valium), when combined with TCAs, can cause CNS depression. Cardiovascular arrhythmias and hypertension can occur when sympathomimetic drugs are taken with TCAs. Phenylpropanolamine, a moderately potent sympathomimetic agent, is present in over 100 over-the-counter (OTC) and prescription anorectics, nasal decongestants, psychostimulants, and treatments for premenstrual syndrome (Dilsaver and others, 1989). To prevent this interaction, parents should be told to discard any unused stimulants if their child is switched from stimulants to TCAs. Additive anticholinergic effects occur when TCAs are combined with other anticholinergic drugs, such as antipsychotics and antihistamines.

Toxicity. TCAs do not produce euphoria, so their potential for abuse is not great. On the other hand, overdosing is very serious and in adults accounts for 25% to 50% of all hospital admissions for overdose (Harsch and Holt, 1988). Toxic levels may result in sedation, ataxia, agitation, stupor, coma, respiratory depression, and convulsions. Any young person suspected of overdosing on these drugs should be taken to a hospital for monitoring.

Parent teaching. The nurse should discuss side effects with the parents and help them to understand how to negotiate the health care system if drug effects warrant their doing so. The nurse should also teach about the potential for interaction. The parent must understand that an abrupt discontinuance of TCAs has been associated with nausea, headache, and malaise. Finally, the nurse must instruct the parent to watch out for the hoarding of TCAs. TCAs have a narrow therapeutic index and are often used as a means of self-injury by adolescent patients. This is extremely important; many young people have died from TCA overdose.

OTHER DRUGS

Use of phenothiazines and haloperidol has also been studied, but these drugs seem less effective than the stimulants. Lithium, diphenhydramine (Benadryl), phenobarbital, and benzodiazepines have also been used with less-than-satisfactory results. In addition, the amino acid phenylalanine has been studied and found ineffective (Zametkin and others, 1987). CNS stimulants remain the drugs of choice for ADHD; however, for the significant group of ADHD sufferers who do not respond to stimulants or in cases in which stimulant abuse is suspected, these alternate drugs remain a viable option.

Psychopharmacological Treatment of Psychotic Disorders

Schizophrenia usually begins to emerge in adolescence or early adulthood. Symptoms include hallucinations, delusions, disordered thoughts, anxiety, inappropriate affect, idiosyncratic speech, morbid thoughts, absence of friends, and concrete thinking. During childhood there is frequently some diagnostic confusion between schizophrenia and autism; however, that confusion is much less prominent during the adolescent years. Autism almost always has its onset before 3 years of age, and schizophrenia often has its onset during adolescence. Autism, in most cases, continues into adolescence, at which time the cardinal symptoms of social and language skills deficit may improve or worsen. Taking a thorough history often precludes misdiagnosis. A reactive depression—that is, a depression caused by the realization that one is "handicapped by autism"—is not uncommon with late-adolescent autism. Schizophrenia, autism, and other psychotic processes share similar psychopharmacological intervention strategies; therefore a general discussion of antipsychotic drugs is essential to understanding the psychopharmacological management of these disorders.

ANTIPSYCHOTIC DRUGS

The goals of intervention with psychotic adolescents are primitive when compared with the goals of drug intervention in ADHD. For the schizophrenic adolescent the goal is to decrease thought disorganization so that restoration to a previous normal level of functioning can occur. In the autistic individual the goal is to decrease behaviors such as biting and head banging or to decrease anxiety. These drugs are used in both groups of patients to manage aggressive, assaultive, or self-destructive behavior. Psychotropic drugs alone are never considered adequate in the treatment of these children. They are but one aspect of a treatment plan that includes therapeutic communication, milieu management, and parental and educational involvement.

Phenothiazines are often the first drugs used to treat adolescent psychoses (Wiener, 1977). The three subclasses of phenothiazines are the aliphatics, the piperidines, and the piperazines. Chlorpromazine (Thorazine), an aliphatic, was the first antipsychotic drug developed and is the antipsychotic prototype. There is little empirical evidence that one antipsychotic is more effective than another.

The phenothiazines are usually taken orally and are absorbed rapidly in the gastrointestinal tract. A tranquillizing effect occurs in about 1 hour with chlorpromazine, which accumulates in fatty tissues and is slowly released. It is highly bound (95% to 98%) to plasma proteins and is extensively metabolized in the liver. It is excreted by the kidney; only 1% is excreted unchanged.

Two prominent desired effects account for the beneficial results of antipsychotic therapy: a *neuroleptic effect* and an *antipsychotic effect.* The neuroleptic effect is characterized by sedation, emotional quieting, and psychomotor slowing. The antipsychotic effect is manifested by normalization of thought, mood, and behavior. The neuroleptic effect may be more significant for the autistic child, and the antipsychotic effect may be more significant for the schizophrenic child. It is thought that the effectiveness of antipsychotic drugs is linked to their ability to block dopamine receptors. The most promising theoretical understanding of schizophrenia involves excessive levels of the neurotransmitter dopamine. Subsequently, as dopamine is blocked, schizophrenic symptomatology is reduced.

Two basic categories of peripheral autonomic side effects relate to these drugs: *anticholinergic side effects* and *antiadrenergic side effects.* (A pharmacology text should provide a review of these concepts if needed.) In addition, these drugs produce central side effects in the extrapyramidal system that are essentially *antidopaminergic side effects.* It is commonly accepted that low-potency antipsychotic drugs such as chlorpromazine and thioridazine (Mellaril)—given in higher doses (100 mg of chlorpromazine equals 2 mg of haloperidol [Haldol])—tend to produce more autonomic side effects; high-potency drugs such as haloperidol and fluphenazine (Prolixin) tend to produce more central side effects or extrapyramidal symptoms (EPS).

Anticholinergic side effects include dry mouth, blurred vision, tachycardia (usually reflexive), constipation, and urinary hesistance. Antiadrenergic side effects include hypotension, reflexive tachycardia, and cardiac stimulation.

Extrapyramidal symptoms include parkinson-like problems such as rigidity, tremors, bradykinesia, akathisia (a subjective complaint about the need to move), and dystonia (an impairment of muscle tone, causing alteration in posture or gait). Young males taking these drugs often experience EPS side effects. Dystonic reactions such as oculogyric crisis, a spasm of the muscles of the neck and eyes resulting in a rigid neck and eyeballs "frozen" in an upward gaze back into the head, can be frightening for the patient and caregivers. The positioning and rigidity of the neck can cause obstruction of the airway; maintaining a patent airway may be a nursing concern.

EPS side effects are caused by an upset of the acetylcholine/dopamine balance brought on by the dopamine-blocking effects of antipsychotic drugs. A balance of the two neurotransmitters is necessary for muscle tone. *Dyskinesia,* an incomplete or jerky muscle action (and yet another EPS side effect) is a major concern in adolescence. Facial muscles become motionless, and the eyes stare ahead without blinking. Although clear-headed, the child may appear dazed. *Tardive dyskinesia,* a serious side effect characterized by uncoordinated, rhythmic movement of the mouth and face, is rare in this age group. Although all the other EPS side effects mentioned are caused by disruptions in the aceytylcholine/dopamine balance, dyskinesias seem to result from a drug-caused sensitivity to dopamine. This sensitivity is irreversible in many people, usually older adults. Because dyskinesias are caused by a sensitivity to dopamine, it is not unusual for the diskinesia to be "hidden" while the patient is taking antipsychotics and to emerge once the drug is withdrawn. Some researchers (Engelhardt and Polizos, 1978) concluded that withdrawal-associated tardive dyskinesia is often reversible.

Neuroleptic malignant syndrome (NMS) is a relatively new but very serious adverse effect of antipsychotic drugs (Keltner and McIntyre, 1985). Approximately 0.5% to 1% of patients taking antipsychotic drugs develop NMS (Lazarus, 1989). NMS is characterized by severe muscle rigidity and high fever, and it frequently results in death. Should an adolescent receiving antipsychotic drugs become rigid or have a high temperature, the drug should be withheld and the physician notified at once.

Finally, sedation and weight gain are side effects of many antipsychotic drugs. Sedation is caused by depression of the CNS. Unfortunately, drowsiness can interfere with other important dimensions of therapy.

The possibilities for interactions with other drugs are numerous. Because drug abuse among adolescents is such a great concern, the nurse must be particularly careful in teaching about these interactions. Common drugs of abuse, such as alcohol and other CNS depressants, cause an increase in sedation and CNS depression. Amphetamines tend to decrease antipsychotic effects. Anticholinergic drugs, including many OTC varieties, increase the risk of anticholinergic side effects. If antipsychotics are given with lithium, a decrease in antipsychotic serum levels occurs; the antiemetic effect of the antipsychotics can mask nausea and vomiting—early signs of lithium toxicity—and the possibility of a neurotoxic reaction exists. When antipsychotic drugs are combined with benztropine (Cogentin), an anticholinergic drug used to treat and prevent EPS side effects, an increase in anticholinergic side effects and a decrease in antipsychotic effects have been reported.

Phenothiazines. As already stated, the phenothiazines were the first antipsychotic drugs on the market, and chlorpromazine was the first phenothiazine. A major drug from each of the three subclasses of phenothiazines—the aliphatics, piperidines, and piperazines—is discussed.

Chlorpromazine (Thorazine) is an aliphatic phenothiazine. If a child is agitated, too excited, or overactive, an aliphatic may be preferable because it will be more sedating than the other antipsychotics. Whether an adolescent (12 to 18 years of age) is given a prescription based on an adult dosage or a child's dosage is related to his or her physical development. Chlorpromazine is usually prescribed at 0.5 mg/kg every 4 to 6 hours and gradually increased up to an oral dosage of 50 mg to 200 mg per day for severely ill and hospitalized children. An initial dosage for a hospitalized adult might be as low as 25 mg t.i.d. and is appropriate for many older adolescents. For children requiring immediate treatment, an intramuscular (IM) dosage of 0.5 mg/kg every 6 to 8 hours as needed is appropriate. Older adolescents may require the adult dosage of 25 mg IM initially, followed by additional chlorpromazine as needed. A 12-year-old child should not receive more than 75 mg IM per day.

Thioridazine (Mellaril), a piperidine phenothiazine, is used by many clinicians. Wysowski and Baum (1989) found it to be the most widely prescribed antipsychotic during the years 1976 to 1985. The usual starting dosage is 50 to 100 mg three times per day for adults. Realmuto and others (1984) gave a mean dosage of 178 mg per day to 21 adolescent schizophrenic patients (ages 11 to 18) and found that half of them showed improvement. Because of significant sedation caused by the thioridazine, they concluded that high-potency agents may be preferable.

Trifluoperazine (Stelazine), a piperazine phenothiazine, is sometimes used to treat both schizophrenia and autistic disorders. The usual starting dosage is 2 to 5 mg twice daily for treating schizophrenia. The lowest effective dosage should be used; the manufacturer states that small or emaciated patients should be started on the lower dosage, so small adolescents should be started at a low dosage. Wolpert and others (1967) gave 13 to 20 mg of trifluoperazine per day to autistic children (ages 8 to 15) and found improvement.

Fluphenazine (Prolixin), is a piperazine commonly used in adults. Clinicians prescribe the drug and find it effective for children over 6 years of age. Werry (1978) recommends a starting dosage of 0.025 to 0.05 mg/kg up to 0.3 mg/kg per day (3 to 6 mg per day). Joshi and others (1988) found that low maintenance dosages of 0.05 mg/kg per day produced significant results.

Thioxanthenes. Thioxanthenes are structurally related to phenothiazines, but they are generally less sedating and cause fewer EPS side effects. There are only two drugs classified as thioxanthenes: thiothixine and chlorprothixene. *Thiothixene (Navane)* is used often in adults but is not recommended for children under the age of 12. For adults and children over age 12, the recommended dosage is 2 mg three times daily or 5 mg two times daily. The optimal maintenance dosage is 20 to 30 mg per day. As with the other drugs, thiothixene is still used by some clinicians in children under 12 years of age. Werry (1978) recommends an average dosage of 0.15 to 0.3 mg/kg per day for these children.

Chlorprothixene (Taractan) is not recommended for children under 6 years of age. For children ages 6 to 12, 10 to 25 mg three or four times per day is recommended. For adolescents over 12 years of age and for adults, 25 to 50 mg three or four times daily is suggested.

Butyrophenone. Haloperidol (Haldol), a high-potency antipsychotic, is structurally unrelated to the phenothiazines. Its antipsychotic use in adolescents causes significant EPS side effects compared with chlorpromazine. It is the least sedating antipsychotic. A dosage of 0.05 to 0.15 mg/kg per day is recommended for children. Joshi and others (1988) found low maintenance dosages of neuroleptics to have a significant effect. They recommend 0.04 mg/kg per day. Pool and others (1976) studied a group of adolescents with schizophrenia and found that a mean dosage of 9.8 mg per day of haloperidol was effective in reducing target symptoms. At somewhat lower dosages, haloperidol is also used to treat adolescent autism.

Dihydroindolone. Molindone (Moban) is not recommended for children younger than 12 years of age. For adults and children over the age of 12, 50 to 75 mg per day is recommended initially for psychotic episodes. Maintenance dosages for mild symptoms are usually 5 to 15 mg three or four times daily.

   Dibenzoxazepines. Loxapine (Loxitane) is not recommended for use in children younger than 16 years of age. However, Pool and others (1976) gave adolescent schizophrenics (ages 13 to 18) a mean dosage of 87.5 mg per day and found loxapine to be safe. Hallucinations, delusions, and other symptoms improved.

Nursing Implications

The nurse needs to understand the variance in bioavailability of antipsychotic drugs. The nurse should not switch to another "brand" if the patient's supply is depleted. Depending on the specific brands involved, switching could cause serum levels to become too high or too low. Compliance is a problem with adult patients and is a potential problem with adolescents. It is important for the patient to swallow the medication. If noncompliance is suspected, a liquid form may be advisable. IM injections should be given deeply because of their potential for drug-induced irritation, and the nurse should always aspirate to avoid IV administration. Contact dermatitis is not uncommon.

   Side effects. EPS effects should be reported to the physician for possible prescription of antiparkinson-anticholinergic drugs, such as benztropine (Cogentin) or trihexyphenidyl (Artane). These antiparkinson-anticholinergic drugs are effective for most EPS effects but are not effective for tardive dyskinesia. The Abnormal Involuntary Movement Scale (AIMS) is an easy-to-use tool for assessment of tardive dyskinesia.

   It should be noted that the antiparkinson-anticholinergic drugs have their own side effects and can add to the anticholinergic effects of the antipsychotic drugs. Anhidrosis, fatal paralytic ileus, exacerbation of psychotic symptoms, and a wide range of anticholinergic effects are possible adverse reactions to these drugs. Because of these potential effects, antiparkinson-anticholinergic drugs are not typically prescribed prophylactically for most age-groups. However, the incidence of EPS effects is so high in teenage boys receiving antipsychotic drugs that prophylactic use of these drugs is relatively common.

   Sedation, weight gain, and the several autonomic side effects described can be treated by dose modification. Sedation, although welcomed at times in the hyperactive child, interferes with other psychotherapeutic interventions. A switch to a less sedating drug such as trifluoperazine (Stelazine) or haloperidol (Haldol) might be required. Drowsiness and weight gain are more common. As a rule, anticholinergic side effects and antiadrenergic side effects can be reduced by dose modification. Antidopaminergic side effects can be resolved by both dose modification and antiparkinson-anticholinergic drugs. Dose modification and the consequent side effect reduction must be weighed against the resultant increase in disturbed behavior.

   Interactions. Adolescents taking antipsychotic drugs should not be given medications containing alcohol, even OTC sleeping aids and cough syrups. Assessment for drowsiness is necessary if such preparations are taken. The nurse should guard against the adolescent's ingestion of OTC anticholinergics such as cold or hay fever medications and should assess for blurred vision and constipation if these drugs are taken. Antiparkinson-anticholinergic drugs prescribed to reduce EPS effects can increase anticholinergic side effects and mask the development of tardive dyskinesia. The nurse should assess for increased anticholinergic effects and question any order combining antipsychotic drugs and lithium.

Toxicity. Deaths from antipsychotic drug overdose alone have been rarely reported in any age group. Overdose usually results in CNS depression, hypotension, and EPS effects. Treatment is symptomatic and supportive. Gastric lavage may help rid the body of unabsorbed drug. Vomiting is not induced because of the potential for dystonic reactions of the head and neck, which might compromise the ability to vomit and cause aspiration. Further information on antipsychotic overdose and treatment can be found in other texts.

Parent teaching. As with all drugs mentioned in this chapter, when the adolescent is living at home, the parents must be committed to compliance to the drug regimen. "Cheeking" of these drugs is common, and drug taking must be closely monitored by the caregiver. Parents must also have a realistic understanding of what these drugs can and cannot do for their child. Holding a frank discussion with the parents regarding side effects, what to watch for, and when to call the physician is imperative. Parents should be taught to assess for muscle rigidity, inability to sit still, vague subjective complaints (such as a "need to move"), and any abnormal involuntary movements. Parents should also be taught to monitor bowel and bladder function and to encourage appropriate fluid intake.

Parents must have permission of the physician or nurse to administer OTC medications. The nurse should be sure parents know that antipsychotic drugs are not addictive. Three general rules regarding antipsychotic medication should be taught: (1) antipsychotic drugs should not be used for nonapproved indications, (2) antipsychotic drugs should be given in the lowest effective dose for maintenance therapy because of the relationship between dose and EPS effects, and (3) adolescents should occasionally be placed on physician-approved drug-free "holidays" (Keltner, 1989).

Psychopharmacological Treatment of Depression and Mania

Depression and mania in adolescents have emerged as significant problems in the 1990s. Adolescent suicide related to depression is the topic of many articles and a source of fear for many parents. In children, depression is more easily recognized than mania is; however, as adolescence approaches, mania takes on the characteristics of the adult manic disorder and is readily detectable. The psychopharmacological treatment of these conditions is important for the psychiatric nurse to understand.

The two major antidepressant drug classes are the tricyclic antidepressants (TCAs) and the monoamine oxidase inhibitors (MAOIs). These two classes of drugs have different mechanisms for accomplishing the same neurophysiological result: an increase in catecholamine (norepinephrine, dopamine, and serotonin) availability at the receptor site. MAOIs have potentially life-threatening side effects and are not recommended for children younger than the age of 16.

TRICYCLIC ANTIDEPRESSANTS

TCAs were developed in the late 1950s and gained acceptance for treatment of childhood depression in the 1960s. Although the clinical effectiveness of TCAs in the treatment of adult depression is clear, little evidence supports the assertion that TCAs are effective in treating major adolescent depression (Puig-Antich and others, 1985).

TCAs are well absorbed from the gastrointestinal tract. The prototype TCA is imipramine (Tofranil). It is highly bound (90% to 95%) to plasma protein and is metabolized in the liver into many other compounds, some of which have their own antidepressant properties. For instance, desipramine (Norpramin, Pertofrane), another TCA, is a naturally occurring metabolite of imipramine. The metabolites of imipramine are excreted in the urine. Physical problems that would cause incomplete metabolism or interfere with excretion can prolong the half-life of imipramine.

TCAs cause both central and peripheral effects by increasing catecholamine availability at the receptor site. The most obvious central response is the *antidepressant effect*. A less obvious central effect is the sedative quality of some TCAs. Peripheral side effects are caused by the increased availability of these same neurotransmitters in the periphery. Increased levels of norepinephrine cause a sympathomimetic response — that is, tachycardia and elevated blood pressure (Table 13-2 on p. 364). TCAs are cardiotoxic, and an overdose can be fatal. Orthostatic hypotension is a common side effect in adults but is not common in adolescents.

An anticholinergic response also occurs with TCAs. All the anticholinergic side effects associated with antipsychotic drugs (including dry mouth, blurred vision, constipation, and urinary hesitance) occur with TCAs. Because of urinary hesitance, TCAs are used in the treatment of enuresis, or bedwetting. Hematological disorders caused by TCAs are not common.

TCAs interact with many other drugs. Drugs with anticholinergic properties (for example, atropine, antihistamines, antiparkinson drugs, and OTC cold and hay fever drugs) increase anticholinergic side effects. Anticholinergic effects can be serious; they include paralytic ileus and urinary retention. Phenothiazines and methylphenidate (Ritalin), psychotropic drugs previously discussed, can cause increased serum levels of TCAs. Sympathomimetics should be used cautiously. These combinations can lead to tachycardia, arrhythmias, and hypertension. CNS depressants combined with TCAs cause increased CNS depression.

The *Physician's Desk Reference (1990)*, or *PDR*, does not recommend any TCA for the treatment of depression in children younger than age 12. The recognized dosage of specific TCAs for adolescent depression is as follows:

Imipramine (Tofranil): A beginning dosage of 10 mg t.i.d. or q.i.d. is appropriate. Dosage should not exceed 100 mg per day.

Desipramine (Norpramin, Pertofrane): The usual dosage is 25 mg, one to four times per day. Dosage should be initiated at a lower level and increased according to tolerance and clinical response. A dosage of 150 mg per day should not be exceeded.

Amitriptyline (Elavil, Endep): The recommended dosage is 10 mg three times per day plus 20 mg at bedtime. This total of 50 mg is usually sufficient. Research has shown use of as much as 200 mg per day with no appreciable reduction in symptoms.

Puig-Antich and others (1985) and Martin and Agran (1988) indicate that serum

Table 13–2 Profile of Related TCAs

Drug	Sedation	Anticholinergic	Neurotransmitter primarily involved	Therapeutic plasma levels* (ng/ml)
Imipramine (Tofranil)	2+	2+	Serotonin	150-240
Desipramine (Norpramin)	1+	1+	Norepinephrine	115
Amitriptyline (Elavil)	4+	4+	Serotonin	100-300

Modified from Pomeroy J and Gadow (1986) Adolescent psychiatric disorders. In Gadow KE, editor, Children on medication, vol 2, San Diego, College Hill Press.
*Data from Puig-Antich and others (1985) and Martin and Agran (1988).

levels are the crucial variable for clinical effectiveness. Imipramine should have a serum level of 150 to 240 ng/ml, desipramine should be 115 ng/ml, and amitriptyline should have a serum level of 100 to 300 ng/ml for a therapeutic effect. As with adults, a period of 3 to 4 weeks is required before clinical improvement is noted. The maximum dosage of imipramine, desipramine, or amitriptyline is 5 mg/kg per day, according to Puig-Antich and others (1985). The *PDR* recommends that a dosage of 2.5 mg/kg per day not be exceeded.

Nursing Implications

Side effects. The nurse must assess for anticholinergic side effects, be prepared to treat symptomatically, and be on guard for anticholinergic toxicity. Dry mouth is alleviated with sugarless candies or sips of water. Good oral hygiene is important. Constipation and urinary hesitance should be monitored as well. A depressed adolescent could develop serious complications from these anticholinergic effects. Since decreased sweating occurs also, adolescents should be guarded from overheating, particularly in hot weather. High activity levels should be cautiously observed. The nurse should assess for a distended bladder or a distended abdomen. Regular measurement of vital signs to assess for elevated blood pressure and tachycardia is routine. A blood pressure greater than 140/90 and a heart rate of more than 130 beats per minute are causes for alarm (Martin and Agran, 1988). Orthostatic hypotension is rare in adolescents. Although hematological disorders are not common, abnormal bruising and bleeding, fever, and sore throat warrant a complete blood count.

Gastrointestinal symptoms such as nausea, vomiting, abdominal pain, diarrhea, and anorexia occur if these drugs are withdrawn abruptly; therefore gradual withdrawal should be practiced. An acute onset of these symptoms along with headache and flu-like symptoms may indicate a lack of compliance to the drug.

Interactions. The nurse should be aware of the many drug interactions with TCAs. Orders for drugs that potentiate anticholinergic or sympathomimetic effects or that elevate TCA serum levels should be questioned.

Toxicity. TCAs have a narrow therapeutic index; the difference between a therapeutic dose and a lethal dose is small. Adolescents are thought to be more sensitive than are adults to overdoses of imipramine. For this reason the prescribed dosage must be carefully maintained and monitored. The potential for suicide or accidental overdose demands that these drugs be kept away from younger adolescents and potentially suicidal older adolescents. Peripheral toxic effects include tachycardia and arrhythmias. Diarrhea or constipation can occur, as can urinary retention. Central toxic effects can include muscle rigidity, hyperactive reflex, sedation, ataxia, respiratory depression, and convulsions. If TCA overdose is suspected, hospitalization is required. Vomiting to rid the body of unabsorbed drug, and activated charcoal to prevent further absorption are emergency treatment measures. The nurse should monitor vital signs for heart rate and rhythm and respirations. Imipramine pamoate (Tofranil-PM) is never ordered for children and may be prohibited for most adolescents because the smallest available unit dose is 75 mg.

Parent teaching. Parents should be taught that a clinical effect takes 3 to 4 weeks to develop. Measures to provide psychotherapeutic support for the parents during this "lag time" is important. Parents must be instructed to administer the exact amount of drug carefully, to keep the drug away from the affected child or any sibling, and never to give other drugs without approval from the physician or nurse. Because adolescents are more sensitive to TCA overdose than are adults, it is important that parents follow these guidelines. In addition, parents must be given an adequate amount of information concerning side effects so that they know to report serious side effects to the nurse.

LITHIUM

Lithium was first reported for treatment of mania by Cade in 1949. Shortly after that, lithium was banned in the United States because of several deaths associated with the drug. Unaware of its low therapeutic index, a number of physicians ordered the use of lithium salt as a salt substitute for cardiac patients. Some of these patients died from lithium toxicity. When the ban was finally lifted in the late 1960s, lithium was used successfully to treat adult manic-depressive patients. Research on its effectiveness in adolescent manic depression is not as substantial.

Of all bipolar patients, 20% to 30% first experienced affective symptoms before the age of 20 (Carroll and others, 1987); Lithium, if effective, is therefore an important drug to consider for adolescent bipolar patients. Most research indicates that children tolerate lithium well (Carroll and others, 1987). Lithium decreases free thyroxine and triiodothyronine, but in euthyroid patients, thyroid-releasing hormone increases to compensate. Children should have baseline thyroid hormone levels taken (Puig-Antich and others, 1985). After the child is stabilized on the drug, monthly serum levels are adequate. A concern exists among clinicians that long-term use of lithium may cause renal damage, but research does not support this concern (Khandelwal and others, 1984). Lithium causes sodium diuresis, and the excretion of lithium is tied to sodium excretion. A decrease in sodium intake can lead to lithium toxicity (which is defined as any level greater than 1.5 mEq/L).

Lithium has been used in children younger than the age of 12 who were diagnosed as manic, but because it is not *PDR*-approved for this use, its use should be carefully reviewed with parents. Dosages of 30 to 40 mg/kg per day have been reported. The effectiveness of lithium is not clear, but best results are likely in patients who have a family history of lithium effectiveness (Carroll and others, 1987). Weller and others (1986) suggest 900 mg per day in divided doses for children weighing 25 to 40 kg, 1200 mg per day in divided doses for children weighing 40 to 50 kg, and 1500 mg per day in divided doses for children who weigh 50 to 60 kg. Puig-Antich and others (1985) recommend that adolescents be started on dosages of 300 mg per day (in divided doses), to be increased by 300 mg per day every 5 to 7 days until a favorable response is obtained. The effective serum level range is 0.6 to 1.2 mEq/L. Carroll and others (1987) found that a dosage of 30 mg/kg per day was sufficient for prepubertal children. Strober and others (1990) found that adolescents who discontinued taking lithium relapsed three times more often than those who continued their treatment.

Nursing Implications

Side effects. Side effects include weakness, tremor, weight gain, stomach ache, and blurred vision. The nurse's role is one of facilitator: helping the patient to deal with minor side effects and closely observing for effects that might indicate toxicity. Many side effects can be treated symptomatically. The nurse should measure and record vital signs at least daily, and if the child experiences tachycardia, the physician should be notified. Nausea can be minimized by giving lithium with meals, and thirst can be relieved by drinking more water. If diarrhea occurs, the adolescent should be observed closely because a loss of sodium through extraurinary routes can lead to lithium toxicity.

Interactions. The most serious interactions are with foods that increase lithium serum levels; these include most diuretics and salt substitutes, which can reduce the amount of sodium ingested, leading to increased levels of lithium. Other drugs — such as alcohol, aminophylline, antacids, caffeine, and sodium bicarbonate — decrease the serum level and should be avoided to gain a consistent therapeutic plasma level. Lithium decreases serum levels of some drugs, such as antipsychotics. Lithium and haloperidol are reported to cause neurotoxicity when used together. The nurse should monitor all drugs to decrease drug interactions.

Toxicity. Lithium has a narrow therapeutic index; consequently, frequent serum level measurements are needed. In some adolescent inpatient programs, daily blood levels are drawn. Lithium levels are at their most accurate in the morning, 8 to 12 hours after the last dose. Toxicity can be precipitated by common conditions that affect fluid and electrolyte balance: excessive sweating, diarrhea, vomiting, and decreased salt intake. There is no pharmacological antidote for lithium poisoning. Nausea and vomiting, slurred speech, and drowsiness may be early indications of toxicity (Puig-Antich and others, 1985). If toxicity is suspected, the nurse should withhold the lithium and notify the physician. Any drug that slows lithium excretion should also be withheld. Hastening lithium excretion through use of mannitol or acetazolamine is a logical treatment plan.

Parent teaching. Parents must be instructed about the signs of lithium toxicity and should be told to withhold the drug and call the physician if a toxic reaction occurs. The fact that lithium has a lag period of up to 10 days is important information for the parent living with a manic child. Medications should be given on time in the accurate prescribed dose. The parent should be instructed to prepare and serve meals in a consistent manner; in particular they must know the basics of sodium-lithium excretion (that depleted sodium will lead to excessive lithium levels and increased sodium will lead to decreased lithium levels). Because of its narrow therapeutic index, parents must carefully assess for "cheeking" and hoarding of lithium. An adolescent that hoards and takes several doses at one time can experience serious and even fatal consequences.

OTHER DRUGS

Clonidine (Catapres). Clonidine has been used successfully in the treatment of manic disorder. Zubenko and others (1984) found that 0.2 mg of clonidine twice daily was effective in relieving manic symptoms after lithium had failed to do so.

Carbamazepine (Tegretol). Lithium is the drug of choice for bipolar disorder; however, up to 40% of these patients do not respond (Wise, 1989). Carbamazepine is used in the treatment of manic disorder when lithium is ineffective. Hematological risks associated with carbamazepine include aplastic anemia and agranulocytosis (Olin, 1990). Fortunately, these adverse affects are rare (Wise, 1989). Serum levels do not guide the clinician in prescribing carbamazepine as they do for lithium. Carbamazepine dosages vary from person to person.

Special Issues

ENURESIS

Enuresis is a developmental eliminative disorder manifested by involuntary urination during sleep in children 5 years old and older. Enuresis is more common in males, and approximately 20% of enuretic children have psychiatric symptoms. A number of approaches have been used. Although behavioral approaches (for example, buzzer pads) are effective for some children, for others a pharmacological approach has been beneficial.

Imipramine (Tofranil). Imipramine is approved for enuresis in children age 6 and over. It is believed that the same anticholinergic effect that causes urinary hesitance and retention in adults is responsible for imipramine's therapeutic effect in enuretic children. In the adolescent enuretic patient, a dose up to 75 mg at bedtime is recommended. Side effects are relatively minor at this dose. At doses greater than 75 mg, side effects increase, although drug effectiveness does not. Early-night bedwetters may benefit from taking imipramine in divided doses, with the first 25 mg given in midafternoon. When it is appropriate to discontinue imipramine, amounts should be reduced slowly to avoid the tendency to relapse. Children should not be given more than 2.5 mg/kg per day. Imipramine pamoate (Tofranil-PM) may be prescribed if the total daily dose is at least 75 mg or greater and one nighttime dose is acceptable. The smallest unit dose is 75 mg; the nurse should be aware of this to avoid an administration error.

TOURETTE'S SYNDROME

Tourette's syndrome (TS) is characterized by involuntary, repetitive, purposeless muscle movements such as gyrating, hopping, clapping, and kicking, accompanied by multiple verbal tics, including screaming and coprolalia (Adkins, 1989). Coprolalia, the excessive utterance of obscene language, can progress to phrases that are filled with cursing and sexually offensive language. The condition occurs in about 40% of patients with TS. Some patients utter profanities as soon as the thoughts enter their minds, without the social restraint most people depend on; upon seeing a person with a big nose, a patient with TS might say something both obscene and offensive about the nose. Social problems can be monumental for the patient and family. Haloperidol and pimozide are the drugs used most often. Shapiro and others (1989) found haloperidol to be more effective but also to have more side effects.

Haloperidol (Haldol). The recommended dosage of haloperidol is 0.05 to 0.075 mg/kg per day for TS children younger than age 12. Shapiro and others (1989) gave a group of adolescents up to 10 mg per day. Bruun (1988) gave 4 to 7 mg per day of haloperidol to patients. Weiden and Bruun (1987) used between 1 and 6 mg per day in their study. Young and others (1985) recommend no more than 3 to 4 mg per day in divided dosages. EPS effects are significant in adolescents. Weiden and Bruun (1987) found that neuroleptic drug–induced akathisia was responsible for suicide, violent outbursts, and a worsening of TS. Since some EPS side effects, such as oculogyric crisis and tremors, are not only frightening but also embarrassing, some physicians order antiparkinson-anticholinergic agents prophylactically, so that the child will not be embarrassed at school. About 80% of the patients treated with haloperidol are helped (Young and others, 1985).

Pimozide (Orap). Pimozide is an antipsychotic drug used for managing severe motor or vocal tics in patients with TS. It is not recommended for use in children younger than 12 years of age. Clinical experience with children is limited at this time, but favorable results have been reported (Adkins, 1989). On the other hand, pimozide is used widely with adolescents. Shapiro and others (1989) gave dosages of up to 20 mg per day in their study, with significant results. They found that patients experienced fewer side effects with pimozide than with haloperidol. Brunn (1988) recommends no more than 8 mg per day of pimozide. Weiden and Bruun (1987) gave between 2 and 6 mg per day of pimozide to adolescents suffering from TS. They believe that at higher dosages, neuroleptic drug–induced side effects can be a serious treatment problem. Olin (1990) recommends an initial dosage of 1 to 2 mg per day in divided doses, then increasing every other day. Maintenance dosage should be less than 0.2 mg/kg per day or 10 mg per day, whichever is less.

Clonidine (Catapres). Clonidine is an antihypertensive, and although it is not FDA approved for use in TS, it is used by many clinicians. It is an alpha-adrenergic agonist that should be initiated at low dosages of 0.05 mg per day and slowly increased for several weeks to 0.15 to 0.30 mg per day. Dosages over 0.4 or 0.5 mg per day lead to side effects (Young and others, 1985; Gallico, 1988). Clonidine has a slower onset of action than haloperidol, taking 3 or more weeks before a therapeutic improvement is noted (Young and others, 1985). Side effects include sedation, dry mouth, and hypotension.

Miscellaneous Drugs

Carbamazepine (Tegetrol). Carbamazepine, an anticonvulsant, is used in a variety of psychiatric diagnoses, including bipolar illness, schizo-affective illness, resistant schizophrenia, and impulse-control problems. Post and others (1987) postulate that a kindling phenomenon, similar to what occurs with epilepsy, may occur in bipolar illness, thus explaining the efficacy of carbamazepine, an anticonvulsant. Carbamazepine is also used in the treatment of conduct disorders. The impulsive and angry outbursts associated with some conduct-disordered children may well respond to carbamazepine for reasons similar to (but not the same as) the reason bipolar patients are helped.

Benzodiazepines. Diazepam (Valium) is a benzodiazepine that has been used in the treatment of separation anxiety, alcohol-withdrawal symptoms, panic attacks, and seizures. It may be used when excessive anxiety occurs; however, concerns related to initiating an early life-style of coping through drugs may overrule its use. Other benzodiazepines used in adolescents are chlordiazepoxide (Librium) and alprazolam (Xanax). Side effects include sedation, disinhibition, and loss of coordination. A withdrawal reaction occurs if benzodiazepines are withdrawn too fast. Withdrawal reactions can include severe anxiety and seizures. Santos and Morton (1989) have found clonazepam (Klonopin) and lorazepam (Ativan) to be effective for managing manic agitation, although they did not specifically mention adolescent cases.

Propranolol (Inderal). Propranolol is a synthetic beta blocker thought to be effective in the treatment of panic and generalized anxiety disorders. Beeber (1989) notes that research has not substantiated these claims.

Clomipramine (Anafranil). Clomipramine is a new tricyclic antidepressant specifically intended for the treatment of obsessive-compulsive disorder (Beeber, 1989). Several studies indicate that it is effective in the treatment of obsessive-compulsive disorder in adolescents. The maximum dosage for adolescents and children is 3 mg/kg per day—up to 200 mg. Somnolence, dizziness, dry mouth, and fatigue are the most often reported side effects in children and adolescents.

Clozapine (Clozaril). Clozapine is a new antipsychotic, which was released for public use in 1990. Dramatic improvement in previously treatment-resistant schizophrenic patients has given great hope to the psychiatric community (Green and Salzman, 1990). Clozapine has the antipsychotic qualities of other neuroleptic drugs but appears to cause substantially less EPS effects. A significant and potentially fatal peripheral side effect is agranulocytosis, which occurs in 1% to 2% of patients. Because of this risk and the associated safeguards it requires, clozapine treatment costs about $9000.00 per year (Griffith, 1990) and is available only through the Clozaril Patient Management System (CPMS). Clozapine use for adolescents of 15 years and younger has not yet been established as safe and effective (Olin, 1990).

REFERENCES AND SUGGESTED READINGS

Adkins AS (1989) Helping your patient cope with Tourette's syndrome, Pediatric Nursing 15:135-137.

American Journal of Nursing (1985) In the case of ritalin, more is not better, American Journal of Nursing 85:526.

American Psychiatric Association (1987) Diagnostic and statistical manual of mental disorders, ed 3, (revised), Washington, DC, The Association.

Beeber LS (1989) Treatment anxiety, Journal of Psychosocial Nursing 27:42-43.

Bradley C (1937) The behavior of children receiving benzedrine, American Journal of Psychiatry 94:577-585.

Brown TR and Sexson SB (1989) Effects of methylphenidate on cardiovascular responses in attention deficit hyperactivity disordered adolescents, Journal of Adolescent Health Care 10:179-183.

Bruun RD (1988) Subtle and underrecognized side effects of neuroleptic treatment in children with tourette's disorder, American Journal of Psychiatry 145:621-624.

Cantwell DP (1977) Psychopharmacologic treatment of the minimal brain dysfunction syndrome. In Wiener J, editor, Psychopharmacology in childhood and adolescence, New York, Basic Books.

Cantwell DP (1985) Hyperactive children have grown up, Archives of General Psychiatry 42:1026-1028.

Carroll JA, Jefferson JW, and Greist JH (1987) Psychiatric uses of lithium for children and adolescents, Hospital and Community Psychiatry 38:927-928.

Clampit MK and Pirkle JB (1983) Stimulant medication and the hyperactive adolescent: myths and facts, Adolescence 18:811-822.

Dilsaver SC, Votolato NA, and Alessi NE (1989) Complications of phenylpropanolamine, American Family Physician 39:201-206.

Engelhardt DM and Polizos P (1978) Adverse effects of pharmacotherapy in childhood psychosis. In Lipton MA, DiMascio A, and Killam KF, editors, Psychopharmacology: a generation of progress, New York, Raven Press.

Gallico RP, Burns TJ, and Grob CS (1988) Emotional and behavioral problems in children with learning disabilities, Boston, College-Hill Press.

Gastfriend DR, Biederman J, and Jellinek MS (1984) Desipramine in the treatment of adolescents with attention deficit disorder, American Journal of Psychiatry 141:906-908.

Green AI and Salzman C (1990) Clozapine: benefits and risks, Hospital and Community Psychiatry 41:379-380.

Griffith EEH (1990) Clozapine: problems for the public sector, Hospital and Community Psychiatry 41:837.

Harsch HH and Holt RE (1988) Use of antidepressants in attempted suicide, Hospital and Community Psychiatry 39:990-992.

Joshi PT, Capozzoli JA, and Coyle JT (1988) Low-dose neuroleptic therapy for children with childhood onset pervasive developmental disorder, American Journal of Psychiatry 145:335-338.

Keltner NL (1989) Antipsychotic drugs. In Shlafer M and Marieb EN, editors, The nurse, pharmacology, and drug therapy, Menlo Park, Calif, Addison-Wesley Publishing Co, Inc.

Keltner NL and McIntyre C (1985) Neuroleptic malignant syndrome, Neurosurgical Nursing 17:362-366.

Khandelwal SK, Vijoy KV, and Murthy RS (1984) Renal function in children receiving long-term lithium prophylaxis, American Journal of Psychiatry 141:278-279.

LaGreca AM and Quay HC (1984) Behavior disorders in children. In Ender NS and Hunt JM, editors, Personality and the behavior disorders, ed 2, New York, John Wiley & Sons, Inc.

Lazarus A (1989) Neuroleptic malignant syndrome, Hospital and Community Psychiatry 40:229-230.

Lerer RJ and Lerer P (1977) Responses of adolescents with minimal brain dysfunction to methylphenidate, Journal of Learning Disabilities 10:223-228.

Martin JE and Agran M (1988) Pharmacotherapy. In Matson JL, editor, Handbook of treatment approaches in childhood psychopathology, New York, Plenum Publishing Corp.

Munoz-Millan RJ and Casteel CR (1989) Attention-deficit hyperactivity disorder: recent literature, Hospital and Community Psychiatry 40:699-707.

Olin BP (1990) Drug facts and comparisons, Philadelphia, JB Lippincott Co.

Physician's Desk Reference (1990) Medical Economics Co, Inc.

Pliszka SR (1987) Tricyclic antidepressants in the treatment of children with attention deficit disorder, Journal of the American Academy of Child and Adolescent Psychiatry 26:127-132.

Pomeroy J and Gadow KE (1986) Adolescent psychiatric disorders. In Gadow KE, editor, Children on medication, vol 2, San Diego, College-Hill Press.

Pool D, Bloom W, Mielke DH, Roniger JJ, and Gallant DM (1976) A controlled evaluation of loxitane in seventy-five adolescent schizophrenic patients, Current Therapeutic Research 19:99-104.

Post RM, Uhde TW, Roy-Byrne PP, and Joffe RT (1987) Correlates of antimanic response to carbamazepine, Psychiatry Research 21:71-83.

Puig-Antich J, Ryan ND, and Rabinovich H (1985) Affective disorders in childhood and adolescence. In Wiener JM, editor, Diagnosis and psychopharmacology for childhood and adolescent disorder, New York, John Wiley & Sons, Inc.

Realmuto GM, Erickson WD, Yellin AM, Hopwood JH, and Greenberg LM (1984) Clinical comparison of thiothixene and thioridazine in schizophrenic adolescents, American Journal of Psychiatry 141:440-442.

Safer DJ and Krager JM (1988) A survey of medication treatments for hyperactive/inattentive students, Journal of the American Medical Association 260:2256-2258.

Santos AB and Morton WA (1989) Use of benzodiazepines to improve management of manic agitation, Hospital and Community Psychiatry 40:1069-1071.

Shapiro E, Shapiro AK, Fulop G, Hubbard M, Mandell J, Nordlie J, and Phillips RA (1989) Controlled study of haloperidol, pimozide, and placebo for the treatment of gilles de la Tourette's syndrome, Archives of General Psychiatry 46:722-730.

Strober M, Morrell W, Lampert C and Burroughs J (1990) Relapse following discontinuation of lithium maintenance therapy in adolescents with bipolar 1 illness: a naturalistic study, American Journal of Psychiatry 147:457-461.

Vincent J, Varley CK, and Leger P (1990) Effect of methylphenidate on early adolescent growth, Am J Psychiatry 147:501-502.

Weiden P and Bruun R (1987) Worsening of Tourette's disorder due to neuroleptic-induced akathisia, American Journal of Psychiatry 144:504-505.

Weller EB, Weller RA, and Fristad MA (1986) Lithium dosage guide for prepubertal children: a preliminary report, Journal of the American Academy of Child Psychiatry 25:92-96.

Werry J (1978) Pediatric psychopharmacology, New York, Brunner-Mazel, Inc.

Wiener JM (1977) Psychopharmacology in childhood and adolescence, New York, Basic Books Inc, Publishers.

Wise SS (1989) Carbamazepine: treatment option for bipolar patients, Hospital and Community Psychiatry 40:123-124.

Wolpert A, Hagamen MB, and Merlis S (1967) A comparative study of thiothixene and trifluoperazine in childhood schizophrenia, Current Therapeutic Research 9:482-485.

Wysowski DK and Baun C (1989) Antipsychotic drug use in the United States—1975-1985, Archives of General Psychiatry 46:929-932.

Young JG, Leven LI, Knott PJ, Leckman JF, and Cohen DJ (1985) Tourette's syndrome and tic disorders. In Wiener JM, editor, Diagnosis and psychopharmacology of childhood and adolescent disorders, New York, John Wiley & Sons, Inc.

Zametkin AJ, Karoum F, and Rapoport JL (1987) Treatment of hyperactive children with D-phenylalanine, American Journal of Psychiatry 144:792-794.

Zubenko GS, Cohen BM, Lipinski JF, Jr, and Jonas JM (1984) Clonidine in the treatment of mania and mixed bipolar disorder, American Journal of Psychiatry 141:1617-1618.

Chapter 14

Nursing Interventions for Common Adolescent Psychiatric Problems

Linda A. Mast
Christina R. Hogarth

STANDARD V. *Intervention*

THE NURSE INTERVENES AS GUIDED BY THE NURSING CARE PLAN TO IMPLEMENT NURSING ACTIONS THAT PROMOTE, MAINTAIN, OR RESTORE PHYSICAL AND MENTAL HEALTH, PREVENT ILLNESS, EFFECT REHABILITATION IN...ADOLESCENCE, AND RESTORE DEVELOPMENTAL PROGRESSION.

STANDARD V-A. *Intervention: Therapeutic Environment*

THE NURSE PROVIDES, STRUCTURES, AND MAINTAINS A THERAPEUTIC ENVIRONMENT IN COLLABORATION WITH THE ADOLESCENT, THE FAMILY, AND OTHER HEALTH CARE PROVIDERS.

STANDARD V-B. *Activities of Daily Living*

THE NURSE USES THE ACTIVITIES OF DAILY LIVING IN A GOAL-DIRECTED WAY TO FOSTER THE PHYSICAL AND MENTAL WELL-BEING OF THE CHILD OR ADOLESCENT AND FAMILY.

STANDARD V-C. *Psychotherapeutic Interventions*

THE NURSE USES PSYCHIATRIC THERAPEUTIC INTERVENTIONS TO ASSIST ADOLESCENTS AND FAMILIES TO DEVELOP, IMPROVE, OR REGAIN THEIR ADAPTIVE FUNCTIONING, TO PROMOTE HEALTH, PREVENT ILLNESS, AND FACILITATE REHABILITATION.

STANDARD V-E. *Health Teaching and Anticipatory Guidance*

THE NURSE ASSISTS THE ADOLESCENT AND FAMILY TO ACHIEVE MORE SATISFYING AND PRODUCTIVE PATTERNS OF LIVING THROUGH HEALTH TEACHING AND ANTICIPATORY GUIDANCE.

STANDARD V-F. *Somatic Therapies*

THE NURSE USES KNOWLEDGE OF SOMATIC THERAPIES WITH THE ADOLESCENT AND FAMILY TO ENHANCE THERAPEUTIC INTERVENTIONS.

General Concepts

ACTING OUT AS OPPORTUNITY

In the adolescent therapeutic milieu, acting out and other negative behaviors of the adolescent are regarded as opportunities for therapeutic intervention rather than obnoxious situations with which the staff must deal. These can be the most opportune times for the adolescent to gain new insight and interrupt old behavior patterns. The nursing process — assessment, planning, intervention, and evaluation — is applicable to every situation. The primary nurse is responsible for gathering data from the adolescent, parents, and school. If applicable, the previous therapist, probation officer, or any other significant person in the adolescent's support system can contribute to the assessment, treatment, and aftercare process. The planning process is individualized for each adolescent's particular problems and issues and is helpful in steering the interventions of the treatment team. The treatment plan keeps the staff focused, and continued evaluation provides the change and flexibility needed in the growth and development of the adolescent.

THE FAMILY AS CLIENT

Because adolescents do not develop their problems in a vacuum, the entire family should be considered as the client base. In addition to biological and social factors, the family system probably still has an influential impact on the adolescent's attitude, judgment, problem-solving, and coping patterns. Because the adolescent is likely to return to this family system, the family will also need treatment. Once the needs of the family system have been assessed, the nurse can begin to educate the parents in consistency, fairness, natural consequences, and limit setting. The nurse also serves as a role model so that parents can learn to recognize and use firm limits and positive reinforcements. Nurse therapists begin the process of change in family therapy sessions.

CONSISTENCE, FAIRNESS, FLEXIBILITY, RIGIDITY, AND LIMIT SETTING

The art of adolescent psychiatric nursing requires balancing consistency, fairness, and flexibility against rigid structure and limit setting. Consistency is extremely important in the management of the adolescent. Part of the purpose of the treatment plan, along with providing a strategy of care, is maintaining consistency. Adolescents need to hear the same therapeutic messages and experience a similar care approach from all staff on a repeated basis before they begin integrating changed behavior. If the plan of care is not consistent and the adolescent receives different messages from different staff members, confusion can result for the adolescent. The staff can be manipulated, thus losing valuable treatment intervention time. If the primary caregiver is not consistent with the adolescent, the message may be conveyed that the caregiver is not credible and does not deserve the trust that the adolescent often seeks to give.

Additionally, the adolescent observes the staff's sense of fairness. Some adolescents will think everything the staff does or says is unfair. Each staff member needs to behave in an unbiased, unprejudiced, equitable manner that accords with the rules or limit-setting strategies of each adolescent's treatment plan. Even though the adolescent may not like the rules and limits established, if the staff is consistent and displays a sense of fairness, the adolescent will begin to trust and know what behaviors are expected.

During the assessment phase the nurse gathers data to help decide how flexible or rigid the interventions for the adolescent should be. An adolescent with poor judgment and little impulse control may need a more rigid structure than an adolescent who tends to be responsible but lacks self-confidence.

Limit setting is needed by adolescents. Limit-setting interventions are never intended to be punitive. If caregivers are seen using limit setting in this manner, staff members may be reflecting their own countertransference, lack of knowledge, or increased stress level. The nurse should respond to the adolescent with clear, firm, nonhostile reinforcement of the limits. It is best to avoid getting caught in a power struggle, because this engages the emotions of the nurse and tends to be detrimental to the therapeutic relationship (Stuart and Sundeen, 1987). The limit-setting process is described in detail in Chapters 8 and 11.

COLLABORATIVE TEAMWORK AND THE THERAPEUTIC USE OF SELF

All staff members must view themselves as part of a team. It is the various team members, with their diverse educational and life experiences, who offer creative ideas and observations of adolescent behaviors that assist in the individualization of treatment. Another important reason for team building is that these same staff members can provide each other with emotional support and constructive feedback for survival and growth in such a demanding environment. There will be times when staff members need to process and change ineffective intervention behaviors or reinforce positive ones. Ideally, all involved staff members need to support the treatment approach by sharing observations and implementing strategies, even when a staff member does not completely agree with those strategies. The psychiatric nurse must constantly assess if interventions are supported by therapeutic use of self or if interventions are guided by individual needs and agendas. Awareness of these sometimes blurred boundaries and reestablishment of professional parameters regarding the treatment approach reflect the nurse's professional growth.

SKILL DEVELOPMENT AND PROGRESSION OF GOAL SETTING

The nurse assists the adolescent to set and achieve goals, progressing from defining problems and acquiring basic communication skills; to identifying behaviors needing change, identifying feelings, and connecting feelings and behaviors; to identifying and practicing new behaviors; and finally to integrating or internalizing the new behaviors. The goal-setting process is described in detail in Chapters 8 and 11. Specific goals for each adolescent problem are described in the following sections and in the nursing care plans provided for each diagnosis.

TEACHING

Adolescents and families gain some benefit from teaching, no matter what the focus of intervention.

SOMATIC THERAPY

Medication is prescribed for many adolescent disorders. Adolescent psychiatric nurses are responsible for administering medications, evaluating their effects and side effects, teaching the adolescent and family about them, and collaborating with the psychiatrist.

Common Adolescent Behaviors and Specific Interventions

ANGER

When an adolescent uses anger or aggression for self-expression, it usually means other more appropriate ways to get needs met have not been learned. Anger and aggression (see box on p. 377) tend to be expressed by physical acting out, for instance, punching walls or other people. Adolescents may destroy their own belongings, raze their rooms, or damage others' property. It is also possible that they may turn their aggression inward and harm themselves. The anger may not be demonstrated physically. Instead, adolescents may use verbal aggression—cursing, name calling, or making threats toward perceived authority figures. When overt aggression is not acceptable, they may emotionally shut down or deny their anger. They hold in or "stuff" these feelings and cover the anger with sad, scared, or glad feelings. They may become passive-aggressive, saying they are not angry, but then undermining, sabotaging, or becoming revengeful.

Another way to display anger is through displacement. Acting out with a staff member or teacher may be more psychologically acceptable than being angry at a mother or father. It is more threatening to be abandoned by parents than by teachers; therefore teachers and staff members are safer targets. When there is failure at school, in extracurricular activities, or within the family, being angry and aggressive may be the only thing the adolescent does well. The anger or aggression may be an artifact of self-esteem. Table 14-1 on pp. 378-379 presents a nursing care plan for adolescents exhibiting aggression.

Anger and aggression can be manifested in adolescents with diagnoses such as attention deficit disorder, learning disabilities, low IQ, and mental retardation, often because of poor coping mechanisms or confusion. An organic source of aggressive outburst may be temporal lobe seizure disorder.

> ### Medical and Nursing Diagnoses Related to Anger
>
> **Medical diagnoses (DSM-III-R)**
>
> 312.   Conduct disorder
> 301.83 Borderline personality disorder
> 296.   Major depression
> V61.20 Parent child problem
> 315.   Learning disabilities
> 309.   Adjustment disorder
> 295.   Schizophrenia
> 317.   Mental retardation
> 314.01 Attention deficit hyperactivity disorder (ADHD)
>
> **Nursing diagnoses (PMH)**
>
> 4.1.2   Altered feeling state
>   4.1.2.1   Anger
> 5.3.2   Altered conduct/impulse processes
>   5.3.2.2   Aggressive behavior toward environment
>   5.3.2.5   Physical aggression toward others
>   5.3.2.6   Physical aggression toward self
>   5.3.2.6.1   Suicide attempt(s)
>   5.3.2.12   Verbal aggression toward others

The adolescent with the diagnosis of borderline personality disorder, conduct disorder, or parent-child problem may demonstrate aggression. Expressing anger may also be a learned pattern. Other diagnoses in which aggression may be a problem are adjustment disorders, depression, and schizophrenia. The most extreme expression of anger or aggression is a suicidal or homicidal attempt.

Nursing Interventions

Limit setting. During the time the adolescent is learning self-awareness and new coping skills (described in the next section), the nurse uses the limit-setting process (presented in Chapter 11) continuously throughout the work with the adolescent. Initially the nurse coaches the adolescent a great deal, but with time, the adolescent can express feelings, needs, and appropriate plans for improved control and coping.

For the extremely violent adolescent, seclusion or restraints may be necessary; if this occurs, a simple plan of what the adolescent needs to do to get out of seclusion should be developed by the nurse and shared with the adolescent.

Remediation after angry outbursts is essential. It is a valuable opportunity for the nurse to help the adolescent achieve some insight, self-awareness, feelings processing, and problem solving. This is often adolescents' most emotionally available time; it can be used for their benefit because they are usually vulnerable and open to trying another way to get their needs met.

Somatic therapy. Medication, in addition to other therapies, can help control aggressiveness, mood swings, impulsiveness, and poor concentration. The adolescent

Table 14-1 Nursing Care Plan for Adolescents Exhibiting Aggression

NURSING DIAGNOSES: Altered feeling state
Anger
Altered conduct/impulse processes
Aggressive behavior toward environment
Physical aggression toward others

GOAL: Decrease anger and aggression toward others and environment

Objectives/Adolescent Outcomes	Nursing Interventions/Adolescent Actions
1. Adolescent will not damage property or harm others during angry outbursts.	A. Place on close observation for 24 hours for his and others' safety.
	B. Adolescent will learn and follow basic unit rules; if he is unable to do this and verbal redirection is ineffective, adolescent should spend quiet time in room doing goal work.
	C. If adolescent becomes aggressive or threatening toward others or property, direct him or her verbally to the time out room. Staff member will have to escort him if he is unwilling to go on his own.
	D. If adolescent becomes extremely aggressive and above measures fail, seclusion is to be considered. To get out, adolescent must • Calm down and not threaten. • Discuss what made him angry. • Devise a plan with staff for what to do when he gets angry again (practice deep breathing; go to his room; go to the time out room).
	E. Adolescent will follow staff redirections the first time he is asked without arguing or showing aggression.
2. Adolescent will take and report side effects of medication.	A. Adolescent will initially take medicine in concentrated form, then pill form as trust is developed.
	B. Nursing staff will monitor for side effects.
	C. Staff will teach adolescent and parents the purpose of medications, their side effects, and the importance of compliance.
3. Adolescent will become aware of angry behavior patterns and their effects on family.	A. Adolescent will list and discuss with primary staff the behaviors/responses that occur when he gets angry (how anger starts, builds up, and ends).
	B. Adolescent will keep a list/journal of events/situations that make him frustrated or angry throughout the day for 2 days.
	C. Adolescent will list and discuss with staff what situations or people make him angry at school and home.
	D. Adolescent will list the consequences of his aggressive behavior and what will he gain if he gives this up.

Continued.

Table 14-1   Nursing Care Plan for Adolescents Exhibiting Aggression — cont'd

Objectives/Adolescent Outcomes	Nursing Interventions/Adolescent Actions
4. Adolescent will identify alternative coping mechanisms that are more socially appropriate.	A. Adolescent will learn and practice progressive relaxation techniques for 2 days. B. Adolescent will learn aggression release techniques and to process his feelings afterwards for 2 days. C. Adolescent and staff will write a deescalation (coping) plan (to include relaxation techniques, timing self out, and remediation) and practice five times a day for 2 days, then p.r.n. D. Adolescent will practice timing self out (in room or time out room) when agitated or when coached by staff for 2 to 3 days, then follow up with use of "I" statements.
5. Adolescent will practice and use new coping behaviors other than anger and aggression.	A. Adolescent will give hourly examples of assertiveness for 2 days. B. Adolescent will teach his parents assertiveness skills, then adolescent and family will give three examples of how they were utilized during visitation for three visits. C. Adolescent will identify situations that trigger anger at home and school and describe what he can do to deescalate himself. He will role play with staff for two days before discussing his progress with the family. D. Adolescent and family will establish house rules, consequences, and privileges — by negotiation. E. Adolescent and family will discuss anxiety and fears about returning to home or school. He will review use of coping strategies. F. Adolescent will review available support systems and role play seeking support.

may need to take medication for a few days before it takes effect and abstract goal work or complex processing can occur. If the adolescent is placed on a medication regimen, medical follow-up is warranted. Medication should be prescribed in routine doses when needed; prn medication should be avoided.

Teaching, role modeling, and therapeutic communication. The nurse also uses *teaching, role modeling* and *effective communication* with the adolescent, groups of adolescents in the milieu, and the family. The nurse will often referee interactions between the adolescent and other adolescents, between parents and adolescents, and — at times — between the adolescent and other staff with less training. Acting as arbitrator is one more way the nurse can role model basic communication techniques, deescalation, and conflict resolution.

Skill development: self-awareness. Early nursing interventions will help the adolescent maintain some degree of self-control and prevent the loss of dignity that is often felt as a result of physical restraint or time out. Adolescents must be made aware of their angry behaviors; this can be accomplished by helping them notice signs such as facial expressions and fist clenching. The daily goals should be used to increase their *self-awareness* of angry feelings. This self-awareness might be demonstrated by their writing a description of what they look like when they are angry. The nurse can coach the adolescent to become aware of his own pattern of escalation: how his angry behavior starts, builds up, and ends. For example, does he begin with pacing or clenching his teeth when he is upset? This may be followed by stomping his feet; clenching his fists; cursing; and harming himself, others, or property. The use of the anger chart (see Figure 11-1 on p. 290) is helpful in this regard.

Nurses will also want the adolescent to identify the covert aspects of passive-aggressive behaviors. The adolescent often does not realize he is being passive-aggressive, and it is important to make him aware so that he can begin to learn to recognize it. Over a period of several days, the adolescent can work on goals that require him to define and identify in himself or others occurrences of passiveness, aggressiveness, and passive-aggressiveness. Because teaching reinforces learning (Pohl, 1978), a follow-up goal could be for this adolescent to teach these definitions to his parents.

Skill development: alternative coping strategies. Besides increasing awareness, the nurse is teaching the client and family a more honest and direct method of *communication.* The adolescent and family are taught "I" statements and active listening. The family will also need to identify ways they display their anger and describe more appropriate methods for managing it. These same concepts of relaxation, time out, and methods of releasing aggression can work effectively for them.

After the adolescent has identified his angry feelings and behaviors, he needs to connect the feeling to the behaviors and identify alternative behaviors. Once the adolescent learns the scope of his angry feelings and what causes them, he can then choose some more appropriate ways of dealing with his feelings or with anger-producing situations.

Some ideas for setting goals to improve coping with feelings and situations are explained in detail in *Skillstreaming the Adolescent* (Goldstein and others, 1980). These include methods of keeping out of fights, responding to teasing, and standing up for individual rights.

Several goals can be centered around learning and practicing aggression-release and relaxation techniques. Teaching relaxation techniques such as deep breathing may help the client to regain control when agitation begins. Removing himself from stimuli for 10 or 15 minutes is another goal that could be practiced the entire day, especially if the adolescent has a significant problem with anger. Another form of aggression release is the use of the *batakkas.* These specially made padded bats are used in a private environment—with staff supervision—to strike an inanimate object to release repressed aggression. If batakkas are not available, throwing a foam ball against a wall or striking a pillow against a bed will help discharge the aggression in a similar way. Thoughts and feelings experienced during these activities must be processed afterward.

The nurse or parent can build in structured aggression-release time throughout the adolescent's day. This may consist of going to the gym and burning off built-up tensions by lifting weights or exercising.

Skill development: integrating. After the adolescent has developed some alternative coping strategies, he must practice them in the milieu, first by role playing and then by actively using the skills. The adolescent should have the opportunity to practice with his family in the milieu and during trial home and school visits if possible. Staff should encourage the adolescent to follow through with his new skills. It is much easier to behave appropriately in an environment with adequate supports than to do so at home or in school.

Supporting the family members through education is a must. They need the same tools their adolescent is being taught. Such skills may include clear communications to get needs met, limit setting, establishing house rules, and establishing age-appropriate consequences. Families may need to be taught when to access the police, court systems, probation officers, and outpatient clinics. If these agencies are concurrently involved with the client, inclusion in treatment planning and discharge planning helps prepare the client for success. Members of this additional support system will know what the client has learned, how well he can use his new skills, and what to reinforce with the adolescent when he begins to slip because of the pressures and stress of his life.

RESISTANCE AND DENIAL

Resistance is the adolescent's attempt to remain unaware of anxiety-producing aspects within herself. A patient's ambivalent attitudes toward self-exploration, in which she both appreciates and avoids anxiety-producing experiences, are a normal part of the therapeutic process (Stuart and Sundeen, 1987).

Manifestations of resistance include intensification of symptoms, acting out, superficial talk, flight into health, verbalizing correctly but not changing, persistent hopeless outlook, transference (Wohlberg, 1967), and defense mechanisms, especially denial and intellectualization.

Resistance (see box on p. 382) is usually encountered in the working phase, or middle part, of treatment. Sometimes an adolescent initially resists because of painful issues and fear of change. Chemically dependent adolescents generally practice denial, projection, and blaming.

Nurses and therapists must assess the reasons for resistance. It may be that milieu or individual and family therapy is moving too quickly and the adolescent has not had enough time to process and express feelings. Also, the primary nurse may not be skilled enough in therapeutic relationships; in this case the adolescent is really not engaged in treatment rather than resistant. Another reason may be that the treatment focus is not on target. These possibilities should be reviewed before a plan for dealing with resistance is developed. Table 14-2 on pp. 383-384 presents a nursing care plan for an adolescent exhibiting resistance and denial.

Nursing Interventions

Multidisciplinary collaboration. The multidisciplinary treatment team should plan a consistent approach for dealing with resistance. Each person's role should be

---

Medical and Nursing Diagnoses Related to Resistance/Denial

Medical diagnoses (DSM-III-R)

　　　　　Resistance occurs in any diagnosis
305.90　Psychoactive substance abuse (denial)

Nursing diagnosis (PMH)

5.5.3　Ineffective individual coping
　　　5.5.3.1　Defensive coping
　　　5.5.3.2　Ineffective denial

---

defined and clearly described in the treatment plan. Part-time staff should receive a thorough explanation. It is also important for parents to have detailed explanations of the therapeutic interventions they may witness being implemented for their child. This is an opportunity for the parents and staff to work together and for the staff to role model limit setting and teach the family about consistence, credibility, and united parenting.

Skill development and goal setting with resistance. Although resistance is met at the working phase, or behavior change point, in the skill progression, it is useful to focus the adolescent's goal setting on the identification of feelings and behaviors relative to the resistance. The nurse can help the adolescent learn about defense mechanisms by reviewing a prepared list (see Chapter 11 for a list) and determining what defense mechanism he is using, then having the adolescent develop a list of examples of these avoidant behaviors by getting feedback from staff, peers, and perhaps parents. The adolescent should then list what resistive behaviors he has a tendency to use, when they most often occur, and what is happening.

Other goals might be to focus on what the adolescent is avoiding or denying, and to deal with his fears and sadness. These goals could be simply stated: "Name three things about myself or my parents that make me sad or scared. Discuss with my primary staff three times today." As appropriate, set goals for exploring feelings—for example, fear, loss, anger, hurt, or abandonment. As the adolescent explores his feelings in difficult situations, he learns that it is alright to have these feelings and that they are bearable if he has support and ways to express the feelings. The adolescent then progresses toward setting goals for identifying ways of expressing or coping with intense feelings and for dealing with the difficult situations that produce them. Some sample skill development scenarios are available in *Skillstreaming the Adolescent* (Goldstein and others, 1980).

Other strategies. Confrontation is a technique available to nursing staff. Confronting the adolescent with the realities of his problems versus his fantasies is often necessary to temper his idealistic perceptions. To do this most effectively, the nurse must establish a relationship with the parents and gather data from them. This information helps the staff to gain a better perspective of what has transpired at home or school, and it can be used to confront the adolescent who is denying his problems.

Table 14-2   Nursing Care Plan for Resistance and Denial

NURSING DIAGNOSES: Ineffective individual coping
                     Defensive coping
                     Resistance
                     Denial

GOAL: Adolescent will identify and use coping mechanisms other than denial and resistance.

Objectives	Nursing Interventions/Adolescent Actions
1. Staff and parents will establish limits for the adolescent.	A. The nurse will establish rapport with the parents and discuss therapeutic interventions to be implemented with the adolescent that support parents' decision to continue treatment. B. The nurse will role model limit setting and educate the family about consistence, credibility, and united parenting concepts—and then coach and support the parents' use of them. C. Adolescent will identify why he is in the program. D. Assign staff to confront the adolescent with the reality that his problem is an unrealistic perception; the primary nurse must be supportive of the adolescent E. Primary nurse will assist the family to identify appropriate limits, rules, and privileges for use at home.
2. Adolescent will increase his awareness of how and when he uses denial/resistance and will begin to verbalize real feelings.	A. Adolescent will learn and review with staff a list of defense mechanisms. B. Adolescent will identify which defense mechanism he uses and also get feedback from three peers, staff, and parents. C. Adolescent will list journal resistive behaviors he uses, identify when he uses them, and describe what is he attempting to avoid. D. Discuss with the primary nurse or staff three times a day his feelings of fear, loss, anger, hurt, or abandonment (for 4 days).

Continued.

When strong confrontation is to be used, the confronters and supporters on the staff are established ahead of time. The staff member may confront the adolescent frequently when specific behaviors are noted, may participate in very confronting role plays with the adolescent, or might insist on repetitive goal activity such as hourly reviews. Confrontation may be used by several staff members during the day. At least one primary caregiver should be supportive of the confrontation but also supportive of the adolescent. The confrontation should not be intimidating or punitive.

Psychodrama and Gestalt therapy techniques can be very effective in working through resistance. These techniques are usually reserved for the nurse therapist or

Table 14-2   Nursing Care Plan for Resistance and Denial—cont'd

Objectives	Nursing Interventions/Adolescent Actions
3. Adolescent will identify alternative coping mechanism to deal with fear and anxiety.	A. Adolescent will practice relaxation techniques—imagery and deep breathing—four times a day to lower anxiety. B. Adolescent will make "I" statements and practice at least once every hour for 2 days. C. Adolescent will utilize the "empty chair" technique to express fears and anger.
4. Adolescent and family will use skills they have learned and establish post-discharge support systems and plans.	A. Adolescent will role play expressing sad or scared feelings with staff prior to sharing with his family. B. Adolescent will review with his family various defense mechanisms, and have them identify which they use. C. Adolescent will teach his family assertiveness and use of "I" statements. Each member will practice using them four times while visiting. D. Primary nurse will reinforce and support parents in being patient, firm, and consistent with the adolescent, and develop other support systems such as Toughlove, outpatient family therapy, and use of school counselor. E. The nurse will review the legal support system and its therapeutic usefulness and also parental guilt feelings associated with the use of this support.

other therapists, but staff nurses who have training and experience may use them with supervision. The "empty chair" technique allows the adolescent to address the person he fears in a soliloquy. This feared person is imagined in an empty chair placed in front of the adolescent. The "two chair" technique is used for the adolescent to play the part of two aspects of himself, that is, old self and emerging self, or to play the part of himself and someone else.

Paradoxical injunction is another technique available to the staff. This technique is not explained to the adolescent and usually not to the family. The adolescent is directed to increase or practice the resistant behavior. For instance, if the adolescent is engaging in silly, distracting behavior, then he is to have a goal of being silly for 15 minutes per hour all day. The result is that the adolescent thinks this is ridiculous and stops the behavior or tires of it and begins to focus on other things. This method is widely used in family therapy.

Isolation is another technique. It consists of isolating the adolescent in his room except for school, goals group, and psychotherapy sessions. During the isolated time, the adolescent has to meet goals regarding his resistance. The adolescent should be placed on close observation (every 15 minutes). This is a last-effort technique and should be viewed as special treatment. It is not really an aversive technique but is very close. Being in isolation for 1 or 2 days should produce the heightened affect needed to mobilize the young person through his resistance.

Family interventions. Parents experience resistance themselves, as well as noticing it in their adolescent. Many parents deny the seriousness of their child's problems. Denial protects parents from experiencing sadness, disappointment, embarassment, or guilt about their child's illness or failure to do well. Other families are not able to change their parenting and communication skills because some defense mechanism interferes. The family therapist may use all of the techniques noted in this section to help a resistant family or family member. During the time the therapist works with the family, the nurse supports the adolescent and the family. The primary nurse may also directly intervene by teaching the family about the adolescent's disorder, encouraging the family to remain in treatment, and serving as cofacilitator in multifamily groups and in family sessions.

The nurse assists parents by teaching about their adolescent's resistance and defense mechanisms. Hearing an explanation of the intensified treatment for their adolescent will reassure them. As the family observes the staff working with the adolescent, the staff role models patience, firmness, consistence, caring, and commitment.

MANIPULATION AND SPLITTING

Manipulation is controlling the behavior of others to achieve one's own purposes. The adolescent and his family both use several types of behavior to get their needs met, either knowingly or unknowingly. The adolescent often learns inappropriate manipulation skills from others. Usually the manipulative behavior is based on a history of not getting needs met through direct expression. Manipulation requires someone to be manipulated. The person being manipulated is naive, uninformed, vulnerable, or wants to be liked or needed by the adolescent.

Manipulative behaviors include aggression toward others; for example, the adolescent may threaten physical harm if his demands are not met. Intimidation, placing guilt, and suicidal gestures are ways to control others when parents and staff set limits the adolescent considers undesirable. Other manipulative behaviors, verbal or nonverbal, can include withdrawal or a display of passivity. For example, an adolescent may agree to communicate and problem solve as long as certain issues are not discussed. Some teens will use "people pleasing" to keep staff or parents from pursuing more sensitive or difficult feelings or to obtain desires. Adolescents sometimes charmingly persuade or negotiate favors.

Splitting is viewing people and situations as either all good or all bad, and failing to integrate personal positive and negative qualities. Splitting (see box on p. 386) is an unconscious mechanism that is one of the hallmarks of the borderline personality disorder. The borderline adolescent quickly establishes intense, clinging relationships with persons who are identified as "all good," and forms highly charged, rejecting relationships with persons identified as "all bad." On an inpatient unit, this has the effect of polarizing staff opinions about the adolescent, with staff and clients beginning to argue and disagree so that the milieu is disturbed and the borderline adolescent intensifies efforts to validate the "good me" or "bad me." Although splitting is not a conscious manipulation, the effect is the same. A staff or family being "split" becomes focused on the adolescent and his good or bad behaviors. When a borderline adolescent becomes focused on "bad me" or fears the loss of a "good" person, he may hurt himself. A very manipulative adolescent rarely hurts himself

---

Medical and Nursing Diagnoses Related to Manipulation/Splitting

Medical diagnoses (DSM-III-R)

301.83   Borderline personality disorder
312.   Conduct disorder
V61.20   Parent child problem
304.90   Psychoactive substance dependence

Nursing diagnoses (PMH)

    5.5.3   Ineffective individual coping
        5.5.3.1   Defensive coping
    5.4.2   Altered family processes
        5.4.2.1   Disabled

---

except through lack of growth, self-responsibility, and intimacy with others.

Individuals diagnosed with borderline personality disorder, conduct disorder, chemical dependence, or parent-child problem will often use manipulative behaviors. Table 14-3 presents a nursing care plan for an adolescent exhibiting manipulation and splitting.

Nursing Interventions

Limit setting and surveillance. As soon as manipulative behavior or splitting is assessed, it is essential to maintain staff-to-staff and staff-to-parent bonds of communication. Consistence must be practiced, and staff members must establish clear guidelines to set limits on the adolescent's behaviors. Very clear instructions should be given to the adolescent, and rigid limits must be maintained. These limits can be altered in accordance with the adolescent's appropriate behavior changes. The adolescent who is splitting or manipulating needs a structured schedule with one-to-one sessions scheduled frequently through the day and evening. In this way the adolescent's needs for attention and caring are met appropriately, anxiety is reduced, and trust develops.

In the milieu the adolescent should be assigned only one primary caregiver and one associate on the alternate shift. The adolescent should always be referred to the same person to get questions answered or needs met. Part-time staff or other staff will also have one person, the adolescent's primary caregiver, to refer to if the adolescent attempts manipulation. Throughout the assessing, planning, and implementation phases of treatment, the staff should frequently and candidly share perceptions of the adolescent's behavior and treatment plan information with parents. This approach helps prevent the parents from being manipulated (turned against the staff) by the adolescent and teaches parents how to confer, share, and plan together and set limits for their child once the child returns home.

Skill development. As the manipulative behavior is reduced by structure and teamwork, the adolescent can begin the process of identifying problems in his life, developing self-awareness, identifying and connecting feelings and behaviors,

Table 14-3 Nursing Care Plan for Manipulation/Splitting

NURSING DIAGNOSIS: Ineffective individual coping
         Defensive coping (manipulation, splitting)

GOAL: Decrease adolescent's manipulation/splitting behaviors and increase direct expression to get needs met.

Objectives	Nursing Interventions/Adolescent Actions
1. Adolescent will have limited opportunity to manipulate and split staff and parents.	A. Adolescent will utilize primary staff to get needs met. B. The nurse will collaborate frequently with the parents regarding course of treatment to minimize splitting. C. Staff members will redirect the adolescent to primary staff PRN. D. Nursing staff will redirect the adolescent to his room when he is manipulating and ask him to examine and identify the inappropriate behavior.
2. Adolescent (with staff assistance) will explore current method of getting needs met.	A. Adolescent will record the times he has manipulated each hour and ask staff to give input also. B. Adolescent will list what he gains and loses because of manipulation/splitting. C. Adolescent will interview staff and parents to get feedback on how they perceive his manipulation/splitting. D. Adolescent will discuss with the primary nurse fears and disappointment of not getting needs met. E. Adolescent will identify when others manipulate and split and review alternative behaviors.
3. Adolescent will use alternative methods to get needs met.	A. Adolescent will learn basic communication skills: "I" statements and active listening. B. The nurse will teach relaxation techniques and have adolescent practice them every hour; he will do the same for frustration, as needed. C. The nurse will identify and confront the adolescent's manipulative behaviors and have the adolescent use direct methods of communication. D. Adolescent will identify age-appropriate rules and privileges; the nurse will determine if these are realistic. E. Adolescent will interview other (similar-age) peers regarding rules and privileges in their homes.
4. Adolescent and family will learn and integrate skills they will need after discharge to maintain gains made.	A. Primary nurse will educate the parents regarding the importance of collaborating, supporting each other and presenting a united front as parents. B. The nurse will role model and assist the parents to learn problem solving techniques. C. Adolescent will identify and list times he has gotten needs met without manipulating. D. Adolescent and family will process follow-up strategies to maintain gains. E. Adolescent and family will discuss fears regarding discharge.

identifying alternatives, and practicing new skills. With the adolescent who is not borderline, some of the strategies for dealing with resistance, especially repeated confrontation, may be used to facilitate treatment. The borderline adolescent's goal setting should focus on behavioral aspects unless the therapist and psychiatrist believe it is appropriate to deal with the underlying emptiness, rage, and fear of abandonment at this time. Goals aimed at developing relaxation and practicing self-soothing activities may be helpful.

Somatic therapy. Medication may be prescribed for the borderline adolescent's associated depression or for severe anxiety and acting out. In these cases, adolescent care measures are instituted.

Teaching. The nurse can assist parents to recognize when splitting or manipulation is happening. The parents should be encouraged to participate in problem solving together. This may help them to remedy any confusion, guilt, or anger the adolescent is creating by the splitting behavior. The parents may need help to pursue therapeutic goals by continuing in family therapy, particularly when their child is being manipulative.

SELF-MUTILATION

Depending on the level of frustration, anger, sadness, or manipulation that causes them, self-inflicted wounds can be minor or devastating. Self-mutilation can be a minor occurrence of superficial scratching and tattooing or may be as extreme as a stab or gunshot wound. There may be a history of self-imposed fractures, bruises, or cigarette burns. Unusual risk-taking, resulting in injuries, may be a form of self-mutilation. Head banging is another type of self-mutilating behavior that may be witnessed in the angry adolescent of average intellect or the adolescent with low intellectual functioning.

Diagnoses most commonly associated with these self-mutilating behaviors (see box) are borderline personality disorder, conduct disorder, and autism. Caregivers may witness these behaviors in autistic youths, as well as in mentally retarded youths. Table 14-4 presents a nursing care plan for self-mutilating adolescents.

Medical and Nursing Diagnoses Related to Self-Mutilation

Medical diagnoses (DSM-III-R)

301.83   Borderline personality disorder
312.   Conduct disorder
299.   Autistic disorder

Nursing diagnoses (PMH)

5.3.2   Altered conduct/impulse processes
      5.3.2.6   Physical aggression toward self

Table 14-4   Nursing Care Plan for Self-Mutilation

NURSING DIAGNOSES: Altered conduct/impulse processes
Physical aggression toward self (self-mutilation)

GOAL: Adolescent will not inflict harm on himself and will learn alternative coping
methods.

Objectives	Nursing Interventions/Adolescent Actions
1. Adolescent will remain safe and not inflict harmful action upon himself.	A. Adolescent will be placed on close observation, maintain close proximity to primary staff, and participate in frequent one-to-one sessions. B. The nurse will physically assess the adolescent for current injuries; record injuries on a body map for comparison against future self-infliction. C. Staff will conduct initial and periodical search of the adolescent's belongings/environment. D. Staff will use a matter-of-fact approach when setting limits on the adolescent's harmful actions. E. Staff will implement natural consequences such as tetanus injection for self-tattooing or appropriate cleansing/disinfecting of wounded area. F. Adolescent and primary staff will explore and write a list of acceptable and unacceptable behaviors and resulting consequences.
2. Adolescent will take medications as prescribed, and learn and report side effects.	A. Observe the adolescent for 30 minutes after medication to avoid hoarding of medications. B. Adolescent will learn side effects and possibilities of organ damage because of overdose. C. Staff will monitor the adolescent for response to chemotherapy as verification of ingestion.
3. Adolescent will begin to manage/control self-harming acts through increased self-awareness.	A. Adolescent and staff will establish a no-harm contract: "I will not do harm to myself today and will check in with my primary staff every hour." B. Adolescent will extend no-harm contract to a written agreement of no-self-harm for 1 day, then 3 days, then 1 week. C. Adolescent will begin to understand why he is in the program. The adolescent will interview primary nurse, family therapist, and parents. D. Adolescent will begin to identify and list feelings and behaviors that result in harming himself, and to discuss them with primary staff. E. Adolescent will identify situations that make him sad, scared, and angry at the unit, at school, and at home; review these with primary staff. F. Adolescent will list behaviors that occur when he is angry, sad, scared, frustrated, or disappointed.

Continued.

Table 14-4   Nursing Care Plan for Self-Mutilation — cont'd

Objectives	Nursing Interventions/Adolescent Actions
3. Adolescent will begin to manage/control self-harming acts through increased self-awareness — cont'd.	G. Adolescent will list gains and losses because of self-harming behaviors, focusing on decreased trust, judgement, and decision making abilities resulting in fewer privileges. H. Adolescent will interview his parents regarding their feelings when he hurts himself, then have him discuss this with his primary nurse.
4. Adolescent will explore and practice alternative means of communicating and coping.	A. Adolescent will learn definitions of behavior that is passive, passive/aggressive, and aggressive (toward self). The nurse will help adolescent to identify which behavior he uses and what triggers it. B. Adolescent will learn "I" statements to get his needs met and will give one example every hour and review these needs with the primary nurse. C. Adolescent will examine unrealistic expectations and develop a list of realistic expectation of parents, school authorities, etc. D. Adolescent will review other sources of support such as teachers, ministers, and relatives. E. Adolescent will identify alternative acceptable behaviors. The nurse will encourage him to substitute these actions for self-harm.
5. Adolescent will integrate and implement new coping methods and behaviors.	A. Adolescent and primary nurse will identify anticipated difficulties at home and school. B. Adolescent will role play difficult situations with nurse. C. Adolescent will contact identified support persons by phone or letter and discuss what kinds of support he needs. D. Adolescent will role play asking for help as the staff slowly withdraws boundaries and support.

Nursing Interventions

Limit setting and surveillance. Initially this adolescent should be placed on close observation until the extent and degree of mutilating behaviors can be assessed. It is wise to keep this adolescent in close physical proximity to staff and schedule frequent one-to-one interactions. Further precautions should be implemented, such as initial and periodic searches of his belongings and environment. This adolescent will sometimes hoard or hide items with which to hurt himself later. The adolescent should be observed for signs of writing on himself or disfiguring and destroying his clothes. The nurse will need to give clear instructions on acceptable and unacceptable behaviors. Staff should avoid giving increased inappropriate attention to the adolescent when he is self-mutilating; they must be matter-of-fact and set limits. It is good for the adolescent to know natural consequences will follow his harmful actions. These might consist of treatment interventions such as tetanus injections, if appropriate; cleansing or soaking the injured area; or antibiotic therapy. If the adolescent is inflicting physical harm on himself and is unable or unwilling to stop the behavior, restraint methods may be implemented.

Somatic therapy. The adolescent will need to be assessed for medication therapy. Purpose and side effects should be explained to the adolescent and his parents. This adolescent must be observed for response to medication; if there is no response, it must be determined if the adolescent is cheeking, hoarding, or throwing out his medication.

Therapeutic relationships. Because self-mutilating behavior is usually indicative of borderline personality disorder, the nurse should carefully structure the adolescent's care with frequent scheduled one-to-one sessions. This reduces the anxiety associated with the fear of abandonment. Because of this adolescent's tendency to cling, split, rage, and cause self-harm, the primary nurse needs support from the staff.

Skill development: self-awareness and problem definition. Initial goal setting will be fulfilling a no-harm contract: "I will not do any harmful actions toward myself today, and I will check in with my primary staff every hour." If this goal is accomplished, then a verbal or written agreement not to harm himself for the next 3 days or 1 week can be made. When this harmful behavior has been stabilized, goal setting can focus on identifying why he is in the treatment setting. After the adolescent determines what problems he has, he should begin to identify the feelings and behaviors that lead to hurting himself. Goals could include listing what behaviors he resorts to when he is sad, angry, frustrated, or not getting his needs met. The adolescent needs to list situations that make him sad, mad, glad, and scared at home or in school and describe what he does when they occur.

Skill development: developing insight; identifying and practicing alternative behaviors. Because the self-mutilating adolescent is usually borderline, identifying and making connections between feelings and behaviors may lead to increased anxiety and acting out. In a short-term treatment setting, nursing interventions should be kept behaviorally focused rather than insight oriented, unless the child's therapist and psychiatrist believe that it is appropriate to begin insight-oriented work. Normally this is a time-consuming process dealt with in outpatient therapy.

Some insight-oriented strategies that do not deal directly with the fear of emptiness and abandonment are listed here:

- Ask the adolescent what he gains or loses when he uses self-harm for coping.
- Help him learn that he loses others' trust and respect for his judgment and decision-making capabilities.
- Ask the adolescent to list nonharmful ways to get his needs met.
- Reinforce basic "I" statements and have the client role play using them; then have him practice using them with staff and peers.
- Help the adolescent identify what he really wants from his family or school; decide together if it is realistic.
- Have the adolescent describe his parent's behaviors when he hurts himself.
- Ask the adolescent to list what he can expect from his parents and what he cannot expect.
- Have the adolescent list and investigate other sources of support, such as

teachers, coaches, ministers, relatives, and neighbors.
- If the self-mutilation is related to lack of self-identity, ask the adolescent to make lists of his likes and dislikes, how he is now, and what he wants to be like.

Skill development: integration. By this stage of treatment the staff will be fairly familiar with the family dynamics and can set up role-playing goals. The adolescent should make a list of anticipated difficulties at home or school, then role play these difficult situations with his primary staff. The adolescent's outpatient support system should be coordinated by the outpatient therapist or school nurse or counselor to maintain gains made and prevent splitting and regression.

RUNNING AWAY

Adolescents run away as an escape from an environment that is perceived to be dangerous. This behavior is often a "scared" reaction. It is usually early in hospitalization or programing, when fear is most prevalent, that runaway behavior occurs. If running away is a usual coping reaction for the adolescent, the nurse will need to reevaluate or set specific objectives to deal with such behavior. Runaway behavior is increasingly likely whenever the adolescent faces additional stress, as in family therapy or because of an abrupt change in status, such as foster care or long-term placement.

Cues the nurse should be aware of include the following:
1. The adolescent may sleep in his clothes so that he is prepared to run.
2. The adolescent may appear very vigilant or suspicious of staff and be observing program routines and patterns to plan his exit.
3. Other adolescents in the program may warn staff of the adolescent's intent to run because the adolescent may boast about his plans.
4. Runaway adolescents may encourage other peers to run with them. (It would be wise therefore for the nurse to assess the adolescents most susceptible to this type of peer pressure.)

Several diagnoses predict runaway behavior (see box on p. 393). Frequently, the adolescent diagnosed with conduct disorder makes attempts to run away. This individual is usually defiant enough and has enough street savvy to succeed. The adolescent with a borderline personality disorder also makes frequent attempts at running away and may have to be physically stopped. The adolescent diagnosed as having a dependent personality, if placed in a setting away from home, will tend to return to his own home, a relative's home, or a friend's house. The adolescent suffering from anxiety disorder usually runs away to cope with the intense anxiety. Adolescents who are being abused verbally, physically, and sexually may run away from home but might not run from a properly managed treatment facility. Table 14-5 on p. 394 presents a nursing care plan for a runaway adolescent.

Nursing Interventions

Limit setting and surveillance. A clear orientation to programing is very helpful to this adolescent; it decreases fear of the unknown and sets up basic expectations. By letting the adolescent know he will be placed on close observation and what he has to do to get off of it, a "no surprises" environment is created that allows for a trusting relationship. The nurse must assess where the adolescent might run (to grandparents,

---

Medical and Nursing Diagnoses Related to Runaway Adolescents

Medical diagnoses (DSM-III-R)

312.   Conduct disorder
301.83 Borderline personality disorder
30.60   Dependent personality
300.   Anxiety disorders
Running away can be associated with many other diagnoses

Nursing diagnoses (PMH)

5.3.2   Altered conduct/impulse processes
        5.3.2.8 Running away
4.1.2   Altered feeling state
        4.1.2.1 Anxiety
        4.1.2.5 Fear

---

boyfriend, or girlfriend) and keep this adolescent in close physical proximity to staff, near the nursing station or office, to help prevent the opportunity for running. Giving this adolescent geographical limits (limiting his space) or placing him in "time out" reduces the potential for running away. Seclusion is certainly the most restrictive method of maintaining safety and should be used only as a last effort to contain the individual.

The adolescent is less likely to run away if he has to turn in his shoes. If the adolescent still attempts to run, then clothing should be confiscated and replaced with hospital gowns and slippers. This intervention should be instituted only after the adolescent has broken staff trust by attempting to run away. The nurse should increase restrictions only as behavior warrants. If this adolescent is being especially resistant, hostile, and unable to practice even minimal active listening skills, then the development of a behavioral contract may be helpful. The contract should include expected behaviors:

1. Adolescent will not attempt to run away.
2. Adolescent will follow all program rules.
3. Adolescent will use basic communication skills of "I" statements or active listening to express himself rather than running away.
4. Adolescent will accomplish daily goals.
5. Adolescent will process goal work every 2 hours with staff.

The contract should also state what the adolescent will earn. He may earn 10 minutes in his room every 2 hours if he completes a designated amount of goal work. (This would be applicable if the treatment plan called for close proximity to staff at all times; if the adolescent is restricted to his room he might earn 10 minutes out of his room.) If the adolescent is able to follow the contract for 24 hours, he may begin to earn street clothing to wear instead of pajamas. Staff should gradually return the personal clothing, based on the degree of cooperation, communication, processing, and trust.

Table 14-5 Nursing Care Plan for the Runaway Adolescent

NURSING DIAGNOSES: Altered conduct/impulse processes
                     Running away

GOAL: Adolescent will not run away as a method of dealing with his problems.

Objectives	Nursing Interventions/Adolescent Actions
1. Adolescent will follow unit rules and individual contract rather than run away.	A. Place the adolescent on close observation for 24 hours and reevaluate daily. B. Remove shoes and coats from his possession when he threatens to run. C. After runaway attempt, give the adolescent only hospital pajamas; he may earn his clothing back based on the behavior contract as trust and safety increase. Behavior contract specifies: • Adolescent must not attempt to run. • Adolescent will follow rules. • Adolescent will work on daily goal. D. Nurse will have frequent one-to-ones to process goal work and assess runaway status.
2. Adolescent will take medications and report side effects.	A. Nurse will observe the adolescent for side effects. B. Adolescent will learn side effects, and the importance of compliance.
3. Adolescent will explore feelings that have led to runaway behavior.	A. Adolescent will list the times he has run away in the past, identify what was happening at the time, and discuss this with his primary nurse. B. Adolescent will explore mad, sad, and scared feelings related to school, home, and parents and discuss them with his primary staff. C. Adolescent will learn relaxation techniques. D. Adolescent will explore and describe personal feelings and make a chart connecting feelings with resulting behavior. E. Adolescent will learn basic communication skills of "I" statements and active listening. The nurse will encourage the adolescent to use them every hour with staff or in therapy group. F. Provide positive reinforcement when the adolescent uses appropriate communication skills and makes good judgments.
4. Adolescent will explore appropriate and alternative behavior to deal with stress.	A. Adolescent will monitor himself against the anger/feelings chart and begin to implement relaxation techniques to gain control. B. Adolescent will identify three or four stressful situations and role play using his new skills to cope and get his needs met. C. Adolescent will explore support systems and establish "parent approach" persons he can turn to when he is extremely stressed. D. Adolescent will contact his support system members and establish "safe houses" to go to.

Therapeutic relationships. During the contract phase, or high-risk phase, the primary nurse should have frequent one-to-one contact to develop the bonding necessary for trust and therapeutic communication. This type of adolescent should have limited time to isolate himself so that he does not have time to plan to run away or to nurse his anger. He should be encouraged to participate in all group activities (except perhaps recreational therapy outings, at least until trust is established).

Somatic therapy. Another consideration for the nurse to assess and monitor is the use of medications. Often adolescents who run away are depressed or suffering the effects of abuse. Drug management can decrease anxiety, reduce depression, and increase the adolescent's ability to process his thoughts and feelings.

Skill development. The adolescent who runs away during the time he is being maintained on a tight contract for runaway behavior should identify what feelings and situations lead to this behavior. As the adolescent begins to develop insight, some very painful issues of abuse may arise that should be dealt with in individual and family therapy. During therapy the adolescent can also develop skills for dealing with his feelings. Appropriate expression of feelings and needs can replace the adolescent's runaway behavior.

Health teaching. The adolescent who has been abused, is sexually promiscuous, or is living "in the streets" may have health problems related to these activities. Sexually transmitted diseases, hemorrhoids, untreated infections, and mononucleosis are typical in these adolescents.

SUICIDAL ADOLESCENTS

Behavior can be overt, such as verbally expressing a desire to kill himself, exhibiting suicidal gestures, or giving away cherished objects and belongings. The family or staff members may also notice more covert actions such as the adolescent's writing letters or poems that deal with death or have themes of "everlasting peace" or "escape." Even if the adolescent with a suicide-related diagnosis (see box on p. 396) is in a safe environment such as an inpatient unit, the nurse must be vigilant during periods of sudden brightness after a depressive episode. It is usually during this "brighter" affect when the adolescent has more energy to follow through on suicidal plans. The nurse should observe for increased isolative behaviors or verbal cues the adolescent might express.

Suicide attempts or gestures are most likely to occur in the adolescent who is diagnosed with depression, bipolar disorder, unipolar disorder, histrionic or borderline personality disorder, conduct disorders, or chemical dependence. Table 14-6 on pp. 397-398 presents a nursing care plan for a suicidal adolescent.

Nursing Interventions

Limit setting and surveillance. When the adolescent is assessed to be a suicidal risk, the nurse will immediately establish a safe environment. The adolescent should be placed on close or constant observation and his room assignment should be moved closer to the nursing station for continuous observation. Contracting with the adolescent to not harm himself for 24 hours and to seek out staff when suicidal thoughts occur is a method of controlling impulses. The nurse assesses the adolescent's degree of impulsiveness and should be aware of sudden changes in affect, either brighter or more depressed. The adolescent's belongings must be

---

Medical and Nursing Diagnoses Related to Suicidal Clients

Medical diagnoses (DSM-III-R)

296.	Major depression
296.6	Bipolar disorder
296.2	Unipolar disorder
301.50	Histrionic
301.83	Borderline personality disorder
312.	Conduct disorder
304.90	Psychoactive substance dependence

Nursing diagnoses (PMH)

8.1.2   Altered meaningfulness
      8.1.2.1   Helplessness
      8.1.2.2   Hopelessness
5.3.2   Altered conduct/impulse processes
      5.3.2.6   Physical aggression toward self; suicide attempts
4.1.2   Altered feeling state
      4.1.2.6   Grief
      4.1.2.7   Guilt
      4.1.2.8   Sadness

---

searched when he is admitted and on a periodic basis. The family and adolescent should know the purpose for these interventions.

Building self-esteem and therapeutic relationships. The nurse must convey the idea that the adolescent is a valuable person and that keeping him safe is a priority. The nurse should model a caring attitude and communicate to the adolescent and his family that their situation is being taken seriously; this begins the process of a bonding relationship between the adolescent and staff. This approach also supports direct and immediate participation of the family. Frequent one-to-one interactions, good eye contact, and gentle touching reinforce the adolescent's feelings of importance. The staff should confront suicidal gestures or ideation directly.

Skill development: self-awareness. Initial goals should focus on identifying feelings. Making lists of sad thoughts and feelings or hurtful incidents and what the adolescent wanted to happen instead are helpful ways to begin to reduce helplessness and gain some control. It is very helpful to have the adolescent process hourly with his primary nurse so that he feels support and the nurse is able to assess suicidal thoughts and plans carefully. The adolescent needs support to get through his emotional pain and must realize that he is not alone and is still accepted by staff. Connecting the suicidal thoughts and behaviors with feelings and events will help the adolescent develop insight into how his depression developed.

Skill development: alternative coping skills. As the adolescent uses and practices "I" statements, he becomes more aware of what he needs and wants. Then daily goals focus on how he can get what he wants or needs in a safe and appropriate manner.

Table 14-6   Nursing Care Plan for the Suicidal Adolescent

NURSING DIAGNOSES: Altered conduct/impulse processes
Physical aggression toward self
Suicide attempts

GOAL: Adolescent will not make suicide attempts and will develop alternative coping mechanisms.

Objectives	Nursing Interventions/Adolescent Actions
1. Adolescent will remain safe from harming himself.	A. Adolescent will be placed on close observation and staff will monitor isolating behaviors.
	B. Staff will assess adolescent impulse to harm self.
	C. Staff will perform initial and periodic searches of the adolescent's belongings and environment.
	D. Adolescent and staff will establish a verbal or written contract not to harm himself. Nurse will assess progress and renew contract every 24 hours.
	E. Adolescent will be maintained close to the nursing station or a staff member until the threat of suicide subsides.
	F. Staff will educate the family regarding what items *not* to bring into the milieu and how to create a safe home environment.
	G. If the adolescent takes medication, nurse will monitor him about ½ hour afterward to ensure that he is not cheeking and hoarding medication.
	H. Educate adolescent and family regarding purpose and side effects of medication.
2. Adolescent and family will verbalize awareness of illness and adolescent's pattern of self-harm.	A. Adolescent will write out thoughts, feelings, and behaviors that led to a past suicide attempt; review this with the primary staff.
	B. Adolescent (with staff support) will share and discuss the list with his family.
1. Adolescent will feel safe and supported in current environment.	A. Ensure that the adolescent maintains close proximity to primary staff and receives frequent one-to-one therapy and positive support.
	B. Adolescent will seek out a primary staff member every hour to discuss his moods and feelings of the previous hour.
	C. Adolescent will take his medication as ordered by the physician.
	D. Adolescent will learn relaxation techniques and to use them when dealing with difficult feelings.
	E. Adolescent will learn basic communication techniques such as "I" statements, and focus on sad, scared, and mad feelings.

Continued.

Table 14-6 Nursing Care Plan for the Suicidal Adolescent — cont'd

NURSING DIAGNOSES: Altered meaningfulness
Helplessness
Hopelessness

GOAL: Adolescent will have decreased feelings of helplessness and hopelessness and increased self-worth.

Objectives	Nursing Interventions/Adolescent Actions
2. Adolescent will explore methods for recognizing hopeless, helpless feelings and will use alternative coping methods.	A. Educate the adolescent and his family about signs and symptoms of depression.
	B. Adolescent and family will list pattern of signs and symptoms particular to adolescent.
	C. Adolescent will list sad thoughts or hurtful incidents in a journal and discuss them with his primary nurse every hour.
	D. Adolescent to identify what he wanted to happen instead of the hurtful incidents and self-harming.
	E. Adolescent will write a description of what he would like his family to be like.
	F. Adolescent to practice seeking out staff to discuss sad feelings when they occur.
3. Adolescent will accept himself as a valuable and worthwhile person.	A. Adolescent will list positive aspects of himself, then ask peers and staff members to point out positives.
	B. Adolescent will interview his parents and ask what they like about him.
	C. Adolescent will ask peers, staff, and parents to write words, songs, or poetry, or choose pictures that depict his strengths, then post them where the adolescent can frequently view them.
	D. Adolescent will role play seeking out staff and asking for support three times a day.
	E. Adolescent will list possible persons who can be part of a support system; he may choose relatives or persons at his school, home, church, or neighborhood.
	F. Adolescent will choose and contact two persons from his list and ask them if they would be part of his support system.

Goal setting should also focus on building self-esteem. Sample goals might include making a list of what peers and staff like or find positive about him, making a list of his positive traits, describing his ideal self, listing what his parents see as his strengths or what they like about him, making a list of his limitations and comparing them with his self-ideal, and discussing with the nurse and in group how realistic his self-ideal is.

Teaching. Because the suicidal adolescent is usually depressed, the adolescent and his parents should be taught the signs and symptoms of depression. If the adolescent is bipolar, he and his parents must learn about the illness and how to manage life-style, medication, and symptoms. However, the teaching should not substitute for family therapy.

Somatic therapy. Suicidal adolescents are usually prescribed antidepressants or lithium carbonate. The nurse should be sure that the adolescent and parents understand the effects and side effects of the medication; the nurse also must carefully monitor the response of the adolescent to the medication.

PSYCHOSIS

Behaviors often seen in an adolescent who is having a psychotic episode can include hallucinations, delusions, loose associations, incoherence, inappropriate affect, paranoid ideas, and ideas of reference. Sometimes the adolescent may have ritualistic and repetitive behaviors. This adolescent will lack judgment, have heightened impulsiveness, and may display activity levels from hyperactivity to catatonia. Initially there is little or no ability to gain insight. Because of his very distorted thought processes, this adolescent has many communication problems and often has difficulties with his peers. The loss of contact with reality may cause inadequate personal hygiene, and the nurse will need to include this type of care in the treatment plan. Because these teenagers require one-to-one supervision, two nursing staff members (ideally on the same team) may have to provide the care every few hours.

Most commonly the diagnosis of a psychotic state (see box on p. 400) is schizophrenia. Psychosis can result from organic causes, head injury, illicit substance abuse, or extreme stress, or it may occur in the manic phase of bipolar disorder. Table 14-7 on pp. 401-403 presents a nursing care plan for an adolescent with psychosis.

Nursing Interventions

Limit setting and surveillance. Because a probability of hallucinations, delusions, or paranoia exists, this adolescent may be harmful to himself or others, and safety is the first priority. The nurse will want to place the adolescent on close observation and have frequent one-to-one contacts. These interactions should be brief and concrete. Until medication begins to take effect, the nurse should avoid or minimize any triggering stimulation. This usually means amending programing or routines and explaining to families that visitation should be kept short. The nurse can support families by encouraging frequent phone calls to the primary nurse to check on the child's condition. This helps create the therapeutic environment of decreased stimuli the adolescent may need, yet it provides support to the family. The nurse may also need to limit this adolescent's space to prevent his wandering from the unit. Keeping the adolescent close to the nursing station when the other adolescents are in groups, and then maintaining him in a quiet, distant room when the milieu is active are other ways of limiting space and decreasing stimuli. In extreme cases of aggressive or violent psychotic behavior, the client may need to be placed in seclusion. The guideline of least restrictive environment should direct the nurse's decision making for physical or mechanical restraints. The adolescent should be allowed out of seclusion and back into the milieu as soon as he can tolerate the stimuli.

Medical and Nursing Diagnoses Related to Psychosis

Medical diagnoses (DSM-III-R)

295.	Schizophrenia
296.4	Bipolar disorder—manic type
298.	Brief reactive psychosis
305.70	Amphetamine intoxication
292.11	Cannabis delusional disorder
	Cocaine delusional disorder
	PCP delusional disorder
305.30	Hallucinogen
	Hallucinosis
293.81	Organic delusional disorder
310.10	Organic personality disorder

Nursing diagnoses (PMH)

6.4.2	Altered sensory perception	
	6.4.2.1	Hallucinations
		6.4.2.1.1 Auditory
2.6.2	Altered thought processes	
	2.6.2.4	Confusion/disorientation
	2.6.2.6	Delusions
	2.6.2.7	Ideas of reference
	2.6.2.8	Magical thinking
	2.6.2.10	Suspiciousness
	2.6.2.11	Thought insertion
5.7.2	Altered social interaction	
	5.7.2.1	Bizarre behaviors
	5.7.2.3	Disorganized social behaviors
	5.7.2.4	Social intrusiveness
	5.7.2.5	Social isolation/withdrawal
	5.7.2.6	Unpredictable behaviors
1.3.3	Altered self-care	
	1.3.3.1	Altered eating
		1.3.3.1.5 Refusal to eat
	1.3.3.5	Altered health seeking behaviors
		1.3.3.5.1 Knowledge deficit
		1.3.3.5.2 Noncompliance
	1.3.3.6	Altered hygiene

Basic physiological needs, including feeding and bathing if necessary, are met under the supervision of the nurse, who should constantly assess the amount of assistance needed. This adolescent often forgets to eat, drink fluids, or rest adequately. Exercise is sometimes a support measure that provides for more restful sleep periods later in the day or helps decrease restlessness. Exercise can consist of a brief walk or playing basketball with his primary staff. If tolerated, brief periods of group recreational therapy may be considered.

Table 14-7   Nursing Care Plan for an Adolescent with Psychosis

NURSING DIAGNOSES: Altered social interaction
Social intrusiveness
Unpredictable behaviors (psychosis)

GOAL: Adolescent will have appropriate social contacts and behavior.

Objectives	Nursing Interventions/Adolescent Actions
1. Adolescent will have decreased unpredictable and inappropriate behavior.	A. Adolescent will be redirected by staff when unpredictable or inappropriate behavior occurs.
	B. Staff to give brief and concrete clarification of appropriate behavior at any given situation.
	C. As medication takes effect adolescent will be asked to identify inappropriate behavior versus appropriate behavior, and tell which is the better choice.
	D. Staff will praise appropriate behavior.
	E. Primary nurse will educate parents regarding symptoms of psychosis.
2. Adolescent will have increased appropriate social interaction with staff and peers.	A. Adolescent will remain in room three fourths of the time when milieu is active, one fourth of the time among peers if tolerated.
	B. Adolescent may be out of room with staff during milieu quiet time or when peers are in therapies.
	C. Adolescent may go to the gym with the primary nurse for physical outlet while peers are in structured groups.
	D. If the adolescent is able to tolerate dessert time with peer group, nurse will then allow him to join for the entire dinner meal.
	E. Adolescent will join peer group for the last 15 minutes of recreational group, with 10 minute increases as tolerated.

Continued.

Until the antipsychotic medication begins to take effect, very little insight work should be done. The adolescent should be reassured that his thinking will improve and that he will begin to feel better. Participation in the structured program must be individualized to the adolescent's tolerance level and assessed needs.

Skill development: basic skills.   Initial daily goals may be as simple as eating half of his meals. Once the adolescent is able to do this, he may be able to progress to having dessert with his peers. Eventually the adolescent will progress to full participation in mealtime with peers. Another first goal may be to have the adolescent focus on what is going on in his current environment. The nurse can ask him each hour to discuss what he observed happening on the unit; this helps keep his thoughts centered on the here and now. If the adolescent is able to tolerate this much redirection and participation, then very basic communication skills and feeling identification can begin.

When the schizophrenic adolescent responds to medication, he and his family can begin a program of education about his illness. The adolescent has daily goals based

Table 14-7 Nursing Care Plan for an Adolescent with Psychosis—cont'd

NURSING DIAGNOSES: Altered thought processes
Delusions
Confusion
Disorientation
Suspiciousness

GOAL: Adolescent will have improved reality-based thought processes.

Objectives	Nursing Interventions/Adolescent Actions
1. Adolescent will accept staff limits to maintain safety and decrease stimuli.	A. Adolescent will be placed on close observation for 24 hours, then nurse will assess, monitor delusions, etc. B. Adolescent will remain out of structured therapies to reduce stimuli. C. Nurse will allow family to visit 20 minutes three times per week; parents to call for phone report daily. D. Adolescent will identify basic unit rules and limits set by staff.
2. Adolescent will take medication as prescribed.	A. Nurse will administer concentrated medicine (later to progress to oral/pill form). B. Nurse will monitor for side effects. C. Nurse will educate the parents about the purpose and side effect of medicine and the importance of compliance.
3. Adolescent will become more aware of environment and self.	A. Nurse will support and reassure the adolescent that his thinking process will clear up. B. Adolescent will review with the primary staff what he has observed in the environment. C. Adolescent will slowly integrate into the group (starting with the last 10-15 minutes of less intense group therapy). D. Adolescent will learn relaxation and stress-reduction activities. E. Adolescent will learn basic communication skills to get needs met or express anxious feelings.

Continued.

on a plan of education with the nurse. The plan includes identifying and naming the symptoms (hallucinations, etc.), identifying situations that exacerbate them, and developing strategies for self-management, including learning about medication and getting help when needed from parents, the psychiatrist, and other support persons such as the therapist or school nurse or counselor. Tarell (1989) recommends a four-phase teaching plan for schizophrenics that is analogous to the four phases of goal-setting progression proposed in this book. The phases are (1) assessment, (2) self-monitoring, (3) self-evaluation, and (4) self-reinforcement. According to Paternostro and others (1989), adolescents respond very favorably to a psychoeducational approach.

Table 14-7   Nursing Care Plan for an Adolescent with Psychosis — cont'd

Objectives	Nursing Interventions/Adolescent Actions
4. Adolescent and family will learn about illness and stress reduction and methods of coping.	A. As thoughts clear, nurse will teach the adolescent the symptoms of his illness. B. Adolescent will identify stressful situations at home, school, etc. C. Adolescent will identify when and how to ask for help when stress or anxiety begins to occur. D. Adolescent will practice relaxation every hour and stress and anxiety reduction techniques as needed. E. Adolescent will use communication skills and "I" statements every hour and as needed. F. Nurse will educate the parents regarding the illness and offer support. G. Nurse will educate the parents regarding adolescent's capabilities and limitations.
5. Adolescent and family will adjust to illness and altered life-style.	A. Nurse will assist the family to reevaluate adolescent's stress within the home and school. B. Nurse will assist the family to reassess and establish simple limits at home. C. Adolescent will identify ways he can ask for help. D. Adolescent to share thoughts and feelings with staff and parents. E. Nurse and parents will review and discuss realistic expectations of the adolescent's capabilities. F. Nurse will assist the family in establishing follow-up family therapy, parent support, and school support for adolescent.

Continued.

The family is included in a psychoeducational program, as well as family therapy. The family is taught to develop patience and a positive-reinforcing approach to the adolescent's gains, which may be small, without encouraging dependence. The family needs support in coping with this seemingly overwhelming change in their teenager. Several excellent books are available for families of mentally ill adolescents (McElroy, 1988; Cantor, 1982; and Torrey, 1988).

ATTENTION DEFICIT HYPERACTIVITY DISORDER

Some parents describe their adolescent's developmental history as one of impulsive and easily distracted behaviors. To diagnose attention deficit disorders (ADDs) (see box on p. 405), the nurse should further assess for patterns of decreased concentration, low frustration tolerance, failure to finish things, poor active listening, and poor organizational abilities. The preadolescent and adolescent may also have poor personal hygiene and have difficulty with activities of daily living. Further investigation may disclose evidence of hyperactivity and fidgety behaviors while

Table 14-7 Nursing Care Plan for an Adolescent with Psychosis—cont'd

NURSING DIAGNOSES: Altered self care
Altered eating
Altered hygiene

GOAL: Adolescent will have improved dietary intake and hygiene.

Objectives	Nursing Interventions/Adolescent Actions
1. Adolescent will have adequate food and fluid intake.	A. Nurse will maintain intake and output daily. B. Ensure adequate nutrition: adolescent will eat half of each meal and drink one carton of milk at each meal with staff supervising in room. If accomplished, adolescent may have dessert. C. If the adolescent can eat meals appropriately at breakfast and lunch, he may join peer group for desserts. D. If adolescent is able to tolerate social stimuli during dessert part of meal time, he may join peers. E. Adolescent will drink one juice or milk between mealtimes. F. Nurse will allow the adolescent to join the peer group for meals as long as three fourths of each meal, including one milk, is consumed appropriately.
2. Adolescent will maintain own daily hygiene.	A. Staff will assist the adolescent with daily shower and oral hygiene and selection of appropriate clothes. B. Adolescent will take his own shower and select his own clothes with staff supervision. C. Adolescent will tidy up his bedroom with staff assistance. D. Adolescent will take a morning shower, incorporate oral hygiene, and tidy his room, then have staff check.

awake or asleep. It is possible for the adolescent to have many of the previously mentioned behaviors without the symptoms of hyperactivity. This adolescent will usually be labeled early in life as the "bad boy" or "bad girl." Behavioral problems will continue to increase if attention deficit disorder (ADHD) goes untreated. This early and ongoing reinforcement of "bad" behavior only strengthens the adolescent's poor self-concept. The assessment may also reveal the adolescent to be very immature and developmentally delayed. If the individual cannot attend to what is going on, then he cannot learn. Peers in the classroom or milieu tend to have low tolerance for this type of adolescent. Rejection by peers further heightens poor school relationships and social participation. This adolescent may begin to develop hostile or aggressive coping mechanisms that set him up for more rejection and poor self-esteem, and this developmental pattern may further increase the adolescent's potential for alcohol or drug abuse.

Although the symptoms of attention deficit hyperactive disorder (ADHD) is often very apparent to the nurse, a careful assessment is still required. Learning disabilities

---

Medical and Nursing Diagnoses Related to Attention Deficits

Medical diagnoses (DSM-III-R)

314.01	Attention deficit hyperactivity disorder
317.	Mental retardation
299.	Pervasive developmental disorder
315.	Developmental disorders
313.	Anxiety disorder
296.	Depression

Nursing diagnoses (PMH)

1.1.2	Altered motor behavior
	1.1.2.6 Hyperactivity
2.6.2.1	Altered abstract thinking
2.6.2.2	Altered concentration
2.6.2.3	Altered problem solving

---

often accompany attention deficit disorder and should be ruled out or diagnosed, as should mental retardation (MR). Pervasive developmental disorder, anxiety disorders, and depression should also be considered when evaluating these adolescents. Table 14-8 on pp. 406-407 presents nursing care plans for a client with ADHD.

Nursing Interventions

Limit setting and surveillance. Patience is probably the most important skill the nurse will need to use with this adolescent. Limits must be concrete and conveyed at the adolescent's level of developmental understanding. Decreasing the stimuli is one of the first strategies that should be implemented. This may be in the form of "quiet time" in the adolescent's room or in a space away from others. It may mean initially keeping the adolescent out of group therapy or the classroom setting because his distracting behaviors are too disruptive to peers. Because the adolescent cannot control his fidgety behaviors, this type of limit setting may help decrease peer rejection and his sense of failure.

Skill development. The primary nurse should build into the treatment plan frequent opportunities for small successes. The focus of daily goals is to provide frequent repetitive reinforcement of the basic communication skills of "I" statements and active listening. The nurse can also teach and have the client practice relaxation techniques that can later be used in the school setting or in group therapy to help maintain control. The staff should remember to keep goals brief, worded in simple language, and very achievable; this may mean breaking one goal into three simple steps and providing a review every 30 to 60 minutes. Use of the "think chair" for 5 minutes helps the adolescent integrate the basic concept of "stop and think" before he acts. The "think chair" is a chair that is placed in an easily observable yet low-stimulus area. The purpose of giving the adolescent time out is to interrupt negative behaviors. Time spent in the think chair allows the adolescent to slow

Text continued on p. 408.

Table 14-8   Nursing Care Plan for Attention Deficit Hyperactivity Disorder (ADHD)

NURSING DIAGNOSES: Altered motor behavior
                     Hyperactivity

GOAL: Adolescent will be less hyperactive and exhibit improved concentration, abstract thinking, and problem-solving abilities.

Objectives	Nursing Interventions/Adolescent Actions
1. Adolescent will begin to rechannel hyperactivity and identify his actions.	A. Adolescent will spend 5 minutes in the "think chair" when he is unable to follow staff redirection. B. Adolescent will identify why he has to use the "think chair" and what he could have done instead. C. Staff will use brief, concrete redirection to interrupt and redirect behaviors. D. Adolescent will remain out of group therapy until medication takes effect.
2. Adolescent will participate in medication program and necessary medical and educational testing.	A. Adolescent will take medication as prescribed. B. Adolescent and parents will learn the purpose of medication, side effects, and precautions. C. Staff will attempt to normalize the routine and need for anti-ADHD medication. D. Explain the purpose of premedication testing (ECG, EEG, or CT scan).
3. Adolescent will use point system to increase awareness of behaviors and implement positive changes.	A. Adolescent will be placed on hourly point system.
4. Adolescent will experience increased self-esteem through better self-control of hyperactivity.	A. Adolescent will identify whether medication helps behavior and will look at before and after behaviors. B. Adolescent will explain and teach the point system to parents. C. Adolescent will give examples of times he used positive behaviors to gain privileges. D. Staff will give frequent *verbal* recognition of positive behaviors in addition to points earned.

Continued.

Table 14-8   Nursing Care Plan for Attention Deficit Hyperactivity Disorder
(ADHD)—cont'd

NURSING DIAGNOSES: Altered concentration
Ineffective individual coping

GOAL: Adolescent will have increased concentration and demonstrate skills for coping
with ADHD.

Objectives	Nursing Interventions/Adolescent Actions
1. Adolescent will learn to follow simple rules of unit and redirections of staff.	A. Staff will *not* expect attentiveness until medication has taken some effect. Staff will use simple redirections and a concrete approach. B. Staff will ask or place the adolescent in the "think chair" for 5 minutes every time he distracts, acts out, or does not follow redirection. C. Adolescent will learn and use "active listening skills" every time he uses the "think chair:" • Look at the person speaking. • Ask questions. • Repeat what he heard.
2. Adolescent will develop better concentration.	A. Adolescent and nurse will develop repetitive unit routine to decrease forgetfulness. B. Adolescent will take medication as described.
3. Adolescent will practice coping skills.	A. Adolescent will learn at least five relaxation techniques and practice one each hour for 2 days. B. Adolescent may take a small ball of clay to group therapy to help control his fidgety behaviors. (Clay should be returned to the nurse each day.) C. Adolescent will practice "stopping and thinking" and asking "will this help me or hurt me?" before making decisions. Adolescent will practice and give examples every hour for 2 days.
4. Adolescent will practice communication skills.	A. Adolescent will learn basic "I" statements to get needs met. Adolescent will use these every hour for 2 days.
5. Adolescent will be able to attend and appropriately participate in unit activities and begin transition to home and school.	A. Adolescent will attend groups (nurse will escort him if necessary). Nurse will have him relay to staff one thing he remembers or learns from the group. B. Adolescent will discuss anxieties of returning to home and school, and role play possible difficulties. C. Staff will maintain the point system but decrease verbal and visual cues to test the adolescent's self-control. D. Parents will learn about ADHD diagnosis and assist them to accept the adolescent's limits and adjust their expectations. E. Adolescent and parents will develop a point system for use at home and school. F. Adolescent will have 4-hour home visits to practice new skills, later to increase to 8 hours.

himself down and to think of what he was doing wrong and what he can do differently to produce a positive outcome. The nurse should use the limit setting–behavior processing protocol described in Chapters 8 and 11 to help the adolescent make more productive choices.

Another method of behavioral control is a point system (Table 14-9). The point system should be based on what is important to the adolescent. The primary nurse should decide with the adolescent what activities or privileges within the structure of the program he would like and what point value each should carry. The adolescent and nurse will also identify desirable behaviors the staff or parents would like to see and how many points he can earn when he exhibits these behaviors. Any sense of accomplishment or positive control over his behaviors should be verbally acknowledged; this contributes to his self-esteem.

Hostility or aggressive outbursts should be confronted directly, and consequences must be delivered. The purpose for this is to interrupt the behavior, reteach, and reinforce the new methods of behavior control until the adolescent can do this for himself.

Structured physical outlets are necessary for the adolescent because they allow him to channel his excess energy. The nurse should make an allowance for distractability during these activities (and to a certain degree in the milieu) at least until medications take effect. Thus careful goal setting and accomplishment, limit setting, positive reinforcement, and logical consequences, along with medication, help the adolescent control disturbing behaviors, improve concentration, and build self-esteem.

Somatic therapy. Medication is a tremendous aid in stabilizing the adolescent so that he can begin to make behavioral changes. Effectiveness and side effects of tricyclics, anticonvulsants, or stimulants must be evaluated. The nurse should educate parents and the adolescent regarding the purpose and side effects of the medications. Parents will need additional education and support to increase their tolerance level and adjust the expectations they have of the child. The adolescent and parents may need education and reassurance if EEGs or CT scans are ordered. Educational testing may be performed to assess for special needs; these results can often aid the nurse's approach to planning and teaching behavioral changes.

Collaboration. To maintain gains made in programing, nursing staff can serve as advocates for the adolescent to the school and teachers. During treatment it is equally important to educate the family and to work with them continually to increase their coping skills and adjustment to the diagnosis. It may be helpful for parents to include respite or quiet time for themselves in their home schedule. The nurse may need to assist parents in developing contracts or point systems to use when the adolescent returns home after discharge.

CHEMICAL DEPENDENCE

The chemically dependent adolescent (see box on p. 410) presents a complex diagnostic and treatment problem. Alcohol abuse (and to some extent, drug abuse) is the norm among adolescents, as are deceit and lying about activities that are "normal" but not likely to be approved by parents. Some parents actually do approve of drinking and early sexual experience of their sons as signs of approaching

Table 14-9   Example of Point System Chart

Desired Behaviors	Earned Points	Privileges	Cost Points
Follow unit rules	1	One hot chocolate (sugar-free)	7
Do what staff asks the first time	1	One soda (sugar-free)	8
Listen in groups	1	One social phone call for 10 minutes	8
Socialize with peers in friendly manner	1	Snack from home	12
Use "I statements" and "active listening skills"	2	Trip to vending machine with staff	12
		Special one-to-one time with staff	10

manhood. Furthermore, many adolescents with emotional disorders and chemical dependence have grown up in alcoholic families, so that when the youngster is referred to treatment, the family does not recognize the problem. The traditional treatment approach based on Alcoholics Anonymous principles requires the adolescent to admit he is "powerless over alcohol" and to turn his "will and life over to the care of God as he understands Him." However, adolescents struggle intensely with issues of dependence and independence and believe they are invincible. A chemically dependent person is well defended, usually by himself and his family, with denial, projection, and rationalization. In addition, the adolescent who began using chemicals around age 11 is probably developmentally delayed and experiencing cognitive disturbances resulting directly from the effects of various drugs.

The chemically dependent adolescent often has a rebellious, argumentative attitude, which may be covered with a charming facade and accompanied by excellent manipulative skills. Underneath the cocky presentation, however, is a frightened adolescent with low self-esteem and possibly other diagnoses. The chemically dependent adolescent needs intensive, acute care. Table 14-10 on p. 411 presents a nursing care plan for a chemically dependent adolescent.

Nursing Interventions

Limit setting and surveillance. The adolescent should have primary nurses to whom he is referred for all requests, as does any manipulative client. The chemically dependent teenager should have a privilege system that incorporates expectations related specifically to his illness and recovery. Depending on his drug of choice, the adolescent is monitored for signs of withdrawal, craving, or depression following cocaine or other stimulant cessation. Craving occurs at intervals for long periods, particularly after cocaine abuse. Running away is a possibility in the beginning and middle of the treatment period, and interventions for running away (described earlier in the chapter) should be instituted. Close observation should be used to prevent

---

Medical and Nursing Diagnoses Related to Substance Abuse

Medical diagnoses (DSM-III-R)

Alcohol
303.90   Dependence
305.00   Abuse
Amphetamine or similarly acting sympathomimetic
304.40   Dependence
305.70   Abuse
Cannabis
304.30   Dependence
305.20   Abuse
Cocaine
304.20   Dependence
305.6   Abuse
Hallucinogen
304.50   Dependence
305.30   Abuse
Inhalant
304.60   Dependence
305.90   Abuse
Nicotine
305.10   Dependence
Opioid
304.00   Dependence
305.50   Abuse
Phencyclidine (PCP) or similarly acting arylcyclohexylamine
304.50   Dependence
305.90   Abuse
Sedative, hypnotic, or anxiolytic
304.10   Dependence
305.40   Abuse
304.90   Polysubstance dependence
304.90   Psychoactive substance dependence not otherwise specified
305.90   Psychoactive substance abuse not otherwise specified

Nursing diagnoses (PMH)

5.3.2   Altered conduct/impulse processes
     5.3.2.9   Substance abuse
5.5.3   Ineffective individual coping
     5.5.3.2   Ineffective denial

---

sexually promiscuous behavior on coeducational units. A toxicology screen, including quantitative marijuana levels, is done at the time of admission and as indicated thereafter. Although a very secure environment and structured approach are needed, the adolescent should be treated with respect, care, and concern for his serious biological and psychosocial needs.

Table 14-10   Nursing Care Plan for a Chemically Dependent Adolescent

NURSING DIAGNOSIS: Substance Abuse

GOAL: The adolescent will demonstrate alternative coping strategies based on the AA
model.

Objective	Nursing Interventions/Adolescent Actions
1. The adolescent will identify aspects of his life that are affected by substance abuse.	A. Adolescent will list in his journal or *Step One** workbook at least three ways that substance abuse has changed his life physically, socially, emotionally, and spiritually. B. Adolescent will discuss his feelings with the group and his primary nurse each day. C. Adolescent will attend a lecture series on chemical dependence.
2. The adolescent will identify triggers that precede usage.	A. Adolescent will list in his journal at least three triggers relative to the physical, social, and emotional aspects in his life. B. Adolescent will discuss these with primary nurse each day.
3. The adolescent will identify strategies to stay sober.	A. Adolescent will list and describe in his journal the 12 Steps, any changes in social relationships and activities that are needed, and a plan for a balanced life. B. Adolescent will discuss these in the group and with his primary nurse and counselor each day. C. Adolescent will attend a lecture series on the 12 steps.
4. The adolescent will practice new strategies in the hospital.	A. Adolescent will attend AA two times per week in the hospital and make plans for attending a home group. B. Adolescent will practice daily meditation. C. Nurse will plan and carry out with adolescent a balanced schedule for therapeutic visits home.

*Naaken J and Van Dyke (1985) Step one for young adults, Minneapolis, Hazelden Publishing.

Skill development. The chemically dependent teenager is assisted with setting
goals in the usual progression of problem definition, self-awareness, connecting
feelings and behaviors, identifying new behaviors, and then practicing them.
However, the self-awareness and problem definition are accomplished through
"step" work. That is, using handouts or workbooks, the adolescent explores
individually with his primary caregiver and in group sessions Step 1 of the Alcoholics
Anonymous (AA) 12 Steps to Recovery (see box on p. 412). His daily goals direct him
to consider and admit that alcohol and drugs are affecting his life in many areas so
that it has become unmanageable. Inexpensive booklets for Steps 1 through 4 are
available from the Hazelden Foundation (Naaken and others, 1985). The Steps are
somewhat parallel to the goal progression described here; Steps 1 and 4 have to do
with self-awareness; and Steps 2, 3, and 5 through 12 offer alternative coping
strategies and life-styles.

During the time the adolescent is working on the steps, he is also developing

---

The Twelve Steps of Alcoholics Anonymous

1. We admitted we were powerless over alcohol—that our lives had become unmanageable.
2. Came to believe that a Power greater than ourselves could restore us to sanity.
3. Made a decision to turn our will and our lives over to the care of God *as we understood Him*.
4. Made a searching and fearless moral inventory of ourselves.
5. Admitted to God, to ourselves, and to another human being, the exact nature of our wrongs.
6. Were entirely ready to have God remove all these defects of character.
7. Humbly asked Him to remove our shortcomings.
8. Made a list of all persons we had harmed, and became willing to make amends to them all.
9. Made direct amends to such people wherever possible, except when to do so would injure them or others.
10. Continued to take personal inventory and when we were wrong promptly admitted it.
11. Sought through prayer and meditation to improve our conscious contact with God *as we understood Him*, praying only for knowledge of His will for us and the power to carry that out.
12. Having had a spiritual awakening as the result of these steps, we tried to carry this message to alcoholics, and to practice these principles in all our affairs.

From Alcoholics Anonymous World Services, Inc, 1976.

---

communication skills and dealing with the feelings that arise as the denial, manipulation, and projection are reduced in intensity.

He and his family make plans for sober living by attending AA or NA and Al-Anon or Better Families Anonymous. A relapse prevention plan and aftercare plan are made carefully and are critical to success after inpatient treatment. Returning to school and not socializing with using teenagers is very difficult. Confrontive role playing practice prepares the adolescent for these events.

The adolescent and his family need specific education about the illness and the treatment for it. Families are often told that the adolescent is responsible for his own recovery, as if the teenager could manage this serious problem on his own. For success in recovery, such as driving and socializing, consequences such as "grounding" or losing driving privileges should be applied if the adolescent fails to meet expectations or uses. Family therapy is often overlooked in aftercare plans and should be set up with appropriately trained therapists.

ANOREXIA NERVOSA AND BULIMIA

Anorexia nervosa and bulimia (see box on p. 413) are often treated in a specific eating disorders program that offers staff expertise and group support. Adolescents may be treated in a psychiatric program on a case-by-case basis if there is sufficient staffing and considerable clinical supervision and training available. The nursing care

Medical and Nursing Diagnoses Related to Eating Disorders

Medical diagnoses (DSM-III-R)

307.5   Bulimia nervosa
307.10   Anorexia nervosa

Nursing diagnoses (PMH)

1.3.3   Altered care
      1.3.3.1   Altered eating
            1.3.3.1.1   Binge-purge syndrome
6.3.2   Altered self-concept
      6.3.2.1   Altered body image
      7.4.2.2   Altered eating processes
            7.7.2.2.1   Anorexia
5.4.2   Altered family processes
      5.4.2.1   Ineffective family coping
            5.4.2.1.1   Compromised
            5.4.2.1.2   Disabled

strategies for the eating and nutritional aspects of both illnesses are the same. However, the interventions for the psychological aspects of each illness depend on the adolescent's behaviors. Usually, after starvation and electrolyte imbalances have been corrected, the anorexic adolescent will be perfectionistic, fearful of identifying and expressing feelings, and fearful of independence and sexuality. The bulimic adolescent may demonstrate characteristics of borderline personality disorder with problems in impulse control and splitting, and coexisting substance abuse, delinquency, or sexual promiscuity (Goldbloom, 1990). Anorexics and bulimics both tend to think in terms of all or nothing. The approaches for dealing with these illnesses range from psychoanalytical to strictly behavioral. The suggested approach described here is eclectic and is based on the model used at Johns Hopkins Medical Institutions (Anderson and others, 1985). Family therapy is especially important.

Nursing Interventions

Limit setting and surveillance. During the first few days (or for as long as necessary), the adolescent is constantly monitored for eating, vomiting, exercise, and stools. The adolescent may choose three foods to exclude, but the rest of the diet is prescribed with no choices. The diet initially includes 1200-1500 calories daily and is low in fats to avoid gastric distress. There are rigid rules about food mixtures, sizes of bites, and other food rituals, as well as length of time spent eating. Talking about food is not permitted during meals. The nurse is supportive and reassures the patient that staff will not allow excessive weight gain or loss of control. If vomiting occurs, the adolescent cleans up and is given a milkshake preparation approximately equal to the volume lost. Otherwise, dietary supplements and nasogastric feedings are not used. The program must be explained thoroughly to the adolescent and family. The anorexic who is not bulimic responds rather quickly to this approach; the bulimic takes longer because of the associated personality factors, especially impulse control. As the adolescent is able to tolerate eating and reduce vomiting, the focus of control is gradually shifted to the adolescent. A goal weight is chosen by staff but is not revealed to the adolescent until well into the program. Clothing that fits appropriately is purchased or brought by the family. Clothing that is too tight will cause the adolescent to feel overweight.

Skill development. Psychotherapy is withheld until the psychological effects of starvation are reduced or eliminated. The adolescent is taught about the illness and the personality traits associated with it; this provides an introduction to self-awareness. The adolescent then begins to identify problem areas that need correction, as does any other adolescent in treatment. Anorexic adolescents will have daily goals geared toward developing or recognizing their identity, developing a normal body image, becoming more independent, and expressing feelings. The adolescent's striving for independence must be coordinated with family therapy. The bulimic adolescent will be working on controlling impulses and identifying, tolerating, and expressing feelings and needs.

Along with the psychosocial skill development, the adolescent is gradually learning to manage the food aspects of the disorder: normal amounts, patterns of eating, food purchasing, preparation, and eating in various situations (such as restaurants).

Somatic therapy. Adolescents may be placed on a mild tranquilizer in small doses to reduce anxiety or severe behavior problems in the first few days. Recent experience has demonstrated that imipramine may be useful for bulimic adolescents (Goldbloom and Garfinkel, 1990).

REFERENCES AND SUGGESTED READINGS

Anderson A, Morse C, and Santmyer K (1985) Inpatient treatment for anorexia nervosa. In Garner D and Garfinkel P, editors, Handbook of psychotherapy for anorexia nervosa and bulimia, New York, The Guilford Press.

Bjorklund P (1985) Step four for young adults, Minneapolis, Hazelden Publishing.

Cantor S (1982) The schizophrenic child: a primer for parents and professionals, Buffalo, NY, Eden Press (distributed by University of Toronto Press).

Goldbloom D and Garfinkel P (1990) Eating disorders: anorexia nervosa and bulimia. In Garfinkel B, Carlson G, and Weller E, editors, Psychiatric disorders in children and adolescents, Philadelphia, WB Saunders Co.

Goldstein AP, Sprafkin RP, Gershaw JJ, and Klein P (1980) Skillstreaming the adolescent, Champaign, Ill, Research Press.

Herskovitz J (1988) Is your child depressed? New York, Pharos Books.

Hodgson W (1986) A parents survival guide: how to cope when your kid is using drugs, Minneapolis, Hazelden Publishing.

Marshall S (1978) Young, sober, and free, Minneapolis, Hazelden Publishing.

Mauren JT (1989) Chronic mental illness: coping strategies, Thorofare, NJ, Slack, Inc.

McElroy E (1988) Children and adolescents with mental illness: a parents guide, Kensington, MD, Woodbine House. (Available from National Alliance for the Mentally Ill (NAMI), 2101 Wilson Blvd., Suite 302, Arlington, VA 22201.)

Mont PM, Abrams OB, Kassen RM, and Cooney NL (1989) Treating alcohol dependence: a coping skills training guide, New York, The Guilford Press.

Naaken J (1985) Step two for young adults, Minneapolis, Hazelden Publishing.

Naaken J and Van Dyke D (1985) Step one for young adults, Minneapolis, Hazelden Publishing.

Paternostro JM, Olah L, and Yurkewicz C (1989) Utilization of professional creativity in relation to initial psychotic episodes in adolescents. Presented at 3-D and beyond: the present and future of child psychiatric nursing, national conference of the Advocates for Child Psychiatric Nursing, White Plains, NY.

Pohl ML (1978) The teaching function of the nursing practitioner, ed 3, Dubuque, Iowa, WC Brown Co, Publishers.

Stuart G and Sundeen S (1987) Principles and practice of psychiatric nursing, ed 3, St Louis, The CV Mosby Co.

Tarell JD (1989) Self-regulation of symptoms in schizophrenia: psychoeducational interventions for clients and families. In Mauren TT, editor (1989) Chronic mental illness: coping strategies, Thorofare, NJ, Slack, Inc.

Tooney EF (1988) Surviving schizophrenia: a family manual (revised edition), New York, Harper & Row, Publishers, Inc.

Van Dyke D (1985) Step three for young adults, Minneapolis, Hazelden Publishing.

Wender PE (1987) The hyperactive child, adolescent, and adult: attention deficit disorder through the life span, New York, Oxford University Press.

Wohlberg L (1967) The technique of psychotherapy, vol 2, New York, Grune & Stratton, Inc.

Chapter 15

Management of the Adolescent Psychiatric Unit

The adolescent inpatient unit is a highly specialized, complex system in a highly competitive environment. The manager of this system must have excellent clinical skills, as well as leadership and communication skills. The ideal mental health professional to fill the program manager role is a psychiatric nurse clinical specialist with management training and experience. If the program manager is not a nurse, it is imperative that a skilled psychiatric nurse provide leadership to the nursing staff. In an ideal program, all staff members report to the program manager, but a matrix system is feasible.

The obligations of the program manager include the following:
1. Provide a quality, cost-effective program for adolescents and their families
2. Ensure the safety of patients and staff
3. Advocate and negotiate with administrators for safety and quality care
4. Ensure continuity of care
5. Provide training and emotional and administrative support to the staff and program
6. Assist with internal and external marketing of the unit

Ensuring Quality Programing

A quality program is described in Chapter 11. The quality of an adolescent psychiatric inpatient program depends on the presence of skilled clinicians and nurses in adequate numbers. The best nurse cannot provide excellent direct care to more than 4 adolescents, and the finest therapist cannot provide group psychotherapy for more than 8 to 10 teenagers, or family therapy to more than 6 or 7 families twice per week. An occupational and recreational therapy staff that is not available evenings and weekends places undue burdens on the nursing staff. Psychiatric units are labor intensive. Because capital expenditures are relatively low, it is easy to generate profits. Inappropriate controls on staffing lead to the hidden costs of staff turnover, especially with registered nurses and nurse managers; patient incidents and acting out; poor follow-through on treatment plan goals; and ultimately staff and patient dissatisfaction.

The program manager should be actively involved with program evaluation. The media, the Joint Commission on Accreditation of Healthcare Organizations (JCAHO) and benefit payors are very concerned about the quality and appropriateness of adolescent inpatient care for psychiatric or substance abuse problems. There is little information available on the effectiveness of inpatient treatment. Outcome-oriented studies based on patient condition before, during, and after treatment, including longitudinal studies, are desperately needed. These studies should also include family treatment. Existing theoretical frameworks, behavior rating scales, nursing diagnoses, and DSM-III-R diagnoses should be used to measure and predict outcomes.

The JCAHO mandate for quality monitoring (JCAHO, 1990) can be very helpful in developing meaningful data to assist the manager in obtaining various necessities for quality care. The most recent quality review standards — if the intent, as well as the letter of the directions, are followed — allow the manager to monitor real problem areas in implementing programs. The considerable time spent in setting up specific outcome indicators to measure progress is well worth the effort. The JCAHO seminar on quality assurance (QA) for psychiatric facilities is very helpful for training managers, and it provides a training manual for use in the hospital. Quality monitoring is a sophisticated process. If the outcome indicators and criteria are beyond the scope of the manager or the QA coordinator, assistance may be sought at the local university, or a consultant can be engaged.

Several widely publicized reports have appeared on television and in newspapers concerning the increase in adolescent inpatient admissions. An editorial (Pothier, 1989) in a psychiatric nursing journal and a recent journal article (Lewis, 1989) joined the list of criticisms by persons and organizations with no direct connections to disturbed adolescents. Although there are some facilities and psychiatric hospital chains admitting adolescents who could be served just as effectively in intensive outpatient situations, the multitude of complex problems and legitimate DSM-III-R axis one diagnoses of many adolescents require intensive treatment. The assessment and treatment of chemically dependent adolescents are particularly problematic (Halikas, 1990). Many adolescents receive an incorrect diagnosis of conduct disorder (Akiskal and others, 1985) or a single diagnosis when two or more problems exist (Lewis, 1990), which further clouds the seriousness of many adolescent emotional disorders. The Academy of Child and Adolescent Psychiatry provides guidelines for utilization review and admission appropriateness (Stevenson and DuPrat, 1989). Program directors must begin to insist on program evaluations that will demonstrate the need and effectiveness of inpatient services and contribute the information needed to plan alternative and after-care services.

Ensuring Safety

Managing violent, suicidal, and self-mutilating adolescents in the least restrictive manner possible requires a safe physical environment and a 1:4 ratio of direct-care staff to adolescents. To teach adolescents impulse management using problem solving and other alternatives, a skilled staff member must be present at all times to instruct and assist the adolescent in the practice of new behaviors. Furthermore, sufficient numbers of registered nurses are required to assess and monitor adolescents receiving medications and to supervise special treatment services such as time out, seclusion, and restraint. The nursing interventions used with adolescents at high risk for injuries include continuous one-to-one observation and interaction. The manager must adjust staffing to provide quality care—not custodial care—for these and the other adolescents admitted to the unit. Careful attention to risk management, needs of high-risk patients, and patterns of intervention, including quality monitoring and direct supervision, provides information for determining staff-to-patient ratios and training.

Advocating for Quality and Safety with Administration

To provide quality programing, the program manager must obtain appropriate budgeting allocations for staffing, materials, physical plant alterations, and training. In private hospital settings, a unit that is producing the desired profit margin can negotiate additional funds. If concrete data that indicate safety problems are available, the administration can be convinced to make changes. Program or staffing deficiencies that can be linked to reduced marketability are bases for negotiating changes as well.

In general hospitals, where the psychiatric unit is administered under nursing service, obtaining changes in staffing patterns is very difficult. In these settings, staffing is based daily or—worse—by shift, on a computerized acuity system that often does not adequately reflect the complexities of the therapeutic milieu, especially primary therapeutic relationships and services that can be provided only by certain specialists. This situation may be compounded by accounting systems that do not provide specific information regarding revenue vs. costs per unit. Cost-control measures are often applied unilaterally, even when a particular unit is profitable. In these cases the manager must determine profitability by other methods and scrupulously monitor safety while establishing positive relationships with the key people in the complex political arena of the general hospital.

In either situation the program manager must supervise clinical and administrative aspects of the program very closely, either directly or through first-line supervisors if the program is fortunate enough to have them. (The elimination of these positions is a cost-cutting device often used when service-line management is initiated.) The manager must also be very assertive and persistent without being offensive to administrators. Having accurate numbers and clear documentation of deficiencies related to licensure, accreditation, quality monitoring, and safety (liability), along with good negotiating skills (Nierenberg, 1981; Nierenberg and Ross, 1985), will help the manager secure needed funds and staffing for the unit.

Ensuring Continuity of Care

The adolescent unit manager oversees the coordination of the patients' inpatient, outpatient, and school programing. Determining follow-up policies and procedures and seeing that they are carried out produces better results for the adolescent and the family and creates a positive public image of the unit in the community. Providing a postdischarge support group requires 1 or 2 hours of staff time without interfering with referral patterns.

Providing Training and Support

Because nurses, therapists, and child care workers often do not receive clinical experiences in adolescent psychiatric nursing and family therapy, the manager must arrange for appropriate training and clinical supervision. Clinical specialists in adolescent psychiatric nursing, especially those who focus on the needs of staff nurses, are scarce. Because the therapists available for employment may not have training and experience in adolescent and family therapy, the entire nursing staff, including the child care workers, should receive paid training that includes in-services, seminars, reading, and networking with others in the field. A consortium with other facilities in the area or a multihospital system should be arranged for providing cost-effective training. The shortage of literature in adolescent psychiatric nursing for the staff nurse has been a serious problem until very recently. The Journal of Child and Adolescent Psychiatric Nursing and this book are the initial resources available for adolescent psychiatric nurses.

Nurses and other staff members who deal with acting out behavior on a daily basis and who must invest themselves in therapeutic relationships with teenagers who are suffering need encouragement and support. An optimal environment is one in which staff members support and appreciate each other and feel valued by the managers. The manager delegates responsibility based on the abilities of each staff member and encourages input and creative problem solving. Time must be designated for staff meetings and meetings between staff and management to deal with patient and staff problems.

Assisting with Marketing

The program manager usually has some responsibility for marketing or selling the unit program to potential referral sources, as well as tracking the results of all marketing efforts. A quality product (program) is the best sales strategy. One of the best ways to avoid census fluctuations and the resultant staffing problems is to carry out a consistent plan of referral source contacts. Although many hospitals engage in mass media campaigns to advertise services, other strategies result in more appropriate referrals. Individual personal visits to pediatricians, family practice physicians, and their office managers; juvenile court personnel; school counselors, nurses, and administrators; children's protective service personnel; and outpatient therapists are all very effective for generating referrals when their clients need inpatient services. Providing an in-service breakfast or lunch and a tour of the facility is another excellent device for developing appropriate referrals. Marketing efforts should aim to elicit legitimate inpatient referrals. Personal contacts by staff to provide continuity of care for a patient who has been referred also serve as an effective marketing tool.

Some program managers feel uncomfortable about marketing and sales roles, but there is a legitimate need to promote quality programs for adolescents and families who require the service. The manager must balance time for program supervision, administrative activities, and marketing.

In a general hospital setting, the manager of the adolescent unit (or other psychiatric unit) may have to teach other managers the nature of adolescent patient behavior and treatment and remind them about special confidentiality laws. The stigma that persists about mental health care exists among hospital personnel as well. Adult psychiatric staff members often need to be taught that acting out is the focus of intervention and that there are good reasons for continuous surveillance of and limit setting for adolescents.

Surviving the Program Manager Role

Staying healthy and effective in this challenging middle management position requires some strategy. Regularly attending the multidisciplinary treatment planning meetings is one of the best ways to manage the day-to-day clinical program. All matters of patient assessment and progress, including discharge planning, are outlined and evaluated at this time. During the meeting the manager can note the appropriateness of admissions, the quality and intensity of treatment, care problems (including use of special treatment), staff relationship problems and morale, and sources of referrals. Some time should be spent observing the milieu at various times of day and directly evaluating personnel performance, even if peer reviews are conducted. Ideally, the manager services a patient or family, or directs a therapy group; this demonstrates the level of consistency and teamwork in the program. Approximately 2 or 3 hours per day are spent "hands on" in these ways. The other 6 or 7 hours are spent on quality assurance and administrative activities, including marketing and staff meetings, which should be held at least once per month. Solving milieu and patient care problems should be delegated to task forces or the appropriate discipline or disciplines, with solutions approved by the manager after the psychiatrist provides appropriate input.

When many problems require the allocation of considerable resources, making a priority list with time limits for tackling the various problems is helpful. Building relationships with key administrative people who can assist in solving problems and influencing others is a necessary activity.

Being available to others as much as possible, including personally answering the telephone, accomplishes two important things. One is that issues are dealt with immediately; this saves time for everyone. The other advantage is that others perceive the manager as available and competent. Accessibility is essential, as is the scheduling of some uninterrupted time each day for paperwork and planning.

A stress management program, including a healthful life-style, an average work day of no more than 10 hours, and at least one supportive relationship at work and home, is helpful for keeping balance in this demanding job. If the hospital exploits patients or staff because of profit motives or because of chronic underfinancing in spite of the manager's reasonable efforts to make changes, alternative career choices should be explored; a qualified, dedicated manager deserves the opportunity to work in a supportive environment.

REFERENCES AND SUGGESTED READINGS

Akiskal HS, Downs J, Watson S, Dougherty D, and Pruitt DB (1985) Affective disorders in referred children and younger siblings of manic-depressives, Archives of General Psychiatry 42:996.

Evans CLS and Lewis SK (1985) Nursing administration of psychiatric–mental health care, Rockville, Md, Aspen Systems Corp.

Halikas J (1990) Substance abuse in children and adolescents. In Garfinkel BD, Carlson GA, and Weller EB, editors: Psychiatric disorders in children and adolescents, Philadelphia, WB Saunders Co.

Joint Commission on Accreditation of Healthcare Organizations (1989) Quality assurance and risk management in psychiatric and substance abuse services under the AMH, Chicago, JCAHO.

Joint Commission on Accreditation of Healthcare Organizations (1990) Accreditation manual for hospitals, Chicago, JCAHO.

Lewis DD (1990) Conduct disorders. In Garfinkel BD, Carlson GA,and Weller EB, editors: Psychiatric disorders in children and adolescents, Philadelphia, WB Saunders Co.

Lewis JE (1989) Are adolescents being hospitalized unnecessarily? Journal of Child-Adolescent Psychiatric and Mental Health Nursing 2(4):134-138.

Nierenberg GI (1981) The art of negotiating, New York, Pocket Books.

Nierenberg J and Ross IS (1985) Women and the art of negotiating, New York, Simon & Schuster, Inc.

Pothier PC (1989) The impact of privatization of psychiatric care on children and adolescents, Archives of Psychiatric Nursing III(3):123-124.

Schiffman JR (1989) Children's wards: teenagers end up in psychiatric hospitals in alarming numbers, The Wall Street Journal Feb 3, p A1, A6.

Stevenson K and DuPrat MM (1989) Child and adolescent psychiatric illness: guidelines for treatment resources, quality assurance, peer review, and reimbursement, Washington, DC, American Academy of Child-Adolescent Psychiatry.

Appendix A

DSM-III-R Diagnoses and Codes

V62.30 Academic problem
309.90 Adjustment disorder NOS
       Adjustment disorder
309.24   with anxious mood
309.00   with depressed mood
309.30   with disturbance of conduct
309.40   with mixed disturbance of emotions and conduct
309.28   with mixed emotional features
309.82   with physical complaints
309.83   with withdrawal
309.23   with work (or academic) inhibition
V71.01 Adult antisocial behavior
300.22 Agoraphobia without history of panic disorder
       Alcohol
305.00   abuse
291.10   amnestic disorder
303.90   dependence
291.30   hallucinosis
291.40   idiosyncratic intoxication
303.00   intoxication
291.00   withdrawal delirium
294.00 Amnestic disorder (etiology noted on Axis III or is unknown)
       Amphetamine or similarly acting sympathomimetic
305.70   abuse
292.81   delirium
292.11   delusional disorder
304.40   dependence
305.70   intoxication
292.00   withdrawal
307.10 Anorexia nervosa
301.70 Antisocial personality disorder
300.00 Anxiety disorder NOS

From American Psychiatric Association (1987) Diagnostic and statistical manual of mental health disorders III-R, ed 3, Washington DC, The Association.

314.01 Attention-deficit hyperactivity disorder
299.00 Autistic disorder
313.21 Avoidant disorder of childhood or adolescence
301.82 Avoidant personality disorder
296.70 Bipolar disorder NOS
        Bipolar disorder, depressed,
296.56   in full remission
296.55   in partial remission
296.51   mild
296.52   moderate
296.53   severe, without psychotic features
296.50   unspecified
296.54   with psychotic features
        Bipolar disorder, manic,
296.46   in full remission
296.45   in partial remission
296.41   mild
296.42   moderate
296.43   severe, without psychotic features
296.40   unspecified
296.44   with psychotic features
        Bipolar disorder, mixed,
296.66   in full remission
296.65   in partial remission
296.61   mild
296.62   moderate
296.63   severe, without psychotic features
296.60   unspecified
296.64   with psychotic features
300.70 Body dysmorphic disorder
V40.00 Borderline intellectual functioning
301.83 Borderline personality disorder
298.80 Brief reactive psychosis
307.51 Bulimia nervosa
305.90 Caffeine intoxication
        Cannabis
305.20   abuse
292.11   delusional disorder
304.30   dependence
305.20   intoxication
V71.02 Childhood or adolescent antisocial behavior
307.22 Chronic motor or vocal tic disorder
307.00 Cluttering
        Cocaine
305.60   abuse
292.81   delirium
292.11   delusional disorder
304.20   dependence
305.60   intoxication
292.00   withdrawal
        Conduct disorder,

312.20	group type
312.00	solitary aggressive type
312.90	undifferentiated type
300.11	Conversion disorder
301.13	Cyclothymia
293.00	Delirum (etiology noted on Axis III or is unknown)
297.10	Delusional disorder
294.10	Dementia (etiology noted on Axis III or is unknown)
291.20	Dementia associated with alcoholism
301.60	Dependent personality disorder
300.60	Depersonalizaton disorder
311.00	Depressive disorder NOS
	Developmental
315.10	arithmetic disorder
315.39	articulation disorder
315.40	coordination disorder
315.90	disorder NOS
315.31	expressive language disorder
315.80	expressive writing disorder
315.00	reading disorder
315.31	receptive language disorder
799.90	Diagnosis or condition deferred on Axis I
799.90	Diagnosis or condition deferred on Axis II
300.15	Dissociative disorder NOS
307.47	Dream anxiety disorder (Nightmare disorder)
302.76	Dyspareunia
307.40	Dyssomnia NOS
300.40	Dysthymia
307.50	Eating Disorder NOS
313.23	Elective mutism
302.40	Exhibitionism
300.19	Factitious disorder NOS
	Factitious disorder
301.51	with physical symptoms
300.16	with psychological symptoms
302.72	Female sexual arousal disorder
302.81	Fetishism
302.89	Frotteurism
307.70	Functional encopresis
307.60	Functional enuresis
	Gender identity disorder
302.85	NOS
302.85	of adolescence or adulthood, nontranssexual type
302.60	of childhood
300.02	Generalized anxiety disorder
	Hallucinogen
305.30	abuse
292.11	delusional disorder
304.50	dependence
305.30	hallucinosis
292.84	mood disorder

301.50	Histrionic personality disorder
780.50	Hypersomnia related to a known organic factor
307.44	Hypersomnia related to another mental disorder (nonorganic)
302.71	Hypoactive sexual desire disorder
300.70	Hypochondriasis
313.82	Identity disorder
312.39	Impulse control disorder NOS
297.30	Induced psychotic disorder
	Inhalant
305.90	abuse
304.60	dependence
305.90	intoxication
302.73	Inhibited female orgasm
302.74	Inhibited male orgasm
780.50	Insomnia related to a known organic factor
307.42	Insomnia related to another mental disorder (nonorganic)
312.34	Intermittent explosive disorder
312.32	Kleptomania
307.90	Late luteal phase dysphoric disorder
	Major depression, recurrent,
296.36	in full remission
296.35	in partial remission
296.31	mild
296.32	moderate
296.33	severe, without psychotic features
296.30	unspecified
296.34	with psychotic features
	Major depression, single episode,
296.26	in full remission
296.25	in partial remission
296.21	mild
296.22	moderate
296.23	severe, without psychotic features
296.20	unspecified
296.24	with psychotic features
302.72	Male erectile disorder
V65.20	Malingering
V61.10	Marital problem
317.00	Mild mental retardation
318.00	Moderate mental retardation
	Multi-infarct dementia,
290.40	uncomplicated
290.41	with delirium
290.42	with delusions
290.43	with depression
300.14	Multiple personality disorder
301.81	Narcissistic personality disorder
	Nicotine
305.10	dependence
292.00	withdrawal
V71.09	No diagnosis or condition on Axis I

V71.09 No diagnosis or condition on Axis II
V15.81 Noncompliance with medical treatment
300.30 Obsessive compulsive disorder
301.40 Obsessive compulsive personality disorder
V62.20 Occupational problem
        Opioid
305.50   abuse
304.00   dependence
305.50   intoxication
292.00   withdrawal
313.81 Oppositional defiant disorder
294.80 Organic anxiety disorder (etiology noted on Axis III or is unknown)
293.81 Organic delusional disorder (etiology noted on Axis III or is unknown)
293.82 Organic hallucinosis (etiology noted on Axis III or is unknown)
294.80 Organic mental disorder NOS (etiology noted on Axis III or is unknown)
293.83 Organic mood disorder (etiology noted on Axis III or is unknown)
310.10 Organic personality disorder (etiology noted on Axis III or is unknown)
        Other or unspecified psychoactive substance
292.83   amnestic disorder
292.89   anxiety disorder
292.81   delirium
292.11   delusional disorder
292.82   dementia
292.12   hallucinosis
305.90   intoxication
292.84   mood disorder
292.90   organic mental disorder NOS
292.89   personality disorder
292.00   withdrawal
V62.81 Other interpersonal problem
V61.80 Other specified family circumstances
313.00 Overanxious disorder
        Panic disorder,
300.21   with agoraphobia
300.01   without agoraphobia
301.00 Paranoid personality disorder
302.90 Paraphilia NOS
307.40 Parasomnia NOS
V61.20 Parent-child problem
301.84 Passive aggressive personality disorder
312.31 Pathological gambling
302.20 Pedophilia
301.90 Personality disorder NOS
299.80 Pervasive developmental disorder NOS
V62.89 Phase of life problem or other life circumstance problem
        Phencyclidine (PCP) or similarly acting arylcyclohexylamine
305.90   abuse
292.81   delirium
292.11   delusional disorder
304.50   dependence
305.90   intoxication

292.84	mood disorder
292.90	organic mental disorder NOS
307.52	Pica
305.90	Polysubstance abuse
304.90	Polysubstance dependence
292.89	Posthallucinogen perception disorder
309.89	Post-traumatic stress disorder
302.75	Premature ejaculation
290.10	Presenile dementia NOS
	Primary degenerative dementia of the Alzheimer type,
290.10	presenile onset, uncomplicated
290.11	presenile onset, with delirium
290.12	presenile onset, with delusions
290.13	presenile onset, with depression
	Primary degenerative dementia of the Alzheimer type,
290.00	senile onset, uncomplicated
290.30	senile onset, with delirium
290.20	senile onset, with delusions
290.21	senile onset, with depression
780.54	Primary hypersomnia
307.42	Primary insomnia
318.20	Profound mental retardation
305.90	Psychoactive substance abuse NOS
304.90	Psychoactive substance dependence NOS
300.12	Psychogenic amnesia
300.13	Psychogenic fugue
316.00	Psychological factors affecting physical condition
298.90	Psychotic disorder NOS
312.33	Pyromania
313.89	Reactive attachment disorder of infancy or early childhood
307.53	Rumination disorder of infancy
295.70	Schizoaffective disorder
301.20	Schizoid personality disorder
	Schizophrenia, catatonic type,
295.22	chronic
295.24	chronic with acute exacerbation
295.21	subchronic
295.23	subchronic with acute exacerbation
295.20	unspecified
	Schizophrenia, disorganized type,
295.12	chronic
295.14	chronic with acute exacerbation
295.11	subchronic
295.13	subchronic with acute exacerbation
295.10	unspecified
	Schizophrenia, paranoid type,
295.32	chronic
295.34	chronic with acute exacerbation
295.31	subchronic
295.33	subchronic with acute exacerbation
295.30	unspecified

	Schizophrenia, residual type,
295.62	chronic
295.64	chronic with acute exacerbation
295.61	subchronic
295.63	subchronic with acute exacerbation
295.60	unspecified
	Schizophrenia, undifferentiated type,
295.92	chronic
295.94	chronic with acute exacerbation
295.91	subchronic
295.93	subchronic with acute exacerbation
295.95	unspecified
295.40	Schizophreniform disorder
301.22	Schizotypal personality disorder
	Sedative, hypnotic, or anxiolytic
305.40	abuse
292.83	amnestic disorder
304.10	dependence
305.40	intoxication
292.00	withdrawal delirium
290.00	Senile dementia NOS
309.21	Separation anxiety disorder
318.10	Severe mental retardation
302.79	Sexual aversion disorder
302.90	Sexual disorder NOS
302.70	Sexual dysfunction NOS
302.83	Sexual masochism
302.84	Sexual sadism
300.29	Simple phobia
307.46	Sleep terror disorder
307.45	Sleep-wake schedule disorder
307.46	Sleepwalking disorder
300.23	Social phobia
300.81	Somatization disorder
300.70	Somatoform disorder NOS
307.80	Somatoform pain disorder
315.90	Specific developmental disorder NOS
307.30	Stereotypy/habit disorder
307.00	Stuttering
307.20	Tic disorder NOS
307.23	Tourette's disorder
307.21	Transient tic disorder
302.50	Transsexualism
302.30	Transvestic fetishism
312.39	Trichotillomania
291.80	Uncomplicated alcohol withdrawal
V62.82	Uncomplicated bereavement
292.00	Uncomplicated sedative, hypnotic, or anxiolytic withdrawal
314.00	Undifferentiated attention-deficit disorder
300.70	Undifferentiated somatoform disorder
300.90	Unspecified mental disorder (nonpsychotic)

319.00 Unspecified mental retardation
306.51 Vaginismus
302.82 Voyeurism

Appendix B

Classification of Human Responses of Concern for Psychiatric Mental Health Nursing Practice

1. HUMAN RESPONSE PATTERNS IN ACTIVITY PROCESSES

1.1   Motor Behavior
    1.1.1   Potential for Alteration
        *1.1.1.1   Activity Intolerance
        1.1.1.2
    1.1.2   Altered Motor Behavior
        *1.1.2.1   Activity Intolerance
        1.1.2.2   Bizarre Motor Behavior
        1.1.2.3   Catatonia
        1.1.2.4   Disorganized Motor Behavior
        *1.1.2.5   Fatigue
        1.1.2.6   Hyperactivity
        1.1.2.7   Hypoactivity
        1.1.2.8   Psychomotor Aggitation
        1.1.2.9   Psychomotor Retardation
        1.1.2.10 Restlessness
    1.1.99 Motor Behavior Not Otherwise Specified (NOS)
1.1   Recreation Patterns
    1.2.1   Potential for Alteration
        1.2.1.1
        1.2.1.2
    1.2.2   Altered Recreation Patterns
        1.2.2.1   Age Inappropriate Recreation
        1.2.2.2   Anti-Social Recreation

From O'Toole AW and Loomis ME (1989) Revision of the phenomenon of concern for psychiatric mental health nursing, Archives of Psychiatric Nursing 3(5):288-299.
*Approved NANDA Diagnoses.

1.2.2.3   Bizarre Recreation
*1.2.2.4   Diversional Activity Deficit
1.2.99   Recreation Patterns NOS

1.3   Self Care
1.3.1   Potential for Alteration in Self Care
*1.3.2   Potential for Altered Health Maintenance
1.3.3   Altered Self Care
*1.3.3.1   Altered Eating
1.3.3.1.1   Binge-Purge Syndrome
1.3.3.1.2   Non-nutritive Ingestion
1.3.3.1.3   Pica
1.3.3.1.4   Unusual Food Ingestion
1.3.3.1.5   Refusal to Eat
1.3.3.1.6   Rumination
*1.3.3.2   Altered Feeding
*1.3.3.2.1   Ineffective Breast feeding
*1.3.3.3   Altered Grooming
*1.3.3.4   Altered Health Maintenance
*1.3.3.5   Altered Health Seeking Behaviors
*1.3.3.5.1   Knowledge Deficit
*1.3.3.5.2   Noncompliance
*1.3.3.6   Altered Hygiene
1.3.3.7   Altered Participation in Health Care
*1.3.3.8   Altered Toileting
*1.3.4   Impaired Adjustment
*1.3.5   Knowledge Deficit
*1.3.6   Noncompliance
1.3.99   Self Care Patterns NOS

1.4   Sleep/Arousal Patterns
1.4.1   Potential for Alteration
1.4.2   Altered Sleep/Arousal Patterns
1.4.2.1   Decreased Need for Sleep
1.4.2.2   Hypersomnia
1.4.2.3   Insomnia
1.4.2.4   Nightmares/Terrors
1.4.2.5   Somnolence
1.4.2.6   Somnambulism
1.4.99   Sleep/Arousal Patterns NOS

2. HUMAN RESPONSE PATTERNS IN COGNITION PROCESSES

2.1   Decision Making
2.1.1   Potential for Alteration
2.1.2   Altered Decision Making
2.1.3   Decisional Conflict
2.1.99   Decision Making Patterns NOS

2.2   Judgment
2.2.1   Potential for Alteration
2.2.2   Altered Judgment
2.2.99   Judgment Patterns NOS

2.3   Knowledge
2.3.1   Potential for Alteration
*2.3.2   Altered Knowledge Processes

2.3.2.1   Agnosia
2.3.2.2   Altered Intellectual Functioning
2.3.99 Knowledge Patterns NOS
2.4   *Learning*
2.4.1   Potential for Alteration
2.4.2   Altered Learning Processes
2.4.99 Learning Patterns NOS
2.5   *Memory*
2.5.1   Potential for Alteration
2.5.2   Altered Memory
2.5.2.1   Amnesia
2.5.2.2   Distorted Memory
2.5.2.3   Long-Term Memory Loss
2.5.2.4   Memory Deficit
2.5.2.5   Short-Term Memory Loss
2.5.99 Memory Patterns NOS
2.6   *Thought Processes*
2.6.1   Potential for Alteration
*2.6.2   Altered Thought Processes
2.6.2.1   Altered Abstract Thinking
2.6.2.2   Altered Concentration
2.6.2.3   Altered Problem Solving
2.6.2.4   Confusion/Disorientation
2.6.2.5   Delirium
2.6.2.6   Delusions
2.6.2.7   Ideas of Reference
2.6.2.8   Magical Thinking
2.6.2.9   Obsessions
2.6.2.10 Suspiciousness
2.6.2.11 Thought Insertion
2.6.99 Thought Processes NOS
3. HUMAN RESPONSE PATTERNS IN ECOLOGICAL PROCESSES
3.1   *Community Maintenance*
3.1.1   Potential for Alteration
3.1.2   Altered Community Maintenance
3.1.2.1   Community Safety Hazards
3.1.2.2   Community Sanitation Hazards
3.1.99 Community Maintenance Patterns NOS
3.2   *Environmental Integrity*
3.2.1   Potential for Alteration
3.2.2   Altered Environmental Integrity
3.2.99 Environmental Integrity Patterns NOS
3.3   *Home Maintenance*
3.3.1   Potential for Alteration
*3.3.2   Altered Home Maintenance
3.3.2.1   Home Safety Hazards
3.3.2.2   Home Sanitation Hazards
3.3.99 Home Maintenance Patterns NOS
4. HUMAN RESPONSE PATTERNS IN EMOTIONAL PROCESSES
4.1   *Feeling States*
4.1.1   Potential for Alteration

4.1.1.1   Anticipatory Grieving
4.1.2   Altered Feeling State
    4.1.2.1   Anger
  *4.1.2.2   Anxiety
    4.1.2.3   Elation
    4.1.2.4   Envy
  *4.1.2.5   Fear
  *4.1.2.6   Grief
    4.1.2.7   Guilt
    4.1.2.8   Sadness
    4.1.2.9   Shame
4.1.3   Affect Incongruous in Situation
4.1.4   Flat Affect
4.1.99   Feeling States NOS
4.2   *Feeling Processes*
4.2.1   Potential for Alteration
4.2.2   Altered Feeling Processes
    4.2.2.1   Lability
    4.2.2.2   Mood Swings
4.2.99   Feeling Processes NOS

5. HUMAN RESPONSE PATTERNS IN INTERPERSONAL PROCESSES

5.1   *Abuse Response Patterns*
5.1.1   Potential for Alteration
5.1.2   Altered Abuse Response
  *5.1.2.1   Post-trauma Response
  *5.1.2.2   Rape Trauma Syndrome
  *5.1.2.3   Compound Reaction
  *5.1.2.4   Silent Reaction
5.1.99   Abuse Response Patterns NOS
5.2   *Communication Processes*
5.2.1   Potential for Alteration
*5.2.2   Altered Communication Processes
    5.2.2.1   Altered Nonverbal Communication
  *5.2.2.2   Altered Verbal Communication
    5.2.2.2.1   Aphasia
    5.2.2.2.2   Bizarre Content
    5.2.2.2.3   Confabulation
    5.2.2.2.4   Ecolalia
    5.2.2.2.5   Incoherent
    5.2.2.2.6   Mute
    5.2.2.2.7   Neologisms
    5.2.2.2.8   Nonsense/Word Salad
    5.2.2.2.9   Stuttering
5.2.99   Communication Processes NOS
5.3   *Conduct/Impulse Processes*
5.3.1   Potential for Alteration
  *5.3.1.1   Potential for Violence
    5.3.1.2   Suicidal Ideation
5.3.2   Altered Conduct/Impulse Processes
    5.3.2.1   Accident Prone
    5.3.2.2   Aggressive/Violent Behavior Toward Environment

            5.3.2.3   Delinquency
            5.3.2.4   Lying
            5.3.2.5   Physical Aggression Toward Others
            5.3.2.6   Physical Aggression Toward Self
                  5.3.2.6.1   Suicide Attempt(s)
            5.3.2.7   Promiscuity
            5.3.2.8   Running Away
            5.3.2.9   Substance Abuse
            5.3.2.10 Truancy
            5.3.2.11 Vandalism
            5.3.2.12 Verbal Aggression Toward Others
        5.3.99   Conduct/Impulse Processes NOS
    5.4   *Family Processes*
        5.4.1   Potential for Alteration
           *5.4.1.1   Potential for Altered Parenting
           *5.4.1.2   Potential for Family Growth
      *5.4.2   Altered Family Processes
           5.4.2.1   Ineffective Family Coping
                *5.4.2.1.1   Compromised
                *5.4.2.1.2   Disabled
        5.4.99   Family Processes NOS
    5.5   *Role Performance*
        5.5.1   Potential for Alteration
      *5.5.2   Altered Role Performance
           5.5.2.1   Altered Family Role
                5.5.2.1.1   Parental Role Conflict
                5.5.2.1.2   Parental Role Deficit
           5.5.2.2   Altered Play Role
           5.5.2.3   Altered Student Role
           5.5.2.4   Altered Work Role
      *5.5.3   Ineffective Individual Coping
           *5.5.3.1   Defensive Coping
           *5.5.3.2   Ineffective Denial
        5.5.99   Role Performance Patterns NOS
    5.6   *Sexuality*
        5.6.1   Potential for Alteration
        5.6.2   Altered Sexual Behavior Leading to Intercourse
        5.6.3   Altered Sexual Conception Actions
        5.6.4   Altered Sexual Development
        5.6.5   Altered Sexual Intercourse
        5.6.6   Altered Sexual Relationships
      *5.6.7   Altered Sexuality Patterns
        5.6.8   Altered Variation of Sexual Expression
      *5.6.9   Sexual Dysfunction
        5.6.99   Sexuality Processes NOS
    5.7   *Social Interaction*
        5.7.1   Potential for Alteration
      *5.7.2   Altered Social Interaction
           5.7.2.1   Bizarre Behaviors
           5.7.2.2   Compulsive Behaviors
           5.7.2.3   Disorganized Social Behaviors

       5.7.2.4   Social Intrusiveness
    *5.7.2.5   Social Isolation/Withdrawal
       5.7.2.6   Unpredictable Behaviors
   5.7.99 Social Interaction Patterns NOS
  6. HUMAN RESPONSE PATTERNS IN PERCEPTION PROCESSES
6.1   *Attention*
   6.1.1   Potential for Alteration
   6.1.2   Altered Attention
       6.1.2.1   Hyperalertness
       6.1.2.2   Inattention
       6.1.2.3   Selective Attention
   6.1.99 Attention Patterns NOS
6.2   *Comfort*
   6.2.1   Potential for Alteration
   6.2.2   Altered Comfort Patterns
       6.2.2.1   Discomfort
       6.2.2.2   Distress
    *6.2.2.3   Pain
           6.2.2.3.1   Acute Pain
         *6.2.2.3.2   Chronic Pain
   6.2.99 Comfort Patterns NOS
6.3   *Self Concept*
   6.3.1   Potential for Alteration
   6.3.2   Altered Self Concept
    *6.3.2.1   Altered Body Image
    *6.3.2.2   Altered Personal Identity
    *6.3.2.3   Altered Self Esteem
        *6.3.2.3.1   Chronic Low Self Esteem
        *6.3.2.3.2   Situational Low Self Esteem
       6.3.2.4   Altered Sexual Identity
           6.3.2.4.1   Altered Gender Identity
   6.3.3   Undeveloped Self Concept
   6.3.99 Self Concept Patterns NOS
6.4   *Sensory Perception*
   6.4.1   Potential for Alteration
  *6.4.2   Altered Sensory Perception
       6.4.2.1   Hallucinations
         *6.4.2.1.1   Auditory
         *6.4.2.1.2   Gustatory
         *6.4.2.1.3   Kinesthetic
         *6.4.2.1.4   Olfactory
         *6.4.2.1.5   Tactile
         *6.4.2.1.6   Visual
       6.4.2.2   Illusions
   6.4.99 Sensory Perception Processes NOS
  7. HUMAN RESPONSE PATTERNS IN PHYSIOLOGICAL PROCESSES
7.1   *Circulation*
   7.1.1   Potential for Alteration
       7.1.1.1   Fluid Volume Deficit
   7.1.2   Altered Circulation
       7.1.2.1   Altered Cardiac Circulation

      *7.1.2.1.1 Decreased Cardiac Output
    7.1.2.2 Altered Vascular Circulation
      *7.1.2.2.1 Altered Fluid Volume
      *7.1.2.2.2 Fluid Volume Excess
      *7.1.2.2.3 Tissue Perfusion
        *7.1.2.2.3.1 Peripheral
        *7.1.2.2.3.2 Renal
  7.1.99 Altered Circulation Processes NOS
7.2 *Elimination*
  7.2.1 Potential for Alteration
  7.2.2 Altered Elimination Processes
    *7.2.2.1 Altered Bowel Elimination
      7.2.2.1.1 Constipation
        *7.2.2.1.1.1 Colonic
        *7.2.2.1.1.2 Perceived
      *7.2.2.1.2 Diarrhea
      7.2.2.1.3 Encopresis
      *7.2.2.1.4 Incontinence
    *7.2.2.2 Altered Urinary Elimination
      7.2.2.2.1 Enuresis
      *7.2.2.2.2 Incontinence
        *7.2.2.2.2.1 Functional
        *7.2.2.2.2.2 Reflex
        *7.2.2.2.2.3 Stress
        *7.2.2.2.2.4 Total
        *7.2.2.2.2.5 Urge
      *7.2.2.2.3 Retention
    7.2.2.3 Altered Skin Elimination
  7.2.99 Elimination Processes NOS
7.3 *Endocrine/Metabolic Processes*
  7.3.1 Potential for Alteration
  7.3.2 Altered Endocrine/Metabolic Processes
    *7.3.2.1 Altered Growth and Development
    7.3.2.2 Altered Hormone Regulation
      7.3.2.2.1 Premenstrual Stress Syndrome
  7.3.99 Endocrine/Metabolic Processes NOS
7.4 *Gastrointestinal Processes*
  7.4.1 Potential for Alteration
  7.4.2 Altered Gastrointestinal Processes
    7.4.2.1 Altered Absorption
    7.4.2.2 Altered Digestion
    *7.4.2.3 Tissue Perfusion
  7.4.99 Gastrointestinal Processes NOS
7.5 *Musculoskeletal Processes*
  7.5.1 Potential for Alteration
    *7.5.1.1 Potential for Disuse Syndrome
    *7.5.1.2 Potential for Injury
  7.5.2 Altered Musculoskeletal Processes
    7.5.2.1 Altered Coordination
    7.5.2.2 Altered Equilibrium
    7.5.2.3 Altered Mobility

    7.5.2.4   Altered Motor Planning
    7.5.2.5   Altered Muscle Strength
    7.5.2.6   Altered Muscle Tone
    7.5.2.7   Altered Posture
    7.5.2.8   Altered Range of Motion
    7.5.2.9   Altered Reflex Patterns
    7.5.2.10   Altered Physical Mobility
    7.5.2.11   Muscle Twitching
  7.5.99   Musculoskeletal Processes NOS
7.6   *Neuro/Sensory Processes*
  7.6.1   Potential for Alteration
  7.6.2   Altered Neuro/Sensory Processes
    7.6.2.1   Altered Level of Consciousness
    7.6.2.2   Altered Sensory Acuity
        7.6.2.2.1   Auditory
       *7.6.2.2.2   Dysreflexia
        7.6.2.2.3   Gustatory
        7.6.2.2.4   Olfactory
        7.6.2.2.5   Tactile
        7.6.2.2.6   Visual
    7.6.2.3   Altered Sensory Integration
    7.6.2.4   Altered Sensory Processing
        7.6.2.4.1   Auditory
        7.6.2.4.2   Gustatory
        7.6.2.4.3   Olfactory
        7.6.2.4.4   Tactile
        7.6.2.4.5   Visual
   *7.6.2.5   Cerebral Tissue Perfusion
   *7.6.2.6   Unilateral Neglect
    7.6.2.7   Seizures
  7.6.99   Neuro/Sensory Processes NOS
7.7   *Nutrition*
  7.7.1   Potential for Alteration
   *7.7.1.1   Potential for More Than Body Requirements
   *7.7.1.2   Potential for Poisoning
  7.7.2   Altered Nutrition Processes
    7.7.2.1   Altered Cellular Processes
    7.4.2.2   Altered Eating Processes
        7.7.2.2.1   Anorexia
       *7.7.2.2.2   Altered Oral Mucous Membrane
    7.7.2.3   Altered Systemic Processes
       *7.7.2.3.1   Less Than Body Requirements
       *7.7.2.3.2   More Than Body Requirements
    7.7.2.4   Impaired Swallowing
  7.7.99   Nutrition Processes NOS
7.8   *Oxygenation*
  7.8.1   Potential of Alteration
   *7.8.1.1   Potential for Aspiration
   *7.8.1.2   Potential for Suffocating
  7.8.2   Altered Oxygenation Processes
    7.8.2.1   Altered Respiration

.

          *7.8.2.1.1   Altered Gas Exchange
          *7.8.2.1.2   Ineffective Airway Clearance
          *7.8.2.1.3   Ineffective Breathing Pattern
        *7.8.2.2   Tissue Perfusion
      7.8.99   Oxygenation Processes NOS

7.9   *Physical Integrity*
      7.9.1   Potential for Alteration
         *7.9.1.1   Potential for Altered Skin Integrity
         *7.9.1.2   Potential for Trauma
    *7.9.2   Altered Oral Mucous Membrane
         *7.9.2.2   Altered Skin Integrity
         *7.9.2.3   Altered Tissue Integrity
      7.9.99   Physical Integrity Processes NOS

7.10   *Physical Regulation Processes*
      7.10.1   Potential for Alteration
         *7.10.1.1   Potential for Altered Body Temperature
         *7.10.1.2   Potential for Infection
      7.10.2   Altered Physical Regulation Processes
         7.10.2.1   Altered Immune Response
            7.10.2.1.1   Infection
         7.10.2.2   Altered Body Temperature
           *7.10.2.2.1   Hyperthermia
           *7.10.2.2.2   Hypothermia
           *7.10.2.2.3   Ineffective Thermoregulation

8. HUMAN RESPONSE PATTERNS IN VALUATION PROCESSES

8.1   *Meaningfulness*
      8.1.1   Potential for Alteration
    *8.1.2   Altered Meaningfulness
         8.1.2.1   Helplessness
        *8.1.2.2   Hopelessness
         8.1.2.3   Loneliness
        *8.1.2.4   Powerlessness
      8.1.99   Meaningfulness Patterns NOS

8.2   *Spirituality*
      8.2.1   Potential for Alteration
      8.2.2   Altered Spirituality
         8.2.2.1   Spiritual Despair
        *8.2.2.2   Spiritual Distress
      8.2.99   Spirituality Patterns NOS

8.3   *Values*
      8.3.1   Potential for Alteration
      8.3.2   Altered Values
         8.3.2.1   Conflict with Social Order
         8.3.2.2   Inability to Internalize Values
         8.3.2.3   Unclear Values
      8.3.99   Value Patterns NOS

Appendix C

Graduate Programs in Child Psychiatric Mental Health Nursing

Wayne State University
College of Nursing
5557 Cars Avenue
Detroit, MI 48202

Vanderbilt University
School of Nursing
500-C Godchaux Hall
Nashville, TN 37240

Medical College of Georgia
School of Nursing
Augusta, GA 30912

Indiana University
School of Nursing
1111 Middle Drive-N 403M
Indianapolis, IN 46202-5107

Georgia State University
School of Nursing
P.O. Box 4019
Atlanta, GA 30302-4019

University of South Florida
College of Nursing
12901 Bruce B. Downs Boulevard
Tampa, FL 33612-4799

Teachers College of Columbia University
525 W. 120th
New York, NY 10027

University of California at Los Angeles
School of Nursing
2/137 Factor
Los Angeles, CA 90024

University of California at San Francisco
School of Nursing
N319X Student-Affairs Office
San Francisco, CA 94143-0602

Yale University
School of Nursing
855 Howard Avenue
New Haven, CT 06520

University of Florida
School of Nursing
Box V197
Gainesville, FL 32611

University of Cincinnati
College of Nursing and Health
Cincinnati, OH 45221-0038

University of Illinois, Chicago
School of Nursing
845 S. Damen
MC 802
Chicago, IL 60612

Index

A

Abdomen, distended, tricyclic antidepressant drugs as cause of, 364

Abnormal Involuntary Movement Scale, tardive dyskinesia measured with, 361

Abortion, legalization of, impact of, 16

Abstraction, intelligence and skills for, 228

Abuse
  drug; *see* Drug abuse
  physical; *see* Physical abuse
  sexual; *see* Sexual abuse
  trauma due to, stress disorder and, 109

Academic achievement
  adolescent assessment and, 145
  conduct disorder and, 170

Academic achievement, poor
  in adolescents, 20
  depression indicated by, 88

Accidents, adolescent, rate of, 17

Acting in, definition of, 72

Acting out
  assessment of, 168
  clinical manifestations of, 72-73
  concept of, 71-74
  definition of, 71
  intervention for, 73-74, 376
  posttraumatic stress disorder and, 116
  sexual, posttraumatic stress disorder and, 117
  therapeutic intervention for, 374

Activities of daily living
  nursing standards and, 12, 273
  standard for intervention and, 373

Adaptation, definition of, in family systems theory, 42

ADHD; *see* Attention deficit hyperactivity disorder

Admission, form for assessment at time of, 156-162

Adolescence; *see also* Adolescent
  definition of, 28
  early, definition of, 29

Adolescence — cont'd
  late, definition of, 29
  law and, 52-55
  problems in
    historical development of, 15-25
    overview of, 16-23

Adolescent; *see also* Adolescence
  alcohol abuse in, assessment of, 178-179
  assessment of, 133-185
    components of, 139-155
    holistic tool for, 152-155
    variations in, 134-135
  biological development of, 35-36
  bonding with nurse by, 321
  chemical dependence in, 106-108
    interventions for, 108
    psychosocial characteristics and, 106
  chemical dependence in, assessment of, 175
  chum relationship in, 319
  clinical disorders in, assessment of, 168-171
  cognitive skills development in, 5-6
  communication with, 216
  community value system and, 7
  compliance difficulties in, evaluation of, 173*t*
  conformity to community standards and, 229-230
  depression in
    assessment of, 174
    rate of, 92
  development of, 27-49
    psychoanalytic theories of, 29-30
    role of community in, 45-46
  disordered, 69-744
  emotionally disturbed
    care for, 187-211
    rights of, 193-194
  freedom and responsibility in, 6
  group behavioral approaches with, 314
  health services for, 206
  high-risk, identification of, 259-260
  identification of, with his/her culture, 337
  as individual, 27-38
  individual behavioral approaches with, 314
  as inpatient, schedule for, 277-280
  interviewing of, 134
    techniques for, 135-138

Entries referring to tables are denoted by an italic *t* following the page number. An italic number indicates an illustration.

443

Adolescent—cont'd
law and, 52-55
legal rights of, 53-54
levels of privilege and, 295
mental health services access for, 55-60
moral development of, 34-35
muscular development in, 37
musculoskeletal growth in, 37
need for commitment in, 3-4
need for love in, 3-4
needs of, 3-7
neuropsychological evaluation of,
155-163
from other cultures, psychotherapy and,
335-336
physical health of, 7
prevalence of mental disorders in, 70-71
problems of
historical development of, 15-25
overview of, 16-23
professional services for, 20-23
psychiatric diagnoses of, tools for, 165
psychiatric disorder in, statistics on, 20
psychiatric problems of, nursing interventions
for, 373-415
psychological evaluation of, 163-168
psychological skills development in, 5-6
psychosocial development of, 27-28
pyschiatric nursing with, 7-11
recreational needs of, 206-207
runaway, 392
nursing care plan for, 394*t*
statistis on, 20
setting limits and, 220; *see also* Limit setting
skeletal development in, 37
social development of, 30-34
social history of, 142, 143-148
social needs of, 206-207
social skills for, 5-6, 223-226
suicidal, nursing care plan, 397*t*-398*t*
suicide rates and, 94-95
teaching programs for, 219-220
Adolescent psychiatric nursing
challenge of, 3-14
common adolescent psychiatric problems and,
373-415
definition of, 7
general concepts of, 374-376
graduate programs in, 441-442
intervention strategies for, 215-243
legal issues in, 51-67
liability and, 62-64
strategies for, 12, 276
strategies for administration of psychopharmacologic agents in, 352

Adolescent psychiatric unit; *see also* Therapeutic
milieu
aggression management in, 288-294
continuity of care in, 419
family programs in, 303
goal setting in, 295-303
inpatient schedule for, 277-280
limit setting in, 288-294
management of, 417-423
manager's role in, 421
marketing of, 420
privilege system in, 295
program of activities in, 275-276
quality control in, 417-418
rules in, 288
safety in, 418-419
staffing of, 276
training of staff in, 420
Adolescent psychotherapy; *see* Psychotherapy,
adolescent
Adulthood
adolescent psychosocial development into, 28
early, definition of, 34
Advocacy
case, 194
case manager and, 210
class, 194
nurse and, 235
system of care and, 193
Advocates for Child Psychiatric Nursing, 235
Affective disorder, 86-94
bipolar, 93-94
suicide associated with, 95
unipolar, 93-94
Aggression
conduct disorder and, 78
intervention for, 376
management of, in adolescent psychiatric unit,
288-294
as manipulative behavior, 385
nursing care plan for, 378*t*-379*t*
Aggression, control of, skills for, 231
Agranulocytosis, clozapine as cause of, 369
AIMS; *see* Abnormal Involuntary Movement
Scale
Akathisia, antipsychotic drugs as cause of, 358
Al-Anon, chemical dependence therapy
and, 412
Alanon/Alateen, address of, 263
Alcohol
antipsychotic drugs interaction with, 361
lithium interaction with, 366
tricyclic antidepressant drugs interaction with,
356
withdrawal symptoms and, diazepam for, 369

Alcohol abuse
  adolescent
    assessment of, 178-179
    rate of, 17
  nursing intervention for, 408-409
  prevention of, Teenage Institute for, 256
Alcoholics Anonymous, treatment program from, 409, 411-412
Alcoholics Anonymous/Narcotics Anonymous, adolescent chemical dependence and, 108
Alcoholism
  attention deficit hyperactivity disorder associated with, 85
  biological basis of, 106
  Diagnostic Statistical Manual of Mental Disorders diagnosis criteria for, 5-39
Aliphatic drugs, psychosis treated with, 358
Allergy, hyperactivity due to, 83
Alprazolam
  adolescent treated with, 369
  school refusal behavior treated with, 101
Amenorrhea, early puberty and, 36
American Academy of Child and Adolescent Psychiatry, guidelines for adolescent hospitalization from, 21
American Academy of Child and Adolescent Psychiatry Peer Review, guidelines on use of restraints from, 295
American Academy of Pediatrics, amphetamine dosage recommendations from, 353
American Humane Association, abuse statistics from, 19
American Nurses Association
  child and adolescent nursing standards from, 8-11
  clinical specialist certification and, 311
  standards for psychiatric nursing from, 62
American Occupational Therapy Association
  occupational therapy certification and, 330
  occupational therapy defined by, 329
American Psychiatric Association
  Diagnostic Statistical Manual of Mental Disorders from, 10, 69
  outpatient commitment and, 58
Aminophylline, lithium interaction with, 366
Amitriptyline, depression treated with, 363
Amnesia, psychogenic, posttraumatic stress disorder and, 116
Amphetamines
  attention deficit hyperactivity disorder treated with, 353
  interaction of, with other substances, 354
  toxicity of, 355
ANA; *see* American Nurses Association
Anafranil; *see* Clomipramine

Androgen, increase in, during pubescence, 36
Anger
  control of, skills for, 231-232
  Human Responses of Concern for Psychiatric/Mental Health Nursing Practice diagnosis and, 377
  intervention for, 376
  limit setting and, 377
  management of, for adolescent, 288-294
  self-awareness of, 380
  somatic therapy for, 377-378
Anger color chart, 289-290
Anhidrosis, antipsychotic drugs as cause of, 361
Animals, killing of, attention deficit hyperactivity disorder assessment and, 172
Anorexia nervosa, 104-105
  central nervous system stimulants as cause of, 354
  nursing intervention for, 412-414
  tricyclic antidepressant drugs as cause of, 364
Antacids, lithium interaction with, 366
Anticonvulsant drugs, tricyclic antidepressant drugs interaction with, 356
Antidepressant drugs
  affective disorders treated with, 93
  tricyclic
    attention deficit hyperactivity disorder treated with, 356-357
    depression and mania treated with, 363-365
    side effects of, 356, 364-365
Antihistamine drugs, tricyclic antidepressant drugs interaction with, 363
Antiparkinson drugs, tricyclic antidepressant drugs interaction with, 363
Antipsychotic drugs, 357-362
  central nervous stimulants affected by, 355
  death from, 362
  nursing implications of, 361-362
  side effects of, 56, 361
Antisocial behavior, oppositional defiant disorder indicated by, 79
Antisocial personality disorder, 75
Anxiety
  behavioral theory and, 313
  diagnosis of, 101
  group procedures for lessening of, 314
  indications of, 321
  prevalence of, in adolescent, 70
  psychoanalysis and, 316
  separation, diazepam for, 369
  suicide associated with, 95
Anxiety disorder, 100-102
  acting out associated with, 73
  depression associated with, 100
Anxiolytic drugs, dependence on, 107

Apathy, schizophrenia indicated by, 96
Arrhythmia, imipramine as cause of, 365
Art therapy, 330
  adolescent psychotherapy and, 312
  description of, 197
Artane; *see* Trihexyphenidyl
Assault, definition of, 63
Assertiveness training, activities for, in adolescent psychiatric unit, 300
Ataxia
  imipramine as cause of, 365
  tricyclic antidepressant drugs as cause of, 356
Ativan; *see* Lorazepam
Atropine, tricyclic antidepressant drugs interaction with, 363
Attention deficit hyperactivity disorder, 81-86
  anger and aggression associated with, 376
  assessment of, 171-174
  biological factors related to, 83
  clinical description of, 83-85
  definition of, 81
  intelligence quotient measurement and, 163
  interventions for, 85-86, 172
  nursing care plan for, 406t-407t
  nursing intervention for, 403-408
  pemoline for treatment of, 354
  psychopaharmacologic treatment of, 351-357
  suicide associated with, 95
  symptoms of, 84
  techniques for treatment of, 231
  theoretical explanation of, 82
  tricyclic antidepressant drugs for treatment of, 356-357
Attention span, attention deficit hyperactivity disorder assessment and, 81, 171
Attitude therapy
  in adolescent psychiatric unit, 306
  therapeutic milieu and, 274
Autism
  psychopharmacological treatment of, 357
  self-mutilation and, 388
Autonomy
  definition of, 61
  local, community structure and, 46
  optimal family relationships and, 43
Avoidance, as defense mechanism, 304

B

Baskethold, aggressive adolescent restrained with, 293
Batakas, anger intervention and, 380
Battery, definition of, 63
Beck Depression Scale for Children, 165
Behavior disorder, assessment of, 169-171

Behavior modification
  behavioral theory and, 314
  description of, 197
Behavior Problems Checklist, description of, 173t
Behavior rating scales, adolescent assessment and, 165
Behavior therapy, school phobia treated with, 100
Behavioral deconditioning, posttraumatic stress disorder treated with, 118
Behavioral theory, adolescent psychotherapy and, 313-315
Bellotti v Baird, 54, 60
Benadryl; *see* Diphenhydramine
Bender Visual-Motor Gestalt Test, description of, 166t
Benzodiazepine drugs
  attention deficit hyperactivity disorder treated with, 357
  tricyclic antidepressant drugs interaction with, 356
Benzodiazepine drugs, psychiatric illnesses treated with, 369
Benztropine
  anticholinergic side effects and, 359
  side effects of, 361
Bethel School District v Fraser, 53
Better Families Anonymous, chemical dependence therapy and, 412
Binge and purge syndrome, bulimia characterized by, 105
Bipolar affective disorder, 86-94
Bipolar affective disorder, acting out associated with, 76
Bipolar disorder
  carbamazepine for, 368
  suicide attempt associated with, 395
  treatment of, 367
Birth control, impact of, 16
Bladder, distended, tricyclic antidepressant drugs as cause of, 364
Blocking, group therapy communication and, 325
Blood pressure, elevated
  central nervous system stimulants as cause of, 354
  tricyclic antidepressant drugs and, 363
  tricyclic antidepressant drugs as cause of, 364
Bonding, lack of, conduct disorder associated with, 77
Borderline personality disorder, 102-104
  anger and aggression associated with, 377
  eating disorders associated with, 413
  self-mutilation and, 388
  suicide attempt associated with, 395

Boy Scouts of America, Students Against Drunk Driving training from, 247

Bradykinesia, antipsychotic drugs as cause of, 358

Brain, pathology of, schizophrenia and, 97

Brain chemistry, psychotherapy and, 331

Brain imaging, neuropsychological evaluation and, 163

Brief Psychiatric Rating Scale, 165

Bulimia, 104-105

Bulimia, nursing intervention for, 412-414

Bupropion, attention deficit hyperactivity disorder treated with, 356

Butyrophenone, psychotic disorders treated with, 360

C

Caffeine, lithium interaction with, 366

California Personality Inventory, description of, 166t

Cannabis, dependence on, 107

Carbamazepine
  bipolar disorder treated with, 367
  psychiatric illnesses treated with, 368-369

Carbohydrates, intolerance to, hyperactivity due to, 83

Cardiac arrythmia, bulimia associated with, 105

Cardiac stimulation, antipsychotic drugs as cause of, 358

Career and vocational services, description of, 203

Carey v Population Services International, 53

Carl Perkins Vocational Education Act, 203

Case management, 207-210
  skills for, 234-235
  system of care and, 193

Catapres; *see* Clonidine

Catatonic behavior, schizophrenia indicated by, 96

Catecholamine, availability of, tricyclic antidepressant drugs and, 363

Cattell 16 Personality Factor Questionnaire, description of, 166t

Central nervous system
  autonomic, psychotherapy research and, 332
  depression of
    stimulants as cause of, 353
    tricyclic antidepressants as cause of, 356
  stimulant drugs and, 352-355
    nursing implications of, 354

CGAS; *see* Children's Global Assessment Scale

Change, in family systems theory, 42

Character disorders, acting out associated with, 73

Cheating, conduct disorder indicated by, 78

Chemical dependence
  acting out associated with, 76
  adolescent, 106-108
  adolescent, assessment of, 176-177
  adolescent, medical and nursing diagnoses related to, 108-109
  assessment of, 175-177
  crisis intervention and, 265-266
  families and, 123
  nursing care plan for, 411t
  nursing intervention for, 408-412
  suicide attempt associated with, 395

Chemotherapy, school phobia treated with, 100

Child
  abused, school support group for, 267
  emotionally disturbed
    care for, 187-211
    early identification of, 192
  health services for, 206
  legal rights of, 54-55
  recreational needs of, 206-207
  social needs of, 206-207
  trauma to, adult denial of, 114

Child abuse, reporting of, nurse's liability and, 62

Child Behavior Checklist, description of, 173t

Child labor laws, history of, 187

Child protection services, professional services for adolescent and, 22

Childhood, middle, 27-28, 33

Children Are People, Inc., address of, 263

Children's Global Assessment Scale, 165

Children's Version of the Schedule for Affective Disorders and Schizophrenia, 165

Chlamydia trachomatis, rate of, in adolescents, 19

Chlordiazepoxide, adolescent treated with, 369

Chlorpromazine
  psychosis treated with, 358
  psychotic disorders treated with, 359-360
  side effects of, 358

Chlorprothixene, psychotic disorders treated with, 360

Chronic illness, high-risk adolescent and, 259

Chum relationship, adolescence and, 319

Churches, prevention strategies and, 246-247

Civil right movement, impact of, 16

Civil rights, use of mechanical restraints and, 293-294

Clarifying, group therapy communication and, 325

Classification of Nursing Diagnoses, 10

Classroom, therapeutic, 304-305

Clinical psychotherapist, training of, 312

Clinical specialist, certification of, 311

Clomipramine, obsessive-compulsive disorder treated with, 102, 369

Clonazepam, mania treated with, 369
Clonidine
  mania treated with, 367
  Tourette's syndrome treated with, 368
Clozapine, schizophrenia treated with, 369
Clozaril; see Clozapine
Clozaril Patient Management System, 369
CNS; see Central nervous system
Cocaine
  adolescent use of, 18
  dependence on, 107
Cocaine abuse, nursing intervention for, 409
Codependence, description of, 108-109
Cogentin; see Benztropine
Cognitive behavior therapy, behavioral theory
  and, 314
Cognitive skills
  description of, 5
  development of, 228-230
  in adolescent, 5-6
Cognitive theory, adolescent psychotherapy and,
  315
Cognitive therapy
  adolescent psychotherapy and, 315
  definition of, 222
Collaboration, adolescent psychiatric nursing
  and, 374-375
Coma, tricyclic antidepressant drugs as cause of,
  356
Commitment
  adolescent need for, 3-4
  definition of, 3
Communication
  adolescent-family, program for, 305
  verbal, development of, 229
Community
  adolescent development and, 7, 45-46
  assessment of
    adolescent social history and, 148
    guide for, 150-151
  standards of, conformity to, 229-230
  system of care and, 193
  troubled, 123-124
Community action, prevention strategies and,
  246-248
Community health system, standard for,
  245, 259
Community Intervention, Inc., address of, 253
Comorbidity, prevalence of, in adolescent, 70
Compensation, as defense mechanism, 304
Computed tomography, 164
  neuropsychological evaluation with, 155
Computerized electroencephalography, neuropsy-
  chological evaluation and, 163
Concentration, poor, depression indicated by, 88

Conduct disorder, 75-80
  academic achievement and, 170
  anger and aggression associated with, 377
  assessment of, 169-171
  depression associated with, 170
  diagnosis of, 76
  intelligence quotient measurement and, 163
  self-mutilation and, 388
  suicide attempt associated with, 95, 395
Conflict
  definition of, in family systems theory, 42
  resolution of, 323
    in optimal family, 43
Confrontation, resistance and denial treated
  with, 382
Confronting, group therapy communication and,
  325
Connors' Parent Rating, description of, 173*t*
Connors' Parent Symptom Questionnaire, 165
Connors' Teacher Rating Scale, 165
Consistence, nursing intervention and, 374-375
Constipation
  antipsychotic drugs as cause of, 358
  imipramine as cause of, 365
  tricyclic antidepressant drugs as cause of, 363,
  364
Constitution of the United States, legal system
  and, 51
Contingency management, definition of, 220
Conversion, as defense mechanism, 304
Convulsions
  imipramine as cause of, 365
  tricyclic antidepressant drugs as cause of, 356
Cooperativeness, skills for development of, 227
Coping, skills for, 230-236
Coprolalia, Tourette's syndrome indicated by,
  367
Corporal punishment, legal basis of, 53
Counseling
  case manager and, 209
  cross-cultural, psychotherapy and, 332
  group, description of, 196
  in home-based programs, 198
  individual, description of, 196
  parental, attention deficit hyperactivity disor-
    der intervention and, 85
  in schools, 201
Countertransference, group therapy and, 324
CPMS; see Clozaril Patient Management
  System
Cramps, early puberty and, 37
Crime
  conduct disorder and, 75
  juvenile, rate of, 19
Crisis center, description of, 267

Crisis intervention
    case manager's role in, 209
    case study of, 264-265
    chemical dependence and, 265-266
    resources for, 263
    skills for, 234
    steps in, 260-266
    strategies for, 198, 259-271
Critical thinking, skills for, 228
CT; *see* Computed tomography
Cultural-specific disorders, 333-340
Culture shock, psychotherapy and, 333
Curiosity, skills for development of, 227
Cylert; *see* Pemoline

D

Daily point sheet, use of, in adolescent psychiatric unit, 281-282
Dance therapy, 331
    adolescent psychotherapy and, 312
DAP; *see* Draw-a-Person test
Day treatment, description of, 196
Death, sudden, bulimia associated with, 105
Decision making, skills for, 228-229
Decision-making skills, development of, 249
Dehydration, bulimia associated with, 105
Delinquency, adolescent, conduct disorder and, 75
Delusions, psychotic episode indicated by, 399
Denial
    diagnosis of, 382
    Human Responses of Concern for Psychiatric/Mental Health Nursing Practice diagnosis of, 382
    nursing care plan for, 383t
    nursing intervention for, 381-385
    posttraumatic stress disorder and, 113, 115
Dental erosion, bulimia associated with, 105
Dependency, satanism related to, 20
Depression, 86-93
    acting out associated with, 76
    adolescent, rate of, 92
    antipsychotic drugs as cause of, 361
    anxiety disorder associated with, 100
    assessment of, 174
    case study of, 92-93
    central nervous system stimulants as cause of, 354
    childhood, treatment of, 363
    conduct disorder associated with, 170
    diagnosis of, 89-91
    episodes of, comparison of, 87-88
    hyperactivity associated with, 84
    major, 88-92
    prevention strategies for, 250

Depression—cont'd
    psychopharmacological treatment of, 362-368
    suicide attempt associated with, 395
Depressive disorder, prevalence of, 70
Desipramine
    depression treated with, 363
    side effects of, 356
Detention facility, description of, 205
Developmental disability, services for, 203-204
Dexedrine; *see* Dextroamphetamine
Dextroamphetamine
    attention deficit hyperactivity disorder treated with, 353
    recommended dosage of, 353
Diagnosis, nursing psychotherapy and, 320
Diagnostic Interview for Children and Adolescents, 165
Diagnostic Interview Schedule for Children, 165
Diagnostic Stastical Manual of Mental Disorders, 69-71
Diagnostic Statistical Manual of Mental Disorders, 10
    anger and related diagnoses in, 377
    anxiety diagnosis and, 101
    attention deficits and related diagnoses in, 405
    criteria of, for defiant and conduct disorders, 78-79
    denial and related diagnoses in, 382
    depression diagnosis and, 89-91
    diagnoses from, interviewing for, 148-155
    diagnosis codes in, 424-431
    eating disorders and related diagnoses in, 413
    hyperactivity described in, 82
    manipulation and splitting diagnosis and, 386
    nursing psychotherapy diagnosis and, 320
    posttraumatic stress and related diagnoses in, 110
    posttraumatic stress disorder diagnosis and, 333
    psychosis and related diagnoses in, 400
    psychosis diagnosis and, 97-98
    resistance and related diagnoses in, 382
    runaway adolescent and related diagnoses in, 393
    schizophrenia and related diagnoses in, 97-98
    self-mutilation and diagnoses in, 388
    substance abuse and related diagnoses in, 410
    suicide and related diagnoses in, 396
Diagnostic Statistical Manual of Mental Disorders criteria, history of present illness and, 140
Diarrhea
    imipramine as cause of, 365
    lithium as cause of, 366
    posttraumatic stress disorder indicated by, 115
    tricyclic antidepressant drugs as cause of, 364

Diazepam, separation anxiety treated with, 369

Dibenzoxazepine drugs, psychotic disorders treated with, 361

Differentiation, definition of, in family systems theory, 42

Dihydroindolone, psychotic disorders treated with, 360

Diphenhydramine, attention deficit hyperactivity disorder treated with, 357

Discrimination, system of care and, 194

Displacement, as defense mechanism, 304

Dissociate Experience Scale, 118

Dissociated personality disorder, acting out associated with, 73

Dissociation, posttraumatic stress disorder and, 116

Diuresis, sodium, lithium as cause of, 365

Divorce
high-risk adolescent and, 259
rate of, 19

Dopamine
affective disorders and, 93
central nervous stimulants affect of level of, 353
dyskinesia related to sensitivity to, 359
schizophrenia related to level of, 98
schizophrenia treatment and, 358

Draw-a-Person Test, adolescent assessment and, 168

Draw-a-Person Test, description of, 166*t*

Drowsiness, antipsychotic drugs as cause of, 361

Drug abuse
adolescent, rate of, 17-18
attention deficit hyperactivity disorder associated with, 85
nursing intervention for, 408-409

Drug-Free Schools Executive Initiative, 22

Drunkeness, adolescent, rate of, 106

DSM III-R; see Diagnostic Statistical Manual of Mental Disorders of Mental Disorders

DSM-III; *see Diagnostic Statistical Manual of Mental Disorders*

Duvall's eight stages of family development, 38-39

Dyes, intolerance to, hyperactivity due to, 83

Dyskinesia
antipsychotic drugs as cause of, 358
tardive, measurement of, 361

Dysphoric mood, depression indicated by, 88

Dystonia, antipsychotic drugs as cause of, 358

E

Eating disorders, 104-106
diagnosis of, 104-105
nursing intervention for, 106, 412-414

Education
ethnocultural identity and, 337
special, 203

Education for All Handicapped Children Act, 134, 200

Educational system, therapeutic care and, 200-203

Ego, psychoanalysis and, 316

Elavil; *see* Amitriptyline

Electrolyte imbalance, bulimia associated with, 105

Electrophysiology computerized electrocephalography, 164

Emancipation, requirements for, 60

Emergency room, crisis intervention at, 267-268

Emergency services, description of, 196

Empathy
definition of, 216
group therapy communication and, 325
lack of, conduct disorder and, 78

Endep; *see* Amitriptyline

Endoscopic retrograde pancreatography, 155

English Common Law, parental rights based in, 54

Entropy, definition of, in family systems theory, 42

Enuresis, treatment of, 367

Environment, control over, 233

Erikson' prototype of psychosocial development, 27, 31-33

ERP; *see* Endoscopic retrograde pancreatography

Estrogen, increase in, during pubescence, 36

Ethnicity, psychotherapy and, 336-340

Ethnocultural assessment, stages of, 334-335

Evaluation, group therapy communication and, 325

Exercise, excessive, anorexia and, 105

Existential therapy, adolescent psychotherapy and, 315-316

Experiential learning, description of, 319

Expressive therapy, 311-350

Eyberg Child Behavior Inventory, description of, 174*t*

F

Facilitating, group therapy communication and, 325

Fairness, adolescent psychiatric nursing and, 374-375

False imprisonment, definition of, 63-64

Families Anonymous, address of, 263

Family
adequate, description of, 44-45
alcoholic, roles and dynamics of, 124*t*
assessment of, guidelines for, 143*t*-145*t*

Family—cont'd
  blended, high-risk adolescent and, 259
  characteristics of, conduct disorders and, 77
  chemical dependence and, 123
  chemically dependent, high-risk adolescent in, 259
  as client, 374
  communication in, program for, 305
  development of, 27-49
  developmental stages of, 38-39
  disordered, 69-74
  dynamics of, acting out related to, 72
  high-risk, 259-260
  historical development of, 15
  midrange
    affective issues in, 120
    autonomy in, 120
    boundaries in, 120
    mental health problems in, 120-121
    power in, 120
  optimal, description of, 42-44
  from other cultures, psychotherapy and, 335-336
  programs for, in adolescent psychiatric unit, 303
  skill development with, 233-234
  structure of, genogram for assessment of, 141-142
  system of care and, 191
  troubled
    affective issues in, 123
    autonomy in, 123
    communication in, 122
    mental health problems in, 121-123
    power in, 123
  value system of, 39-40
Family disorders, 119-123
Family history
  family interview and, 140-142
  hyperactivity and, 83
Family resource services, description of, 204
Family systems theory, 41
Family therapy, 326-329
  in adolescent psychiatric unit, 303
  for anorexic adolescent, 413
  description of, 197
  minors treated with, 61
  nurse's role in, 328
  posttraumatic stress disorder treated with, 118
  psychotic adolescent and, 403
  quality control of, 417
  school phobia treated with, 100
  techniques of, 328
Federal court, common law and, 51

Feedback, group therapy communication and, 325
Fever, antipsychotic drugs associated with, 359
Fidelity, definition of, 28
Fire setting, conduct disorder indicated by, 78
Flashback experiences
  drug-related, posttraumatic stress disorder and, 117
  posttraumatic stress disorder and, 110
Flexiblity, adolescent psychiatric nursing and, 374-375
Fluphenazine
  psychotic disorders treated with, 360
  side effects of, 358
Foster care, therapeutic, 198
Foster parent, role of, in therapeutic foster care, 198-199
4-H Clubs, prevention strategies and, 248
Freedom, adolescent need for, 6
Friendliness, skills for development of, 223-226
Frontal lobe, deficit in, schizophrenia related to, 98

G

Game therapy, posttraumatic stress disorder treated with, 118
Gatehouse levels system, 284-287
Genogram, family history organized through, 141-142
Gestalt therapy
  adolescent psychotherapy and, 315-316
  resistance treated with, 383
  self-awareness and, 316
Ginsberg v New York, 53
Glucose, metabolism of
  obsessive-compulsive disorder and, 101
  psychotherapy research and, 332
Goal setting
  adolescent psychiatric nursing and, 376
  in adolescent psychiatric unit, 295-303
  description of, 221-223
  group therapy communication and, 325
  resistance intervention and, 382
Goss v Lopez, 53
Government agencies, prevention strategies and, 246-247
Group home, therapeutic, 199
Group home services, description of, 198
Group therapy
  communication in, 325
  didactic, 326, 327
  inpatient, 326
  multifamily, 329
  phases of, 326

Group therapy—cont'd
  posttraumatic stress disorder treated
    with, 118
  practice of, 324-325
Growth, retardation of, central nervous system
    stimulants as cause of, 354
Guilt
  parental, attention deficit hyperactivity disor-
    der and, 171
  posttraumatic stress disorder and, 117, 119
Gynecomastia, causes of, 37

H

Haldol; see Haloperidol
Hallucinations
  psychotic episode indicated by, 399
  schizophrenia indicated by, 96
Hallucinogenic drugs
  adolescent use of, 18
  dependence on, 107
Haloperidol
  attention deficit hyperactivity disorder treated
    with, 357
  lithium interaction with, 366
  psychotic disorders treated with, 360
  side effects of, 358
  Tourette's syndrome treated with, 368
Havighurst's Developmental Stages and Tasks,
    30-33
Hazelden Foundation, chemical dependence
    therapy and, 411
Head banging, self-mutilation and, 388
Health
  mental; see Mental health
  physical; see Physical health
Health Care Financing Agency, 295
Health teaching, standard for, 374
History of present illness, interviewing
    techniques for, 139-140
Home and School Questionnaire, description of,
    173t
Home-based services, description of, 197
Home-bound instruction, description of, 203
Homemaker services, description of, 204
Homicide
  assessment of potential for, 265
  nurse's liability for, 62
Hopelessness
  depression indicated by, 88
  suicide associated with, 95
Horowitz and Davidson, 56
Hospitalization
  primary uses of, 199-200
  psychiatric, 199
HPI; see History of present illness

*Human Responses of Concern for
    Psychiatric/Mental Health Nursing Practice*,
    10, 432-440
  anger diagnosis in, 377
  interviewing skills for, 148-155
  manipulation diagnosis in, 386
  resistance diagnosis and, 382
  runaway adolescent and, 393
  self-mutilation and, 388
  splitting diagnosis in, 386
*Human Responses of Concern for
    Psychiatric/Mental Health Nursing Practice*
  denial diagnosis in, 382
Human services, description of, 204-205
Humanistic theory, adolescent psychotherapy
    and, 315-316
Hyperactive reflex, imipramine as cause of, 365
Hyperactivity
  attention deficit hyperactivity disorder assess-
    ment and, 171
  clinical description of, 83-85
  conduct disorder and, 75
  dopaminergic, schizophrenia associated with,
    98
  medication for, 353
  nursing care plan for, 406t-407t
  nursing intervention for, 403-408
  theoretical explanation of, 82
Hyperkinesis, theoretical explanation of, 82
Hypnosis, posttraumatic stress disorder treated
    with, 118
Hypnotic drugs, dependence on, 107
Hypomania, oppositional defiant disorder indi-
    cated by, 79
Hypomanic behavior, 94
Hypotension
  antipsychotic drugs as cause of, 358, 361
  tricyclic antidepressant drugs and, 363
Hypothalamus, function of, during pubescence,
    36

I

"I" statements
  attention deficit hyperactivity disorder therapy
    and, 405
  nursing intervention for anger and aggression
    and, 380
  one-to-one communication and, 306
  skill development and, 300
  therapy for suicidal adolescent and, 396
Id, psychoanalysis and, 316
Idealization, as defense mechanism, 304
Ideas of reference, psychotic episode indicated
    by, 399
Identification, as defense mechanism, 304

IEP; *see* Individualized Education Plan
Imipramine
    depression treated with, 363
    dosage of, 365
    enuresis treated with, 367
    school refusal behavior treated with, 101
Imipramine pamoate
    contraindications for, 365
    enuresis treated with, 367
Impulsiveness, control of, 231-233
In Re Gault, 53, 54
Inappropriate affect, psychotic episode indicated
        by, 399
Inattentiveness, schizophrenia indicated by, 96
Incest, posttraumatic stress disorder and, 116
Incoherence, psychotic episode indicated by, 399
Incoherence, schizophrenia indicated by, 96
Incomplete sentence test, adolescent assessment
        and, 164
Inderal; *see* Propranolol
Individualized Education Plan, 197
Industry versus inferiority, psychosocial develop-
        ment theory and, 27-28
Infant, experience of trauma in, 113
Informed consent, description of, 59-60
Ingraham v Wright, 53
Inhalant drugs, dependence on, 107
Inpatient treatment, adolescents in, statistics on,
        20-21
Insight therapy, description of, 317
Insomnia, central nervous system stimulants as
        cause of, 354
Intelligence, ability to abstract and, 228
Intelligence quotient
    disorders and, 163
    low, anger and aggression associated with, 376
Intermediate care facility, description of, 204
Interpersonal theory, psychotherapy and, 318
Interpreting, group therapy communication and,
        325
Intervention
    for adolescent psychiatric problems, 373-415
    for anorexia nervosa, 412-414
    for attention deficit hyperactivity disorder, 403-
        408
    for bulimia, 412-414
    for chemical dependence, 408-412
    crisis; *see* Crisis intervention
    culturally sensitive, 336-340
    definition of, 265
    health teaching and, standard for, 245
    for hyperactivity, 403-408
    for psychosis, 399-403
    psychotherapeutic, standards for, 245, 259,
        274, 373

Intervention — cont'd
    resources for, 252-253
    for self-mutilation, 390-392
    somatic therapy, standard for, 351
    steps in, 265-266
    for suicidal adolescent, 395-399
Interviewing
    assessment, 135-138
        objectives of, 136
    clinical assessment, 135
    family, 140-142
    family intake, 136
    psychotherapeutic, 135
        objectives of, 136
    resistance to, 138
    techniques checklist for, 180-181
    techniques for, 135-138
    types of, 134
IQ; *see* Intelligence quotient
Irritability
    depression indicated by, 88
    oppositional defiant disorder indicated by, 79
    posttraumatic stress disorder indicated by, 115
Isolation, resistance treated with, 384

J

JCAHO; *see* Joint Commission on Accreditation
        of Healthcare Organizations
Joint Commission on Accreditation of Health-
        care Organizations, 295
    quality control of psychiatric unit and, 418
Joint Commission on Hospital Accreditation,
        nursing care plan mandated by, 11
Juvenile court, professional services for adoles-
        cent and, 21
Juvenile court system, history of, 187
Juvenile crime, rate of, 19
Juvenile justice system, 205
Juvenile offender, residential placement of, 205

K

Klonopin; *see* Clonazepam
Knowledge
    adolescent need for, 4
    definition of, 4
Kohlberg's cognitive theory of moral develop-
        ment, 34-35

L

Lactate, level of, panic disorder and, 100
Law
    adolescent psychiatric nursing and, 51-67
    child's rights basis in, 54-55
    common, 51-52
    constitutional, 51

Law—cont'd
  parental rights basis in, 54-55
  sources of, 51-55
  statutory, 52
Learning disability
  anger and aggression associated with, 376
  attention deficit hyperactivity disorder co-
      existing with, 86
Leninger's transcultural nursing theory, 332
Lessard v Schmidt, 56
Liability, legal, adolescent psychiatric nursing
      and, 62-64
Librium; *see* Chlordiazepoxide
Limit setting
  adolescent psychiatric nursing and, 374-375
  in adolescent psychiatric unit, 288-294
  for adolescent with eating disorders,
      413-414
  anger intervention and, 377
  for attention deficit hyperactivity dis-
      order, 405
  chemical dependence therapy and, 409
  description of, 220-221
  manipulation intervention and, 386
  psychosis therapy and, 399-400
  runaway adolescent and, 392-393
  self-mutilation therapy and, 390-391
  for suicidal adolescent, 395-396
Listening, active, 229
  attention deficit hyperactivity disorder therapy
      and, 405
  group therapy communication and, 325
  skill development and, 300
Lithium
  affective disorders treated with, 93
  attention deficit hyperactivity disorder treated
      with, 357
  mania treated with, 365-367
  nursing implications of use of, 366-367
  parent teaching about, 366-367
  poisoning from, 366
  toxicity of, 359
Locus of control, internal, development
      of, 231
Loose associations, psychotic episode in-
      dicated by, 399
Lorazepam, mania treated with, 369
Love
  adolescent need for, 3-4
  definition of, 3
Loxapine, psychotic disorders treated with, 361
Loxitane; *see* Loxapine
Loyalty, adolescent psychosocial development
      and, 28
Lying, conduct disorder indicated by, 78

M
Magnetic resonance imaging, 164
  neuropsychological evaluation and, 163
Mainstreaming Act, description of, 52
Malpractice
  common law as basis of, 51
  description of, 62-63
Mania
  drugs for treatment of, 369
  psychopharmacological treatment of, 362-368
Manic personality disorder, acting out associated
      with, 76
Manipulation
  diagnosis of, 386
  *Human Responses of Concern for Psychiatric/
      Mental Health Nursing Practice* diagnosis
      of, 386
  nursing care plan for, 387t
  nursing intervention for, 385-388
MAPI; *see* Milton Adolescent Personality Inven-
      tory
Marijuana, adolescent use of, 18
Marital distress, adolescent conduct disorder
      and, 169
Marketing, adolescent psychiatric unit and, 420
Marriage, rate of, by adolescents, 20
Massachusetts Adolescent Level of Functioning
      Scale, 165
Maturation, hyperactivity and, 82
"Mature minor" rule, 60
MBD; *see* Minimal brain damage
Mediation, ethnocultural identity and, 337
Medical history, adolescent assessment and, 140
Medication, right to refuse, 57
Mellaril; *see* Thioridazine
Menarche, onset of, 36
Menstrual water retention, early puberty and, 37
Mental health facility, commitment to, adoles-
      cent rights and, 55-59
Mental health facility, crisis intervention and,
      267
Mental Health Planning Act of 1986, 58-59
Mental health services
  access to, 55-60
  description of, 194-200
Mental retardation
  anger and aggression associated with, 376
  services for, 203-204
Mental status examination, 142, 146-148
Methylphenidate
  attention deficit hyperactivity disorder treated
      with, 353
  recommended dosage of, 353
  tricyclic antidepressant drugs interaction with,
      363

Meyer v Nebraska, 55
Millon Adolescent Personality Inventory, 165
    description of, 166*t*
Minimal brain damage, hyperactivity and, 82
Minnesota Multiphasic Personality Inventory,
    165
    description of, 166*t*
Minor
    emancipated, 60
    family therapy and, 61
    informed consent and, 59
    legal status of, 51
    mature, 60
Mitral valve prolapse, panic disorder associated
    with, 100
MMPI; *see* Minnesota Multiphasic Personality
    Inventory
Moban; *see* Molindone
Modeling, adolescent psychotherapy and, 314
Molindone, psychotic disorders treated with, 360
Monoamine oxidase inhibitor drugs, interaction
    of, with central nervous system stimulants,
    355
Mood disorder, 86-94
    Diagnostic Statistical Manual of Mental Disor-
        ders diagnoses of, 89-91
Mouth, dry
    antipsychotic drugs as cause of, 358
    tricyclic antidepressant drugs and, 363
    tricyclic antidepressant drugs as cause of, 364
MRI; *see* Magnetic resonance imaging
MSE; *see* Mental status examination
Multiple personality disorder, satanism related
    to, 20
Murder, conduct disorder indicated by, 78
Music therapy, 331
    adolescent psychotherapy and, 312
    description of, 197
Mutilation; *see* Self-mutilation

N
NALSAP; *see* National Association of Leader-
    ship for Student Assistance Programs
NarAnon Family Groups, address of, 263
Narcotics Anonymous, chemical dependence
    therapy and, 412
National Association of Leadership for Student
    Assistance Programs, address of, 263
National Institute of Mental Health
    address of, 263
    child mental health research and, 22
National Parents Resource Institute for Drug
    Education, address of, 253
Nausea
    lithium as cause of, 366

Nausea—cont'd
    tricyclic antidepressant drugs as cause
        of, 364
Navane; *see* Thiothixene
Negentrophy, definition of, 42
Neglect, crisis intervention and, 262*t*
Neisseria gonorrhoeae, rate of, in adolescents, 19
Nervous system; *see* Central nervous system
Nervousness, central nervous system stimulants
    as cause of, 354
Neurobiology, psychotherapy and, 331
Neuroleptic malignant syndrome, antipsychotic
    drugs and, 359
Neuropsychological evaluation, 155-163
Neurosis, behavioral theory and, 313
Neurotransmitters
    affective disorders and, 93
    dysfunction in, obsessive-compulsive disorder
        associated with, 101
New York-London survey, description of, 174*t*
Newborn, experience of trauma in, 113
Nicotine, dependence on, 107
Nightmares, posttraumatic stress disorder and,
    110
NIMH; *see* National Institute of Mental Health
NMS; *see* Neuroleptic malignant syndrome
Nocturnal emissions, onset of, 36
No-harm contract, self-mutilation therapy and,
    391
Norepinephrine
    affective disorders and, 93
    regulation of, obsessive-compulsive disorder
        associated with, 101
    tricyclic antidepressant drugs effect on, 364*t*
Norepinephrine, central nervous stimulants af-
    fect of level of, 353
Norpramin; *see* Desipramine
NPA; *see* Nurse Practice Act
Nurse
    adolescent psychiatric
        adolescent bonding with, 321
        advocacy role of, 60-61
        family therapy and, 328
    advocacy role of, 60-61
    characteristics of, 8
    emergency room, crisis intervention by, 268
    prevention strategies promoted by, 248-249
Nurse generalist, certification of, 311
Nurse Practice Act, 52
Nursing, adolescent psychiatric, challenge of,
    3-14
Nursing admission, form for assessment at time
    of, 156-162
Nursing care plan
    for aggression, 378*t*-379*t*

Nursing care plan—cont'd
for attention deficit hyperactivity disorder,
406t-407t
for chemical dependence, 411t
description of, 11
for hyperactivity, 406t-407t
for manipulation and splitting, 387t
for psychosis, 401t-404t
for resistance and denial, 383t
for runaway adolescent, 394t
for self-mutilation, 389t-390t
for suicidal adolescent, 397t-398t
Nursing diagnosis (psychiatric mental health)
attention deficits and related diagnoses in, 405
eating disorders and related diagnoses in, 413
psychosis and related diagnoses in, 400
substance abuse and related diagnoses
in, 410
suicide and related diagnoses in, 396

O

Obsessive-compulsive disorder, 101-102
treatment of, 369
Occupational therapy, 329-330
adolescent psychotherapy and, 312
definition of, 329
OCD; *see* Obsessive-compulsive disorder
O'Conner v Donaldson, 57
ODD; *see* Oppositional defiant disorder
Operant group therapy, definition of, 314
Opioid drugs, dependence on, 107
Oppositional defiant disorder, 74-75, 79
interventions for, 79-80
Oppositional disorder, prevalence of, 70
Orap; *see* Pimozide
Outpatient commitment, legal considerations of,
57-59
Outpatient services, description of, 195
Outreach services, description of, 195
Overanxious disorder, prevalence of, 70

P

Panic attack, diazepam for, 369
Panic disorder, 100
Paradoxical injunction
family therapy and, 327
resistance treated with, 384
Paralytic ileus, antipsychotic drugs as cause of,
361
Paranoia, psychotic episode indicated by, 399
Parens patriae, description of, 54
Parent
behavior of, conduct disorders and, 77
counseling of, for attention deficit hyperactivity
disorder adolescent, 85

Parent—cont'd
emotionally ill, high-risk adolescent and, 259
guilt feelings of, attention deficit hyperactivity
disorder and, 171
inept discipline from, 169
inept monitoring by, 169
legal rights of, 54-55
responsibility of, in administration to central
nervous system stimulants to adolescent,
355
therapeutic milieu and, 303
Parental counseling, posttraumatic stress disorder treated with, 118
Parents Anonymous, address of, 263
Parham v J.R., 58
Passive-aggressive behavior, nursing intervention
for, 380
Peer group, adolescent psychosocial development
and, 28
Peer pressure, adolescent drinking and, 106
Peer therapy, adolescent psychotherapy and, 314-
315
Pemoline
attention deficit hyperactivity disorder treated
with, 354
recommended dosage of, 354
Peplau's theory of nurse-client interpersonal re-
lationship, 319
Personality inventory, adolescent assessment and,
164
Personality Inventory for Children, 165
Personality test, adolescent assessment and, 163
Pertofrane; *see* Desipramine
PET; *see* Positron emission tomography
PGH; *see* Pituitary growth hormone
Phencyclidine, dependence on, 107
Phenobarbital, attention deficit hyperactivity dis-
order treated with, 357
Phenothiazine drugs
attention deficit hyperactivity disorder treated
with, 357
psychosis treated with, 358
psychotic disorders treated with, 359
tricyclic antidepressant drugs interaction with,
363
Phenylpropanolamine, tricyclic antidepressant
drugs interaction with, 356
Physical abuse, child, rate of, 19
PIC; *see* Personality Inventory for Children
Pica, 104
Pimozide, Tourette's syndrome treated with, 368
Piperazine drugs, psychosis treated with, 358
Piperidine drugs, psychosis treated with, 358
Pituitary gland, function of, during pubescence,
36

Pituitary growth hormone, function of, during pubescence, 36
Planned Parenthood of Missouri v Danforth, 53, 54
Play therapy, posttraumatic stress disorder treated with, 118
PMH; *see Human Responses of Concern for Psychiatric/Mental Health Nursing Practice*
Point system, attention deficit hyperactivity disorder therapy and, 408, 409
Positron emission tomography, 164
Positron emission tomography, neuropsychological evaluation and, 163
Posttraumatic stress disorder, 109-119, 333
  assessment of symptoms of, 110
  diagnosis of, 112
  interventions for, 118-119
  symptoms of, 115-117
Postvention, definition of, 267
Poverty, number of children in, 19
Power, personal, 233
Preadolescence, definition of, 29
Pregnancy, teenage
  crisis intervention and, 262*t*
  prevention strategies for, 250
  rate of, 18-19
Premenstrual syndrome, early puberty and, 36
President's Commission on Mental Health, 184
Prevention
  primary, definition of, 245
  resources for, 252-253
  strategies for, 245-257
Prevention services, description of, 195
PRIDE, address of, 253
Prince v Massachusetts, 55
Privilege system, behavior therapy and, 315
Probation officer, function of, 205
Problem-solving skills, 228-229
Problem-solving skills, development of, 249
Professional Code of Ethics, 64
Prognosis, nursing psychotherapy and, 320
Project Re-Ed, 200
Projection, as defense mechanism, 304
Prolixin; *see* Fluphenazine
Promiscuity, posttraumatic stress disorder and, 117
Propranolol, description of, 369
Prostitution, posttraumatic stress disorder and, 117
Protective services, description of, 204
Psychiatric disorder, in adolescent, statistics on, 20
Psychiatric facility, commitment to, adolescent rights and, 55-59
Psychoanalysis
  description of, 316

Psychoanalysis—cont'd
  Freudian, 316
  psychotherapy and, 316-318
Psychoanalytical theory, psychotherapy and, 316-318
Psychodrama
  acting out treated with, 73
  resistance treated with, 383
Psychological evaluation, adolescent assessment and, 163-168
Psychological skills, development of, in adolescent, 5-6
Psychological tests, description of, 166*t*-167*t*
Psychomotor behavior, poor, depression indicated by, 88
Psychopathology, suicide associated with, 95
Psychopharmacology, 351-371
Psychosis
  nursing care plan for, 401*t*-404*t*
  nursing intervention for, 399-403
  psychopharmacological treatment of, 357-362
  satanism related to, 20
Psychosocial development, adolescent, 27-28
Psychotherapy, 311-350
  adolescent
    behavioral theory and, 313-315
    schools of thought on, 313
    theoretical approaches to, 312
  attention deficit hyperactivity disorder treated with, 85
  brief, description of, 317
  as component in nursing standards, 12
  cross-cultural counseling and, 332
  culturally sensitive, 337-338
  group, 322-326
    in adolescent psychiatric unit, 417
    inpatient, 326
    quality control of, 417
  integrative, 340-343
  interpersonal theory and, 318
  investigative nurse, 318-322
  nursing, 339-340
    components of, 320
    definition of, 312
  posttraumatic stress disorder treated with, 118
  professional accountability and, 312
  psychoanalytical, 316-318
  psychoanalytical theory and, 316-318
  somatopsychic, 339-340
  standards for, 311
  strategic principles of, 340-343
  trends in, 331-343
Psychotropic drugs
  psychiatric patient restraint with, 56

Psychotropic drugs—cont'd
   tricyclic antidepressant drugs interaction with, 363
PTSD; *see* Posttraumatic stress disorder
Puberty, definition of, 36
Pubescence, definition of, 36
Public Law 94-142, 134, 200
Public Law 98-524, 203
Public Law 94-142, description of, 52

Q

Questioning, group therapy communication and, 325

R

Random movements, attention deficit hyperactivity disorder indicated by, 81
Rape, conduct disorder indicated by, 78
Rationalization, as defense mechanism, 304
Reaction formation, as defense mechanism, 304
Reality therapy
   definition of, 220
   description of, 315
   limit setting process and, 290
Recreational therapy, 330-331
   adolescent psychotherapy and, 312
   description of, 197
Reexperiencing, posttraumatic stress disorder and, 110
Reflection
   ethnocultural identity and, 337
   group therapy communication and, 325
Reflex, hyperactive, imipramine as cause of, 365
Regression, as defense mechanism, 304
Rehabilitation Act of 1973, description of, 52
Reinforcement
   definition of, 221
   differential, 221
   token, 221
Relationship therapy, description of, 317
Relaxation techniques, anger intervention and, 380
Rennie v Klein, 56
Repression
   as defense mechanism, 304
   psychoanalysis and, 316
Residential treatment
   conduct disorders treated with, 79
   description of, 200
Resistance
   diagnosis of, 382
   Human Responses of Concern for Psychiatric/Mental Health Nursing Practice diagnosis and, 382
   nursing care plan for, 383*t*

Resistance—cont'd
   nursing intervention for, 381-385
Respect
   adolescent need for, 4
   definition of, 4
Respiratory depression
   imipramine as cause of, 365
   tricyclic antidepressant drugs as cause of, 356
Respite care, description of, 199
Respondeat superior, malpractice and, 51
Response cost contingency management, 221
Responsibility
   adolescent freedoms linked to, 6
   definition of, 4
   skills for development of sense of, 229
Restating, group therapy communication and, 325
Restraint
   manual, in adolescent psychiatric unit, 293
   mechanical, in adolescent psychiatric unit, 293
Right to refuse treatment, 56, 57
Rigidity
   adolescent psychiatric nursing and, 374-375
   antipsychotic drugs associated with, 358, 359
Risk-taking, self-mutilation and, 388
Ritalin; *see* Methylphenidate
Rogers v Commissioner of the Department of Mental Health, 57
Rogers v Okin, 57
Role modeling, 219
   anger intervention and, 379
   group therapy communication and, 325
   therapeutic milieu and, 307
Role playing, acting out treated with, 73
Roles, alternate, 227
Rorschach test, 165
Rosenzweig Picture Frustration Test, description of, 167*t*
Rouse v Cameron, 55
Rumination disorder, 104
Runaway children, statistics on, 20
Running away
   Human Responses of Concern for Psychiatric/Mental Health Nursing Practice diagnosis of, 393
   nursing care plan for, 394*t*
   nursing intervention for, 392-395

S

SADD; *see* Students Against Drunk Driving
Safety, adolescent psychiatric unit and, 418-419
Satanism, statistics on, 20
SBH; *see* Severely behaviorally handicapped child
Schizo-affective illness, carbamazepine for, 368

Schizophrenia, 96-100
  carbamazepine for, 369
  diagnosis of, 97-98
  indications of, 79
  interventions for, 100
  psychopharmacological treatment of, 357-362
  psychotic episode and, 399
  symptoms of, 99
School
  abused child program in, 267
  adolescent development and, 7
  assessment services in, 201
  attendance of, adolescent assessment and, 145
  counseling services in, 201
  crisis intervention in, 266-267
    following successful suicide, 267
  prevention strategies and, 247-248
  professional services for adolescent and, 22
  psychotherapeutic intervention in, 312
  support groups in, 267
School nurse, prevention strategies promoted by, 248
School phobia, description of, 100
Screaming, Tourette's syndrome indicated by, 367
SCT; *see* Symonds Picture Story Test
Sculpting, description of, 327
Seclusion, aggressive behavior managed with, 293
Seclusion room, adolescent psychiatric unit and, 292-293
SED; *see* Severely emotionally disturbed child
Sedation
  antipsychotic drugs associated with, 358, 359, 361
  imipramine as cause of, 365
  tricyclic antidepressant drugs as cause of, 356
Sedative drugs, adolescent use of, 18
Sedative drugs, dependence on, 107
Sedgewick's holistic assessment tool for adolescents, 149
Seizure, diazepam for, 369
Self system, definition of, 319-320
Self-awareness
  anger intervention and, 379
  definition of, 215
  development of, 230
  gestalt therapy and, 316
  self-mutilation therapy and, 391
  suicidal adolescent and, 396
Self-blame, posttraumatic stress disorder and, 119
Self-Control Rating Scale, description of, 174*t*
Self-depreciation, depression indicated by, 88
Self-esteem
  attention deficit hyperactivity disorder and, 404

Self-esteem—cont'd
  building of, 219
  chemical dependence and, 409
  development of, 230-231
  low
    attention deficit hyperactivity disorder assessment and, 172
    depression indicated by, 88
    hyperactivity associated with, 84
    suicidal adolescent and, 396
Self-image, adolescent psychosocial development and, 28
Self-mutilation
  Human Responses of Concern for Psychiatric/ Mental Health Nursing Practice diagnosis, 388
  nursing care plan for, 389*t*-390*t*
  nursing intervention for, 388-392
Self-Report Rating Scales for Children, description of, 173*t*
Self-worth, adolescent, chum relationship and, 319
Sense of humor, nurse's need for, 8
Sensitivity, interpersonal, 226
Sentence completion test, description of, 167*t*
Separation anxiety, posttraumatic stress disorder indicated by, 115
Separation anxiety disorder, 100-101
  interventions for, 100-101
Serotonin
  affective disorders and, 93
  central nervous stimulants affect of level of, 353
  regulation of, obsessive-compulsive disorder associated with, 101
  tricyclic antidepressant drugs effect on, 364*t*
Severely emotionally disturbed child, system of care and, 203
Severely behaviorally handicapped child, system of care and, 203
Sex drive, acting out related to, 71
Sexual abuse
  child, rate of, 19
  crisis intervention and, 262*t*
  posttraumatic stress disorder and, 116
Sexual intercourse, adolescent, statistics on, 18
Sexual organization, psychoanalysis and, 316
Sexual promiscuity
  eating disorders associated with, 413
  prevention strategies for, 250
Sexually transmitted disease, adolescent, rate of, 19
Silence, group therapy communication and, 325
Sill development, eating disorders therapy and, 414

Single photon emission computed tomography, 164

Single photon emission computed tomography, neuropsychological evaluation and, 163

Skill building, home-based programs and, 198

Skill development
adolescent psychiatric nursing and, 376
anger intervention and, 379
chemical dependence therapy and, 411-412
description of, 221-223
four-phase sequence of, 300
prevention strategies and, 249-254
for psychotic adolescent, 401-403
resistance intervention and, 382
runaway adolescent and, 395
self-mutilation therapy and, 391-392

Sleep disorder, posttraumatic stress disorder indicated by, 115

Sleeping, problems in, depression indicated by, 88

Smith v Seibly, 60

Social function, poor, schizophrenia indicated by, 96

Social groups, prevention strategies and, 246-247

Social history, adolescent, 142, 143-148

Social learning theory, therapeutic milieu and, 274

Social skills
development of, 5-6, 223-228, 249
sources for, 239-240
Structured Learning approach to, 300
training for, 314

Sociodrama, acting out treated with, 73

Sodium bicarbonate
amphetamines interaction with, 354
lithium interaction with, 366

Somatic therapy
as component in nursing standards, 12
standard for nursing intervention and, 374

Somatopsychic therapy, 339-340

Special education, system of care and, 203

Special education services, description of, 197

SPECT; *see* Single photon emission computed tomography

Splitting
definition of, 385
diagnosis of, 386
Human Responses of Concern for Psychiatric/ Mental Health Nursing Practice diagnosis of, 386
nursing care plan for, 387t
nursing intervention for, 385-388
posttraumatic stress disorder and, 116-117

SQ; *see* Vineland social quotient

Staffing, adolescent psychiatric unit and, 418-420

Standards
child and adolescent nursing and, 8-11
for psychotherapy, 311

Standards of Child and Adolescent Psychiatric and Mental Health Nursing Practice, 8, 62

Standards of Child and Adolescent Psychiatric and Mental Health Nursing Practice, 245, 259, 273
health teaching and, 374
psychotherapy and, 373
somatic therapy and, 351, 374
therapeutic environment, 373
therapeutic milieu and, 273

Stanton-Schwartz syndrome, 72

State's rights, parental rights and, 54-55

Stealing, conduct disorder indicated by, 78

Stelazine; *see* Trifluoperazine

Stepfamily Association of America, address of, 253

STEP-Teen Program, 233

Stimulant drugs
adolescent use of, 18
central nervous system affected by, 353-355

Stomach ache
central nervous system stimulants as cause of, 354
lithium as cause of, 366

Stress, coping with, 233

Stress management program, adolescent psychiatric unit staff and, 421

Structure, adolescent need for, 5

Structured Learning, social skills development and, 30

Students Against Drunk Driving, 246, 247-248

Stupor, tricyclic antidepressant drugs as cause of, 356

Sublimation, as defense mechanism, 304

Substance abuse
acting out associated with, 76
crisis intervention and, 261t
prevention strategies for, 250
satanism related to, 20
suicide associated with, 95

Substitute care, description of, 204

Suicide, 94-95
acting out and, 73
adolescent, rate of, 17
assessment of potential for, 265
crisis intervention and, 261t
crisis intervention for survivors at school following, 267
danger of, in depressed adolescent, 86
incidence of, 95
nurses' liability for, 62
nursing care plan for, 397t-398t

Suicide—cont'd
  nursing intervention for, 395-399
  prevention strategies for, 250
  risk factors for, 95, 265
Suicide prevention center, 267
Sullivan's interpersonal theory, 318
Summarizing, group therapy communication and, 325
Superego, psychoanalysis and, 316
Supportive therapy, description of, 317
Supreme Court, common law and, 51
Surveillance
  adolescent need for, 4-5
  in adolescent psychiatric unit, 288
  for adolescent with eating disorders, 413-414
  for attention deficit hyperactivity disorder, 405
  chemical dependence therapy and, 409
  definition of, 4
  description of, 216-219
  manipulation intervention and, 386
  psychosis therapy and, 399-400
  runaway adolescent and, 392-393
  self-mutilation therapy and, 390-391
  for suicidal adolescent, 395-396
Symonds Picture Story Test, 164
  description of, 167t
System of care
  basic assumptions of, 191-194
  case management and, 193
  definition of, 188
  description of, 188-194
  education system and, 200-203
  planning strategies in, 192

T

Tachycardia
  antipsychotic drugs as cause of, 358
  central nervous system stimulants as cause of, 354
  imipramine as cause of, 365
  lithium as cause of, 366
  tricyclic antidepressant drugs and, 363
Talk therapy, psychotic adolescent treatment and, 321
Talking with Kids About Alcohol, address of, 253
Taractan; see Chlorprothixene
Tarasoff v Regents of the University of California, 62
TAT; see Thematic Apperception Test
TCA; see Antidepressant drugs, tricyclic
Teacher, therapeutic classroom and, 304-305
Teaching
  anger intervention and, 379
  prevention strategies and, 248-249
  therapeutic milieu and, 307

Teamwork, adolescent psychiatric nursing and, 375
Teenage Institute
  address of, 252
  case study from, 255
  description of, 249-251
Teenage pregnancy
  crisis intervention and, 262t
  prevention strategies for, 250
  rate of, 18-19
Tegretol; see Carbamazepine
Television, impact of, 15-16
Temporal lobe seizure disorder, anger and aggression associated with, 376
Terminating, group therapy communication and, 325
Testosterone, testicular enlargement due to, 37
Thematic Apperception Test, 163
  description of, 167t
Therapeutic classroom, 304-305
Therapeutic communication, techniques for, 216, 217-218
Therapeutic environment
  as component in nursing standards, 12
  nursing standards and, 273
  standard for intervention for, 373
Therapeutic milieu
  basic principles of, 274-275
  concept of, 200
  definition of, 275
  historical background on, 274
  nursing standards applicable to, 273
  role modeling as factor in, 307
  strategies for, 273-309
  structured elements of, 275-305
  teaching in, 307
  unstructured aspects of, 306-307
Therapeutic privilege, informed consent and, 59
Therapeutic relationship, description of, 215-216
Thioridazine
  psychotic disorders treated with, 360
  side effects of, 358
Thiothixine, psychotic disorders treated with, 360
Thioxanthene drugs, psychotic disorders treated with, 360
Thorazine; see Chlorpromazine
Thyroid-releasing hormone, effect of lithium on level of, 365
Thyroid-stimulating hormone, function of, during pubescence, 36
Thyroxine, effect of lithium on level of, 365
Tic, verbal, Tourette's syndrome indicated by, 367
Time out
  adolescent use of, 221

Time out—cont'd
 description of, 291-292
Tinker v Des Moines Independent School District,
 53
Tofranil; *see* Imipramine
Tort, intentional, 62-63
Toughlove
 address of, 263
 description of, 268
Tourette's syndrome
 obsessive-compulsive disorder and, 102
 psychopharmacologic treatment of, 367-368
Toxicology screen, chemical dependence diagno-
 sis and, 410
Tranquilizer drugs, adolescent use of, 18
Transference, group therapy and, 324
Tremors
 antipsychotic drugs as cause of, 358
 lithium as cause of, 366
Trifluoperazine, psychotic disorders treated with,
 360
Trigger factor, posttraumatic stress disorder and,
 115
Trihexyphenidyl, side effects of, 361
Triiodothyronine, effect of lithium on level of,
 365
True self/false self, posttraumatic stress disorder
 and, 116-117
TS; *see* Tourette's syndrome
TSH; *see* Thyroid-stimulating hormone
TWIKA; *see* Talking with Kids About Alcohol

U

Unipolar disorder, suicide attempt associated
 with, 395
United Learning, critical thinking skills
 and, 228
Urinary hesitance, tricyclic antidepressant drugs
 as cause of, 363, 364
Urinary retention, antipsychotic drugs as cause
 of, 358

V

Valium; *see* Diazepam
Vandalism, conduct disorder indicated by, 78
Vietnam War, impact of, 16
Vineland Social Maturity Scale, 165
Vineland social quotient, 165
Violence
 acting out and, 73
 adolescent or child, attention deficit hyperac-
 tivity disorder assessment and, 171

Vision, blurred
 antipsychotic drugs as cause of, 358
 lithium as cause of, 366
 tricyclic antidepressant drugs and, 363
Voluntary admission to psychiatric facility,
 adolescent rights and, 55
Vomiting
 self-induced, bulimia characterized by, 105
 tricyclic antidepressant drugs as cause of, 364

W

Weakness, lithium as cause of, 366
Wechsler Adult Intelligence Scale, description
 of, 167*t*
Wechsler Intelligence Scale for Children
 description of, 167*t*
 Revised, 163
Wechsler Preschool and Primary Scale of Intelli-
 gence, description of, 167*t*
Weeping, depression indicated by, 88
Weight
 change in, depression indicated by, 88
 loss of, central nervous system stimulants as
 cause of, 354
Weight gain
 antipsychotic drugs as cause of, 361
 antipsychotic drugs associated with, 359
 lithium as cause of, 366
Wellbutrin; *see* Bupropion
Wet dreams, onset of, 36
White House Conference on Children, history of,
 187, 188
Wisconsin v Yoder, 53
WISC-R; *see* Wechsler Intelligence Scale for
 Children, Revised
Withdrawal
 chemical dependence and, 409
 as defense mechanism, 304
 depression indicated by, 88
 schizophrenia indicated by, 96
Word association technique, description of, 167*t*
Work, capacity to, development of, 227-228

X

Xanax; *see* Alprazolam

Y

Yalom's therapeutic factors, 324*t*
YAVIS syndrome, 319
Youth charter, community value system and, 7
Youth organizations, prevention strategies and,
 247

Mosby–Year Book's 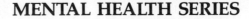 # MENTAL HEALTH SERIES

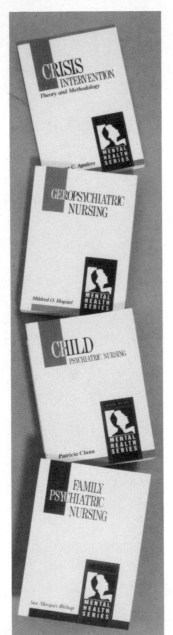

CRISIS INTERVENTION:
THEORY AND METHODOLOGY, *6th Edition*
Donna C. Aguilera, Ph.D., F.A.A.N.

Both students and professionals will rely on this highly respected classic for the most up-to-date information on the basic theory and principles of crisis intervention.

1990. 308 pages, 25 illustrations. ISBN 0-8016-0063-4

GEROPSYCHIATRIC NURSING
Mildred O. Hogstel, Ph.D., R.N., C.S.

A new text that provides a comprehensive overview of geropsychiatric nursing by focusing on the mental health problems, psychosocial needs, and special care of the elderly.

1990. 392 pages, illustrated. ISBN 0-8016-3331-1

CHILD PSYCHIATRIC NURSING
Patricia Clunn, Ed.D., A.R.N.P., C.S.

This comprehensive reference is designed for practicing psychiatric nurses and specialists who care for children with mental disorders. It provides a strong theory base and thoroughly discusses practical patient care strategies.

October 1990. Approx. 600 pages, illustrated.
ISBN 0-8016-0363-3

FAMILY PSYCHIATRIC NURSING
Sue Marquis Bishop, Ph.d., R.N.

June 1991. Approx. 375 pages, 40 illustrations.
ISBN 0-8016-0159-2

PSYCHIATRIC NURSING:
A PSYCHOTHERAPEUTIC APPROACH
Norman L. Keltner, R.N., Ed.D.

December 1990. Approx. 300 pages, 50 illustrations.
ISBN 0-8016-5840-3

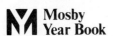
Mosby Year Book

To order, ask your bookstore manager or call toll free: 800-633-6699.
We look forward to hearing from you!   NMA-008